# Congenital Heart Defects - Recent Advances

*Edited by P. Syamasundar Rao*

Published in London, United Kingdom

Congenital Heart Defects - Recent Advances
http://dx.doi.org/10.5772/intechopen.98012
Edited by P. Syamasundar Rao

Contributors
Jiuann-Huey Lin, Jose Da Silva, Luciana Da Fonseca Da Silva, William Devine, Justin Yeh, Tarek Alsaied, Maria Giovanna Russo, Fiorella Fratta, Antonia Giudicepietro, Marina De Marco, Fortuna Del Gaizo, Carmela Morelli, Laura di Pietto, Ludovica Spinelli Barrile, Federica De Fazio, Rakesh Donthula, P. Syamasundar Rao, Animisha Rudra, Shaad Abqari, Arpit Agarwal, Harinder Singh, Daniel Nento, Si Hui Wong, Osama Elshazali, Abdelmoniem Elseed, Murtada Ibrahim, Aimann Surak, Teja Senekovič Kojc, Nataša Marčun Varda, Unnati Doshi, Elizabeth Wang-Giuffre, Ikechukwu Andrew Nwafor, Josephat Maduabuchi Chinawa, John Chukwuemeka Eze, Fidelis Anayo Onyekwulu, Yolandee Bell-Chedder, Mario Castro-Medina, Raymond Morales, XinXiu Xu, Cecilia W. Lo



First published in London, United Kingdom, 2022 by IntechOpen
IntechOpen is the global imprint of INTECHOPEN LIMITED, registered in England and Wales, registration number: 11086078, 5 Princes Gate Court, London, SW7 2QJ, United Kingdom

British Library Cataloguing-in-Publication Data
A catalogue record for this book is available from the British Library

Additional hard and PDF copies can be obtained from orders@intechopen.com

Congenital Heart Defects - Recent Advances
Edited by P. Syamasundar Rao
p. cm.
Print ISBN 978-1-80356-080-9
Online ISBN 978-1-80356-081-6
eBook (PDF) ISBN 978-1-80356-082-3

For EU product safety concerns:
IN TECH d.o.o., Prolaz Marije Krucifikse Kozulić 3, 51000 Rijeka, Croatia,
info@intechopen.com or visit our website at intechopen.com.

# Meet the editor

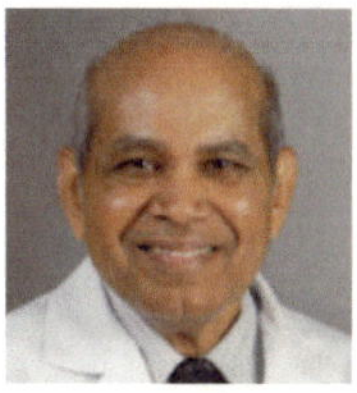

Dr. P. Syamasundar Rao is a Professor of Pediatrics and Medicine, and Emeritus Chief of Pediatric Cardiology at the McGovern Medical School, University of Texas at Houston. Dr. Rao received his medical degree from Andhra Medical College, Visakhapatnam, India where he also received initial pediatric training. He trained in pediatric cardiology in the United States at Stanford University, Case-Western Reserve University, and University of California at Los Angeles. He has held faculty positions at the Medical College of Georgia, USA; King Faisal Specialist Hospital and Research Center, Riyadh, Saudi Arabia; University of Wisconsin, USA; and Saint Louis University School of Medicine/Cardinal Glennon Children's Hospital, USA. Dr. Rao has authored 420 papers, 15 monographs/books, and 150 book chapters.

# Contents

**Preface** **IX**

**Section 1**
Introduction **1**

**Chapter 1** **3**
Introductory Chapter: Introduction to Recent Advances in the Diagnosis and Management of Congenital Heart Defects
*by P. Syamasundar Rao*

**Section 2**
Fetal Ultrasound **7**

**Chapter 2** **9**
The Impact of Fetal Echocardiography on the Prognosis of Congenital Heart Disease
*by Maria Giovanna Russo, Fiorella Fratta, Antonia Giudicepietro, Carmela Morelli, Fortuna Del Gaizo, Laura di Pietto, Marina De Marco, Ludovica Spinelli Barrile and Federica De Fazio*

**Section 3**
Echocardiography **21**

**Chapter 3** **23**
Clinical Benefits of New Echocardiographic Methods
*by Teja Senekovič Kojc and Nataša Marčun Varda*

**Section 4**
Prevention of Sudden Cardiac Death in the Athlete **41**

**Chapter 4** **43**
Pre-Sports Participation Cardiac Screening Evaluation – A Review
*by P. Syamasundar Rao*

**Section 5**
Individual Heart Defects 71

**Chapter 5** 73
Ventricular Septal Defects: A Review
*by Unnati Doshi and Elizabeth Wang-Giuffre*

**Chapter 6** 91
Atrioventricular Septal Defects
*by Rakesh Donthula, Animisha Rudra and P. Syamasundar Rao*

**Chapter 7** 113
Hypoplastic Left Heart Syndrome
*by Yolandee Bell-Cheddar, William Devine, Mario Castro-Medina, Raymond Morales, XinXiu Xu, Cecilia W. Lo and Jiuann-Huey Ivy Lin*

**Chapter 8** 139
Ebstein's Anomaly
*by Luciana Da Fonseca Da Silva, William A. Devine, Tarek Alsaied, Justin Yeh, Jiuann-Huey Ivy Lin and Jose Da Silva*

**Section 6**
Therapy 175

**Chapter 9** 177
Pharmacological Treatment of Patent Ductus Arteriosus in Preterm Infants
*by Aimann Surak*

**Chapter 10** 187
Right Ventricular Outflow Tract Stenting
*by Shaad Abqari*

**Chapter 11** 197
Advances in the Management of Congenital Malformations of the Aortic Valve
*by Si Hui Wong, Daniel Nento, Harinder Singh and Arpit Agarwal*

**Section 7**
International Issues 221

**Chapter 12** 223
Management of Congenital Heart Disease in Low-Income Countries: The Challenges and the Way Forward
*by Osama Elshazali, Murtada Ibrahim and Abdelmoniem Elseed*

**Chapter 13** 235
Establishing Sustainable Pediatric Cardiac Surgery Program in Nigeria: Challenges and Prospects
*by Ikechukwu Andrew Nwafor, Josephat Maduabuchi Chinawa, John Chukwuemeka Eze and Fidelis Anayo Onyekwulu*

# Preface

This book presents some of the advances that have occurred in pediatric cardiology over the last 50 years for healthcare personnel involved in caring for infants, children, and adults with congenital heart disease (CHD).

The book is divided into seven sections. The first section introduces the book. In the introductory chapter, I review the evolution of pediatric cardiology over the last 50 years and summarize developments during this period. Then, I outline how this book is organized.

In Section 2 on fetal ultrasound, Dr. Russo et al. address the impact of fetal echocardiography on the prognosis of CHDs in Chapter 2. The authors state that CHD is one of the most common birth defects discovered both in utero and immediately following birth. They opine that current advances in the diagnosis and management improved the prognosis of babies born with CHD such that a large number of these babies are reaching adulthood. Then, they review historical aspects of fetal echocardiography since its early phases in the late 1980s. They assert that the diagnostic accuracy of fetal echocardiography is high, permitting the identification of most types of CHDs in the fetus. This facilitates fetal cardiac interventions when indicated; enables voluntary interruption of pregnancy, if necessary; simplifies pregnancy and delivery management; provides fetal and genetic counselling; identifies babies that need emergent neonatal management (ductal dependent lesions); and most importantly has a positive impact on improving long-term outcomes.

In Section 3 on echocardiography, Drs. Kojc and Varda review the clinical benefits of new echocardiographic methods in Chapter 3. The authors state that the chief objectives of echocardiography are the precise evaluation of myocardial function and accurate demonstration of cardiac morphology. The authors review some of the new echocardiographic approaches, including functional echocardiography, cardiac deformation imaging, and three-dimensional echocardiography with a focus on the key advantages, clinical utility, and chief limitations of each technique. Functional echocardiography, also called targeted echocardiography, is different in newborns compared to older children. It involves evaluation of cardiac function, assessment of the degree of pulmonary hypertension, detection of pericardial effusion and its adverse effects, and assessment of the magnitude of shunts (such as hemodynamically significant patent ductus arteriosus [hsPDA] in premature babies). Functional echocardiography permits real-time assessment of cardiac function recognizes the type of cardiovascular compromise, guides therapy, and monitors response to therapy. Myocardial deformation imaging includes assessment of strain and strain rate change, which helps evaluate both global and regional functions of both ventricles and helps circumvent disadvantages of load-dependent ventricular function parameters such as fractional shortening, ejection fraction, and fractional area shortening. Three-dimensional speckle-tracking offers an additional inclusive assessment of ventricular function. While strain imaging is well studied in adult subjects, its use appears limited in pediatric patients. Three-dimensional echocardiography along with real time imaging (four-dimensional) is a relatively recent invention in ultrasound of the heart. It may be useful in subjects with CHD because it provides an appreciation of intricate spatial relationships. These new modalities may have advantages over the other existing imaging techniques such as magnetic resonance imaging (MRI) and computed tomography (CT), which are expensive, require anesthesia, or have increased radiation exposure. The disadvantages of three-dimensional imaging are low temporal and spatial resolution and the need for offline processing.

In Section 4, on the prevention of sudden cardiac death (SCD) in the athlete, I review in Chapter 4 issues related to sudden death associated with sports participation of athletes with a particular focus on pre-participation screening. SCD in sports, although rare, is a disastrous event. Sudden death in athletes often has a cardiac etiology and the most frequent causes are hypertrophic cardiomyopathy (HCM) and congenital coronary artery (CA) anomalies. I present a brief description of the anatomy, pathophysiology, and clinical features of HCM, aberrant CAs, Marfan's syndrome, arrhythmogenic right ventricle, and other entities responsible for SCD. The current recommendations are to perform a pre-spots participation screening consisting of complete personal and family history and a thorough physical examination. If abnormalities are detected during history or physical examination, further studies should be performed to define the etiology of the abnormalities. Using an electrocardiogram, echocardiogram, or MRI as a routine screening method is not recommended in the United States. I suggested that the pre-spots participation screening be undertaken at the primary care physicians' office as a part of routine annual physical (instead of mass screening but should include the fourteen-element history and physical examination. The justification of pre-participation screening is to allow as many athletes as feasible to take part in sports instead of being excluded from participation.

Section 5 consists of Chapters 5–8 on individual heart defects. Chapter 5 by Drs. Doshi and Wang-Giuffre discusses ventricular septal defect (VSD). The authors state that VSDs constitute up to 30% of all CHDs and that they are the most frequent heart defects seen in everyday clinical practice. The causation of CHDs, including VSDs, is largely explained based on multifactorial inheritance, although chromosomal abnormalities may sometimes be involved. Symptomatology is largely related to the magnitude of the shunt across the VSD. Echocardiographic studies are the chief modes of investigation to define the defects and their clinical significance. The natural history of VSDs involves spontaneous closure, development of pulmonary vascular obstructive disease (PVOD), onset of infundibular stenosis, and evolution to aortic insufficiency. Spontaneous closure is one of the main features of VSD; when that happens, no treatment is necessary. Hemodynamically significant shunts require surgical repair. Surgery is also recommended in patients with aortic valve leaflet prolapse and aortic insufficiency, irrespective of the degree of shunting across the VSD. The outcome following surgical correction is excellent, although an occasional patient may develop complete atrioventricular block or worsening aortic valve regurgitation. New methods of transcatheter and hybrid device closures are useful in patients with large muscular VSDs. Large, unrepaired VSDs may go on to develop irreversible PVOD, leading to Eisenmenger's syndrome, although this is uncommon in developed countries. Patients with Eisenmenger's syndrome may be treated with endothelin receptor antagonists, phosphodiesterase 5 inhibitors, and prostacyclins; such treatment modalities appear to improve functional capacity. Patients with PVOD are not candidates for closure of VSD but may require eventual lung transplantation. In Chapter 6, Dr. Donthula and I review the issues related to atrioventricular septal defects (AVSDs). AVSDs are defects in the atrioventricular (AV) septum and AV valves. AVSD is the most common defect seen in patients with Down syndrome. They are classified into complete, intermediate, partial, and transitional forms. Complete forms of AVSDs are further divided into balanced and unbalanced defects. Echo-Doppler studies are the main imaging methods used for the diagnosis and assessment of AVSDs. Subjects with complete and intermediate types manifest early in infancy and surgical repair is needed, also in early infancy, while partial and transitional varieties develop symptoms in early childhood and need surgical intervention at that time. Babies who can't undergo complete surgical correction (because of their weight or comorbidities) are addressed by palliation with pulmonary artery banding. Surgical treatment of unbalanced AVSDs is more complicated. These patients are addressed with either single ventricle, one-and-a-half ventricle, or bi-ventricular repair, depending upon their anatomy and physiology. Prognosis following surgery is generally good for balanced AVSDs and residual mitral valve insufficiency is the most frequent reason for repeat surgery. For the unbalanced AVSDs, the selection of the type of procedure is more complex and the long-term outcome is less than ideal. In Chapter 7, Dr. Bell-Cheddar et al. tackle issues related to hypoplastic left heart syndrome (HLHS). The authors define HLHS as a complex CHD consisting of the hypoplastic left ventricle (LV), aorta (Ao), and mitral valve. This defect resulted in the uniformly fatal outcome prior to the description of the Norwood procedure in the early 1980s, but now, with the use of a three-stage surgery including Fontan, prognosis has improved remarkably. Nevertheless, a high morbidity and mortality still exist in 25% of babies with HLHS who either need heart transplantation or die within one year following the Norwood procedure. While the reasons for such high morbidity/mortality were not clearly defined, they appear to be related to cardiovascular/hemodynamic abnormalities. In the remaining part of the chapter, the authors focus on the studies of a mouse model of HLHS. The studies demonstrate metabolic dysfunction resulting in the arrest of cell cycle and defects in cardiomyocyte differentiation. It is hypothesized that these intrinsic cell defects contribute to cardiac abnormalities of HLHS. In addition, the association of HLHS with chromosomal anomalies and high recurrence rates support the genetic etiology of HLHS. Finally, Chapter 8 by Dr. Da Silva et al. is on Ebstein's anomaly. The authors characterize Ebstein's anomaly of the tricuspid valve (TV) as downward displacement of the septal and inferior leaflets of the TV. In addition, there is a redundancy of the anterior leaflet with a sail-like morphology, dilatation of the true right AV valve annulus, TV regurgitation, and dilation of the right atrium and right ventricle (RV). They also describe a similar abnormality of the left-sided morphologic tricuspid valve in patients with congenitally corrected transposition of the great arteries. Then they review the existing classifications and pathophysiology of Ebstein's anomaly. This is followed by a description of diagnostic studies such as echocardiography, cardiac MRI, and CT for evaluation of Ebstein's. The authors also examine the historical evolution of surgical management. They comment that the wide variability of anatomic and pathophysiologic characteristics of Ebstein's anomaly resulted in not securing uniformly good results following surgical repair; this resulted in the development of several surgical repair techniques. Then, they provide a detailed description of the cone procedure, which was developed by one of the authors of this chapter. The Da Silva technique of cone reconstruction of the TV involves the creation of a cone-like structure from all available TV leaflet tissue; the result simulates normal TV structure. The authors contend that the cone procedure for Ebstein's anomaly has low mortality/morbidity with effective and long-lasting results in most patients. They also discuss the relative advantages of valved atrial septal defect (ASD) closure vs. bidirectional Glenn procedure in patients with inadequate RV to support pulmonary circulation. They then address surgical management of Ebstein's anomaly in the neonate. In the final section, they discuss post-operative management in detail. They conclude that given the advances in diagnostic techniques, surgical management, and peri-operative care, most Ebstein's anomaly patients are likely to have two-ventricle repair with good long-term results.

Section 6 reviews therapy. In Chapter 9, Dr. Surak reviews the pharmacological management of patent ductus arteriosus (PDA) in preterm infants. The author states that PDA is responsible for several morbidities in preterm infants and that there is an inclination toward a more conservative treatment of PDA instead of surgical therapy. He discusses the utility of targeted neonatal echocardiography in the detection of hsPDA. He then reviews the results of pharmacological therapy of PDA in preterm babies with non-steroidal anti-inflammatory drugs (NSAIDs) such as indomethacin and ibuprofen as well as acetaminophen. He also refers to the usefulness of combined therapy (ibuprofen and acetaminophen) in occluding the ductus. Finally, he mentions device closure of PDA and quotes safety and efficacy data of device occlusion of PDA. It is concluded that pharmacological therapy, while causing ductal constriction, does not guarantee the elimination of the shunt and that additional research is necessary to see if the device closure approach would produce added favorable outcomes in the premature. In chapter 10, Dr. Abqari discusses right ventricular outflow tract (RVOT) stenting. The standard management option in children with CHDs with diminished pulmonary blood flow is the creation of systemic-to-pulmonary artery shunt such as a modified Blalock-Taussig (BT) shunt. However, RVOT stenting has recently been used for palliation. The author asserts that RVOT stenting results in fewer complications and achieves physiological growth of pulmonary arteries (PAs). The latter may have a positive impact during final corrective surgery. Usually, RVOT stenting is undertaken in the neonate, but in some institutions, it is being used in older children. The author presents indications for RVOT stenting and provides a detailed description of RVOT stent procedure. The author also presents modifications, complications, challenges, and outcomes of the procedure. Two-point fixation of the stent guarantees the prevention of stent embolization. However, covering only the infundibular region, and sparing the pulmonary valve may prevent future trans annular patches, although removing the stent may be challenging. The author believes that RVOT stenting is a safer alternative in some pediatric cardiac programs, although several programs opt for primary surgical correction. The author concludes that RVOT stenting is expected to garner greater acceptance amongst other palliative procedures as larger experience with this procedure is gained. In Chapter 11, Dr. Wong et al. review the advances in the management of congenital malformations of the aortic valve. The authors state that congenital malformations of the aortic valve are life-long ailments that may need many catheters and/or surgical procedures. The bicuspid aortic valve may be seen in 1%–2% of live births, whereas aortic valve stenosis is much less common. The authors review management options, including balloon aortic valvuloplasty, surgical valvotomy, surgical repair of the aortic valve, and aortic valve replacement. The options of bicuspidization and tricuspidization types of reconstruction and materials used for the reconstruction of the aortic valve are also reviewed in detail. Then, the authors address aortic valve replacement with mechanical valves and bioprosthetic valves (bovine or porcine valves, homografts, and allografts) or by Ross procedure (patient's own pulmonary valve is relocated to the aortic valve position and a tissue valve replaces the pulmonary valve). They also review the relative advantages of repair vs. replacement. In general, the described techniques carry their own benefits and have their own limitations regarding growth potential, longevity of repair, need for repeat surgery, anticoagulation requirement, risk of infection, and morbidity/mortality risks. The authors conclude by presenting a basic algorithm for the management of aortic stenosis.

Section 7 reviews international issues. In Chapter 12, Dr. Elshazali et al. discuss the management of CHD in low-income countries (LICs) and low-middle-income countries (LMICs). They review the epidemiology of CHD in the LICs and compare it with that in high-income countries (HICs). Although the overall prevalence of CHD is similar (8 to 9 per 1,000 live births), higher fertility and birth rates in LICs than in HICs result in 90% of babies with CHDs being born in countries with limited resources in caring for these babies. Pediatric cardiac services are considered to be a burden and a challenge in LICs and are a challenge as well in LICs. The currently available pediatric cardiac services in most LICs are difficult to access and not affordable for most and there is an absence of awareness of the necessity for quality pediatric cardiac services. Healthcare planners should recognize that pediatric cardiac services are essential services and are not a luxury. The authors recommend collaboration and partnerships among international organizations, national and local governments, and non-governmental organizations. They also assert that patient and family advocates are required to assure that children around the world have access to quality and dependable pediatric cardiac care. They quote some shining examples of countries such as Cuba, India, and China which accomplished providing pediatric cardiac services with strategic planning and leadership. They conclude that capacity building to accomplish the eventual objective of self-sufficient LIC and LMIC programs will necessitate a paradigm change by the leadership of the respective countries, better alliance among stakeholders, and facilitate data sharing and research expansion. In Chapter 13, Dr. Nwafor et al. review issues similar to those dealt with in the preceding chapter, but with a focus on Nigeria. They state that the delivery of cardiovascular services to children and adults with CHDs in Nigeria is grossly inadequate. They also opine that there is no accurate statistical data on CHD in Nigeria, but suggest that the prevalence of CHD is comparable to that reported in other countries (8 per 1,000 live births). They first review historical aspects of the development of surgery for CHD in Nigeria. The problems of inadequate surgical resources are presently improved by medical tourism and cardiac surgery missions from foreign countries, but the authors' assessment is that such services are still not adequate. They opine that there is a need for the government to share resources between non-communicable diseases such as CHD and communicable diseases. When this is accomplished with the help of international partners and humanitarian organizations, a sustainable pediatric cardiac surgery program is likely to be established. They conclude that such efforts will definitely improve the care of patients with CHD.

The last five decades have witnessed a great many advances in the diagnosis and management of CHD that have resulted in increased survival of children with heart disease. This book discusses some of these advances and is a useful resource on diagnostic and therapeutic methods for healthcare professionals in providing quality care to their patients with cardiac disease.

**P. Syamasundar Rao, MD, DCH, FAAP, FACC, FSCAI**
Children's Heart Institute,
University of Texas at Houston McGovern Medical School,
Children's Memorial Hermann Hospital,
Houston, Texas, USA

Section 1

# Introduction

Chapter 1

# Introductory Chapter: Introduction to Recent Advances in the Diagnosis and Management of Congenital Heart Defects

*P. Syamasundar Rao*

## 1. Introduction

Congenital heart defects (CHDs) are defined as anatomic malformations of either the heart or great vessels, which occur while intrauterine development of the heart is taking place [1]. This is regardless of the age at which the CHD manifests. Typical examples of CHDs are ventricular septal defect and coarctation of the aorta. Many studies were performed to determine the incidence of CHDs; these investigations indicate an incidence of 0.8% of live births [2]. This would result in the birth of approximately 40,000 babies in the United States alone, and over 1,000,000 babies are born with a heart defect worldwide. There is no evidence for any differences in the prevalence of CHD among continents or between racial groups [3]. Recent description of pulse oximetry screening of newborn babies prior to discharge from the hospital has resulted in early identification of critical CHDs [4–6]. This adds to the early detection strategies offered by fetal echocardiography [7]. Approximately half of the patients with CHDs may be addressed by providing ordinary medications and clinical follow-up without major therapeutic interventions. Nevertheless, the outstanding half formerly needed surgery, and some requiring open-heart procedures through cardiopulmonary bypass. Subsequently, following the development of percutaneous methods [8–12], half of these children (i.e., 25% of the total) are being addressed by percutaneous, transcatheter techniques that are less invasive than surgery.

Availability of highly sensitive noninvasive diagnostic tools such as echo-Doppler studies [13–16], magnetic resonance imaging (MRI) [17, 18], computed tomography (CT) [19, 20]; identification of CHD in the fetus by echo [7]; early detection of neonates with serious heart disease [21, 22], including pulse oximetry screening of the neonates prior to discharge from the hospital [4–6] and their rapid transport to tertiary care centers [21, 22]; advances in transcatheter interventional procedures [8–12]; improvements in pediatric cardiac anesthesia [23, 24]; and extension of complicated surgical procedures to treat children with complex CHDs [25] have resulted in the successful management of all children with heart disease. Consequently, almost all CHDs are diagnosed and "corrected." Defects that cannot be completely corrected can be effectively palliated [26] or cardiac transplantation performed [27–29]. The last five decades have seen a great many advances and as mentioned above, these resulted in the increased survival of children with CHD. The purpose of this book on


IntechOpen

"Congenital Heart Defects: Recent Advances" is to present some of these advances in an easily readable format for the physicians and other health-care personnel interested in the care of infants, children, and adults with congenital heart disease.

While a number of chapters were contributed to this book, not all the advances that occurred during the last 50 years could be included; this is largely related to the method by which the authors were recruited and chapter titles were selected and limitations of the space. Yet, the authors of the book chapters and I hope that the discussed matter is helpful to the reader and help him/her in the care of the patients that they are involved in.

## Author details

P. Syamasundar Rao
Children's Heart Institute, University of Texas McGovern Medical School and Children's Memorial Herman Hospital, Houston, Texas, USA

*Address all correspondence to: p.syamasundar.rao@uth.tmc.edu

## References

[1] Rao PS. Congenital heart defects – A review. In: Rao PS, editor. Congenital Heart Disease - Selected Aspects. Rijeka, Croatia: InTech; 2012. pp. 3-44

[2] Hoffman JI, Kaplan S. The incidence of congenital heart disease. Journal of the American College of Cardiology. 2002;**39**:1890-1900

[3] Rao PS. Demographic features of tricuspid atresia. In: Rao PS, editor. Tricuspid Atresia. 2nd ed. NY, Mt. Kisco: Futura Publishing Co.; 1992. pp. 23-37

[4] Hoke TR, Donohue PK, Bawa PK, et al. Oxygen saturation as a screening test for critical congenital heart disease: A preliminary study. Pediatric Cardiology. 2002;**23**:403-409

[5] Diller CL, Kelleman MS, Kupke KG, et al. A modified algorithm for critical congenital heart disease screening using pulse oximetry. Pediatrics. 2018;**141**(5):e20174065. DOI: 10.1542/peds.2017-4065

[6] Vidyasagar D, Beligere N. Pulse oximetry screening for detecting congenital heart defects in the newborn. In: Rao PS, Vidyasagar D, editors. A Multidisciplinary Approach to Perinatal Cardiology. Vol. 1. New Castle upon Tyne, UK: Cambridge Scholars Publishing; 2021. pp. 268-291

[7] Randall P, Brealey S, Hahn S, et al. Accuracy of fetal echocardiography in the routine detection of congenital heart disease among unselected and low risk population, a systemic review. BJOG: An International Journal of Obstetrics & Gynaecology. 2005;**112**:24-30

[8] Rao PS. Balloon Angioplasty and Valvuloplasty in Infants, Children and Adolescents. Current Problems in Cardiology. Chicago: YearBook Medical Publishers, Inc.; 1989;**14**(8):417-500

[9] Rao PS. Transcatheter Therapy in Pediatric Cardiology. New York: Wiley-Liss, Inc.; 1993

[10] Rao PS. Interventional pediatric cardiology: State of the art and future directions. Pediatric Cardiology. 1998;**19**:107-124

[11] Rao PS, Kern MJ, editors. Catheter Based Devices for Treatment of Noncoronary Cardiovascular Disease in Adults and Children. Philadelphia, PA: Lippincott Williams & Wilkins; 2003

[12] Rao PS. Stents in the management of vascular obstructive lesions associated with congenital heart disease. In: Vijayalakshmi IB, editor. Cardiac Catheterization and Imaging (from Pediatrics to Geriatrics). New Delhi, India: Jaypee Publications; 2015. pp. 573-598

[13] Tworetzky W, McElhinney DB, Brook MM, et al. Echocardiographic diagnosis alone for the complete repair of major congenital heart defects. Journal of the American College of Cardiology. 1999;**33**:228-233

[14] Rao PS. Echocardiography: An overview - part I. Vessel Plus. 2021;**11**:2. DOI: 10.20517/2574-1209.2021.91

[15] Rao PS. Echocardiography: An overview - part II. Vessel Plus. 2022;**6**:25. DOI: 10.20517/2574-1209.2021.92

[16] Rao PS. Echocardiography: An overview - part III. Vessel Plus. 2022;**6**:26. DOI: 10.20517/2574-1209.2021.93

[17] Kellenberger CJ, Yoo SJ, Buchel ER. Cardiovascular MR imaging in neonates and infants with congenital heart disease. Radiographics. 2007;**27**:5-18. DOI: 10.1148/rg.271065027

[18] Occleshaw C. Technical aspects of pediatric cardiac MR. In: Fogel MA, editor. Principles and Practice of Cardiac Magnetic Resonance in Congenital Heart Disease: Form, Function and Flow. 1st ed. UK: John Wiley & Sons Ltd; 2010. pp. 20-21

[19] Kawano T, Ishii M, Takagi J, et al. Three-dimensional helical computed tomographic angiography in neonates and infants with complex congenital heart disease. American Heart Journal. 2000;**139**:654-660

[20] Long YG, Yang YY, Huang IL, et al. Role of multi-slice and three-dimensional computed tomography in delineating extracardiac vascular abnormalities in neonates. Pediatrics and Neonatology. 2010;**51**:227-234. DOI: 10.1016/S1875-9572(10)60043-5; 10.1016/S1875-9572(10)60043-5

[21] Vincent WR, Rao PS. Early identification of the neonate with suspected serious heart disease. Paediatrician. 1973;**2**:239-250

[22] Rao PS, Strong WB. Early identification of the neonate with heart disease. Journal of the Medical Association of Georgia. 1974;**63**: 430-433

[23] Kambam J, editor. In: Cardiac Anesthesia for Infants and Children. St. Louis, MO: Mosby-Year Book; 1994

[24] Gautam NK, Hubbard R. Anesthesia for the neonate with congenital heart disease. In: Rao PS, Vidyasagar D, editors. A Multidisciplinary Approach to Perinatal Cardiology. Vol. 2. New Castle upon Tyne, UK: Cambridge Scholars Publishing; 2021. pp. 1-20

[25] Greenleaf CE, Salazar JE, Douglas WI. Cardiac surgery in the neonate. In: Rao PS, Vidyasagar D, editors. A Multidisciplinary Approach to Perinatal Cardiology. Vol. 2. New Castle upon Tyne, UK: Cambridge Scholars Publishing; 2021. pp. 21-50

[26] Rao PS. Single ventricle—A comprehensive review. Children. 2021;**8**:441. DOI: 10.3390/children8060441

[27] Bailey LL, Concepcion W, Shattuck H, et al. Method of heart transplantation for treatment of hypoplastic left heart syndrome. The Journal of Thoracic and Cardiovascular Surgery. 1986;**92**:1-5

[28] Dipchand AI. Current state of pediatric cardiac transplantation. Annals of Cardiothoracic Surgery. 2018;7(1):31-55

[29] Aggarwal A. Cardiac transplantation infants and children. In: Rao PS, Vidyasagar D, editors. A Multidisciplinary Approach to Perinatal Cardiology. Vol. 2. New Castle upon Tyne, UK: Cambridge Scholars Publishing; 2021. pp. 51-74

Section 2

# Fetal Ultrasound

Chapter 2

# The Impact of Fetal Echocardiography on the Prognosis of Congenital Heart Disease

*Maria Giovanna Russo, Fiorella Fratta, Antonia Giudicepietro, Carmela Morelli, Fortuna Del Gaizo, Laura di Pietto, Marina De Marco, Ludovica Spinelli Barrile and Federica De Fazio*

## Abstract

Congenital heart disease (CHD) represents the group of the most common malformations detected both prenatally and after birth. Although progress in the management and treatments of CHD, it still remains a significant cause of neonatal morbidity and mortality. However, the recent improvement in the diagnosis and therapy of CHD represents one of the most important successes of cardiac surgery and medical treatment. Accordingly, in the last twenty years, the number of patients with CHD who have reached adulthood has increased significantly and even surpass the number of affected pediatric patients, due to the extraordinary progress in the diagnostic, clinical, and surgical technologies. In particular, the ultrasound study of the fetal heart allows a diagnosis of CHD in the prenatal period, significantly improves perinatal outcomes in infants with critical CHD, and enables a reduction in stillbirth.

**Keywords:** Congenital heart disease, fetal echocardiography, invasive fetal cardiac intervention, counseling

## 1. Introduction

Congenital heart disease (CHD) is the most common malformation detected prenatally and at birth. Generally, estimated incidence is approximately 10/1000 of live births and is significantly higher in premature infants and in stillborn [1]. Although remarkable progress has been made in the diagnosis and treatment of this condition, it still remains a significant cause of neonatal morbidity and mortality. Congenital malformations of the heart are a broad spectrum of defects varying from mild lesions that produce only minimal or no symptoms and might be incidentally detected in adult life to severe anomalies that cause premature death. There are many factors that increase the risk of having a child with CHD. The etiology of CHD can be separated into genetic and non-genetic forms. Epidemiological studies have suggested that a genetic or environmental cause can be identified in approximately 30% of CHD cases [2]. Approximately 17% of CHD occurs in association with a well-defined syndrome such as trisomies 13, 15, 18, 21 and Turner syndrome [3]. Some environmental factors have been identified as responsible for CHD such as congenital rubella infection or teratogenic drugs [2]. However, the majority of cases remain unexplained, probably due to some combination of genetic and environmental factors [4].

The main classification of CHD includes:

- Left-to-right shunt leading to an increased pulmonary flow
- Reduced pulmonary blood flow
- Transposition of the great arteries
- Left and right heart obstruction
- Duct dependent pulmonary or systemic circulation

In this chapter, we will discuss in detail the importance of fetal echocardiography and the fundamental impact of early detection and interventions during fetal life on postnatal outcomes. We will also discuss the importance of adequate counseling in order to allow parents to understand the condition, to support them in the most difficult decision to interrupt or keep pregnancy, to offer extensive information on available therapeutic options, and prevision of data on outcome and quality of life.

## 2. Fetal echocardiography, impact on the prognosis

Fetal echocardiography is born in the late 80s, when the improvement of ultrasound technology has made possible to focus attention on the characteristics of the fetal heart. Huhta JC, one of the pioneers of this method, raised the question if, without the possibility of treating in utero CHD, is it useful or advisable to make the diagnosis in advance, before birth [5]. It is clearly demonstrated that a team consisting of an expert gynecologist and a pediatric cardiologist can make diagnosis of a number of congenital heart defects in the fetal stage with very high degree of accuracy [6]. The prenatal diagnosis of CHD in the last 30 years has reached a high degree of diagnostic accuracy allowing to identify of almost all forms of CHD during fetal life; this is true in most expert centers since the interpretation of fetal echocardiography requires advanced skills. Accordingly, a suspected cardiac abnormality should then always be referred to a fetal cardiology specialist in a tertiary level center for further evaluation. Prenatal diagnosis rates for CHD increased from 23.0% in 1983–1988 to 47.3% in 1995–2000 [6]. Similarly, termination rates increased from 9.9% (between 1983 and 1989) to 14.7% (between 1989 and 2000) [6]. The spectrum of CHD observed before birth appears similar to the spectrum of CHD postnatally detected [6]. Early diagnosis of CHD during fetal echocardiography can influence the prognosis because it can permit the parents and clinicians to treat the defect. In this chapter, we will address pregnancy and delivery management, issues related to voluntary interruption of pregnancy, and fetal interventions.

## 3. Pregnancy and delivery management

Prenatal diagnosis has an impact on morbidity and mortality for most severe conditions because it allows an appropriate referral and planning of delivery and immediate assistance in expert centers resulting in improving short-term outcomes. However, its influence on long-term outcomes are still not clarified. In particular, prenatal diagnosis of conditions that constitute a neonatal emergency, such as duct dependent lesions, allows for manage the delivery in a tertiary care center. This strategy improves survival significantly and reduces preoperative morbidity and risk of neurological compromission [7]. CHD patients diagnosed postnatally that were born at non-tertiary centers, without specialist neonatal or cardiac services, presented later and required much higher levels of cardio-respiratory support during transfer from geographically distant locations [8]. Of note, clinical instability in postnatally diagnosed infants with CHD is an established risk factor for morbidity and mortality [8]. Moreover, it has also been proven that prenatally diagnosed infants undergo significantly earlier surgery [8].

## 4. Voluntary interruption of pregnancy

It has been documented that a parallel increase in pregnancy interruption occurred with fetal CHD diagnosis [9]. Thus, early diagnosis of CHD permits parents to make the difficult choice of eventual interruption of pregnancy. The rates of prenatal diagnosis of CHD were 47,3% in France, 49% in USA, and 52,8% in Australia [10]. In our center, our 21 years' experience is in accord with the one of Khoshnood [6]: the spectrum of prenatally diagnosis CHD is getting similar to the one observed after birth. This is due to the great number of detected cases. Other than hypoplastic left heart syndrome (HLHS), pregnancy termination was exceptional. Early neonatal mortality in patients with severe CHD decreased to less than 1/3 in the period 1995–2000 [6]. The curve of survival shows a slightly worse survival for neonates with the prenatal diagnosis but this is likely to be related to the composition of the population and selection bias since fetal echocardiography is performed only when there is a high index of suspicion for more severe CHD [11].

### 4.1 Fetal cardiac intervention

Several fetal studies reported that structural heart disease, in particular aortic stenosis, evolves in utero, hindering the growth of the left ventricle [12]. Fetal cardiac intervention (FCI) is a novel and advanced technique that allows in utero treatment of a subset of congenital heart disease. Fetal cardiac intervention with valvuloplasty, is based on the principle that intervention will modify the natural history of the disease process [13]. To prove an eventual favorable impact of FCI, we must first gain a full understanding of the unaltered progression of heart disease in utero. Referral centers that have performed the most procedures have shown that in utero valvuloplasty can be performed successfully, with limited risk to the mother and encouraging outcomes for fetuses, especially in those with aortic stenosis at risk of evolving to HLHS [14].

Fetal intervention is technically feasible only in a small specific subset of congenital heart defects.

The three most commonly performed FCI are [15]:

1. **Fetal aortic stenosis** with risk factors for evolving into hypoplastic left heart syndrome (HLHS).

2. **HLHS** with intact or restrictive atrial septum.

3. **Pulmonary atresia/stenosis with intact ventricular septum,** with concern for worsening right ventricular (RV) hypoplasia.

- **Fetal aortic stenosis.** In Linz center between October 2000 and February 2020, 115 fetal aortic valvuloplasties (FAV) were undertaken in 95 fetuses. All patients but one had at least one technically successful procedure. An overall success rate of 82.4% (14/17 procedures) was reported by Tulzer et al. [16]. Similarly, Pickard et al. reported in a period from 2000 to 2017 that fetal aortic valvuloplasty was technically successful in 84% of 143 fetuses, while fetal demise was observed in 8%. Biventricular circulation was achieved in 50% of the remaining 111 live-born infants with successful fetal aortic valvuloplasty, while only 16% of the 19 patients with unsuccessful valvuloplasty achieved biventricular circulation [17].

- **HLHS with intact or restrictive atrial septum.** The incidence of intact atrial septum in HLHS is approximately 6%, with restrictive atrial septum occurring in up to 22% [18]. Survival for patients with HLHS and intact atrial septum remains poor, with a 1-year survival rate of ~ 30% [19]. The rationale for FCI in HLHS with intact or restrictive atrial septum is to avoid severe neonatal hypoxia and death and to prevent worsening of the lung disease that frequently occurs as a result of chronic in utero pulmonary venous hypertension. Postnatal management involves atrial septostomy, the Rashkind procedure, to open the atrial septum and enhance atrial mixing. Some selected centers performing this type of FCI, have attempted to maintain patency of the atrial septal defect until the time of delivery, with an atrial septal stent. In the largest cohort of patients undergoing FCI on the atrial septum (n = 47) from the International Fetal Cardiac Intervention Registry, technical success was reported in 77% of cases, with 65% success in atrial stent placement [20].

- **Pulmonary atresia/stenosis with an intact ventricular septum.** Even lesions like pulmonary atresia with intact ventricular septum and severe pulmonary stenosis can progress to significant right ventricular dysplasia and evolve to unfavorable univentricular circulation at birth which will require complex and multiple interventions in the follow-up. These fetuses are potential candidates for pulmonary balloon valvuloplasty in utero. Fetal cardiac intervention offers the potential for improved right ventricle and tricuspid valve growth, less damage to the myocardium, potential for biventricular circulation, and improved morbidity and mortality [21].

The International Fetal Cardiac Intervention Registry (IFCIR) has published data from multiple institutions that provide FCI for PA/IVS [22]. In this study, 16 patients enrolled underwent FCI with 11 successful procedures. The procedure success rate was 11/16 (69%). Of the 11 technically successful cases, five (45%) had postnatal biventricular repair [22]. The group at the Children's Hospital Heart Center in Linz has published a large cohort of patients at a single center [23]. They performed 35 FCI on 25 maternal-fetal pairs for either PA/IVS (n = 15) or critical pulmonary valve stenosis (n = 8). They report either partial or successful FCI in 21/23 maternal-fetal pairs. In the successful intervention group, 15 had a predicted biventricular surgery (70%), three a one and a half ventricle surgery and three an indeterminate outcome. No patients that had a successful FCI were predicted to have a single ventricle outcome [23]. A study performed at Boston Children's Hospital describes their experience [24]. FCI was performed in ten fetuses with PA/IVS. The first four procedures were technically unsuccessful and the following six procedures were successful. Compared with control fetuses (n = 15) with PA/IVS who did not undergo prenatal intervention and had univentricular outcomes after birth, the tricuspid valve annulus, right ventricle length, and PV annulus grew significantly more from midgestation to late gestation in the six fetuses who underwent successful interventions. Nine fetuses were liveborn; one fetus was terminated after an unsuccessful attempt at FCI. All nine patients required postnatal interventions. Of the six successful FCIs, five had a predicted biventricular outcome (83%) and one had a predicted single-ventricle outcome [24].

FCI also includes transplacental drug therapy, such as maternal antiarrhythmic drugs in case of fetal arrhythmias and steroids [25].

### 4.2 Termination of pregnancy

FCI techniques have made possible to improve the success rates of cardiac interventions in utero, obtaining better postnatal outcomes. However, it is inevitable to consider the consequences of a diagnosis of CHD in the prenatal period, leading to a set of complex emotional states in parents who move away from the concept of "healthy condition" of their future child. Discussion with parents on the long-term prognosis constitutes a fundamental element of adequate counseling. Appropriate counseling is ideally composed of an interdisciplinary team: obstetrician, pediatrician, pediatric cardiologist, and heart surgeon [26]. Counseling to parents following the diagnosis of congenital heart disease should take into account: the severity of CHD, the association with extracardiac malformations, and the presence of an associated genetic syndrome. All of these factors influence the parents' decision regarding pregnancy continuation or interruption.

In recent decades, the study of the heart in the prenatal period through fetal echocardiography, associated with a marked improvement in ultrasound technologies, and a greater competence of the operators, has significantly increased detection of the prenatal CHD. The incidence cardiac anomalies diagnosed at prenatal ultrasound screening differs from that observed at birth, due to intrauterine fetal demise and the recourse to termination of pregnancy (TOP). Indeed, in countries where prenatal evaluation is considered as standard of care, the incidence of CHD births is even lower [27]. As mentioned before, the main advantages of an early diagnosis of cardiac malformation are the possibility of adequate preparation for childbirth and neonatal care and early interventions in utero. However, it is inevitable to consider the consequences of a diagnosis of cardiac malformation have in the prenatal period, leading to a set of complex emotional states in parents who have to move away from the concept of "healthy condition" of their future child and eventually undertake the difficult choice of TOP [6]. Annually in the European Union, it has been estimated that 36000 children are live-born with CHD [28]. Increasing prenatal detection may lead to a reduced birth incidence of severe complex CHD through a high rate of TOP, even if this trend is not universal [29]. In the EUROCAT registry, a total of 31% of prenatally diagnosed nonchromosomal CHD resulted in TOP [28]. The parent's choice to TOP is conditioned by several factors as listed below [30–32]:

1. ethical and/or religious reasons;
2. current legislation;
3. severity of cardiac malformation;
4. impact of heart disease on quality of life;
5. possibly associated extracardiac malformations;
6. underlying genetic condition;
7. complexity of cardiac surgery;
8. prediction of survival to adulthood and long-term quality of life;

Additional components that influence the couple's decision-making process include the socioeconomic status, the age of the parents, and the overall family context (caregivers) [33]. It is also reported in the literature that the "pressure" regarding the choice to terminate a pregnancy following multidisciplinary counseling is greater when listening to gynecologists than to pediatric cardiologists and cardiac surgeons [34]. A French study reports an interesting analysis of isolated CHD fetuses; concluding that more than half of the choices for termination of pregnancy were based on the "complexity" of heart disease as HLHS, univentricular heart, pulmonary valve atresia, aortic stenosis [6]. It is, therefore, essential to transfer adequate and precise counseling to the couple without limiting the decision-making process. Thus, considering the information that is offered to parents by pediatric cardiologists and cardiac surgeons regarding the diagnosis of hypoplastic left heart syndrome, it is not surprising that the choice for TOP will increase in this condition because this CHD has a poor post-natal outcome with an impact on the quality of life of the newborn, given the multistage palliative surgery and the surgical risks associated with each intervention [35]. After these considerations, we should if fetal echocardiography should be performed ignoring the consequence of such acts [36]. This debate is still ongoing today, asking questions about the impact that prenatal ultrasound diagnosis can have on the future of humanity [37, 38].

### 4.3 Fetal counseling

Since the prenatal diagnosis of fetal malformation has improved and it's now possible to detect or suspect a fetal malformation from the mid-gestation, it has been necessary to improve the counseling, paying attention to the ethical and psychological aspects related to this issue [39–42]. This is an important issue raised by the large and growing scientific literature on this argument [39–42]. As a consequence of these observations, many authors [43, 44] suggest that is necessary that counseling is performed by a multidisciplinary team comprising the obstetrician, the cardiologist, the surgeon, and the psychologist, in order to provide a fully comprehensive information to the parents. The passage from *paternalistic medicine* to *defensive medicine,* which recognizes the patient's right to have full information, incites the doctor to tell the truth, even in the case of the inauspicious diagnosis of a life-threatening illness. During counseling, at the communicative level, the challenge is not "*whether to tell the truth, but* rather, *how to tell it*". Since CHD is a significant cause of morbidity and mortality in the newborns, its diagnosis may lead to a huge crisis in the affected families, considering the perceived implications of having an abnormality of such vital an organ. The severity of the crisis depends not only on the nature of the abnormality, but also upon its perceived seriousness and whether the defect is correctable. During the pregnancy, parents idealize the newborn and give him/her qualities, feelings, and capacities that they wish. The birth of a baby with a malformation is a sorrow including the death of the imagined child.

The majority of the diagnosis of fetal congenital heart disease occurs after the 18th week of gestation, when the mother already feels the first fetal movements, and the baby is part of her body [45]. During counseling, parents need to know if there is a possibility of repair and what is the risk of the procedures, and how will be the child's quality of life. Some authors analyzed the mother's desire for more information on prenatal diagnosis of fetal abnormality [46]. Some mothers preferred to have increased information upfront in order to "wrap their head around the disease," while other mothers felt that too much information upfront increased anxiety and would rather "cross that bridge when they came to it."

The explanation should possibly be given with both parents present, allowing each to provide support to the other, considering that the impact may be different on either parent, since each may perceive the abnormality differently.

### 4.4 Genetic counseling

The etiology of congenital heart disease is currently the focus of intense research. The ideal genetic counseling for cardiovascular malformations includes a thorough understanding of the anatomy, management, and outcome of the particular defect, identification of other affected family members, and careful pedigree analysis for prediction of familial risks, identification of associated malformations or syndromes, and options for prenatal diagnosis [2]. Preferably, genetic counseling should be provided both by a clinical geneticist with adequate knowledge about cardiac defects and outcomes and by a pediatric cardiologist who has good knowledge and skills in genetic issues.

In the past, genetic counseling for isolated congenital cardiovascular malformations (i.e., without extracardiac malformations or syndromic diagnosis) was transmitted as an advice, with the use of overall recurrence risk for first-degree relatives of 2–5%. These malformations were reputed to be *multifactorial*, but recent studies suggest that specific *genetic* influences may be more important than previously recognized, and that certain malformations are more likely to have a stronger genetic component [47, 48].

A common genetic defect or pathogenetic mechanism may cause several apparently different forms of congenital cardiovascular malformations, as, for example, in case of chromosome 22q deletion, that cause a variety of conotruncal malformations and aortic arch anomalies [49, 50].

## 5. Conclusions

The prenatal diagnosis of CHD in the last 30 years has reached a high degree of diagnostic accuracy allowing identification of almost all the main forms of CHD during fetal life, in expert centers. In particular, prenatal diagnosis of conditions that constitute a neonatal emergency, such as duct dependent lesions, allows to manage the delivery in a tertiary care center. This strategy improves survival significantly, and reduces preoperative morbidity, and the risk of neurological compromise. While some CHD may have a successful surgical correction in postnatal life, a small selective subset of these defects can progress during intrauterine life and be susceptible to early interventions in the uterus. Fetal cardiac interventions might prevent in utero worsening from a simple, potentially correctable lesion to a complex cardiac condition in selective patients. FCIs are most commonly and successfully performed in the setting of 1) fetal aortic stenosis with risk for evolving to hypoplastic left heart syndrome, 2) HLHS with intact or restrictive atrial septum 3) pulmonary atresia/ stenosis with intact ventricular septum, with specific features associated with risk for worsening right ventricular hypoplasia. FCI also includes transplacental therapy, including maternal antiarrhythmic drugs in case of fetal arrhythmias and steroids. FCI is a procedure that has maternal and/or fetal risks, which must be well explained to parents at the time of counseling, to be sure that they fully understand the possible complications.

Moreover, fetal early diagnosis allows to program earlier clinical management and surgery after birth, improving outcomes. The improvement in the diagnosis and treatment of these conditions, due to extraordinary advances in imaging and cardiac surgical and interventional technologies in the last twenty years, has led to a significant increase in survival rate in patients with CHD, and accordingly, the number of patients with CHD who have reached adulthood has increased significantly and even surpass the number of affected kids.

## Author details

Maria Giovanna Russo*, Fiorella Fratta, Antonia Giudicepietro, Carmela Morelli, Fortuna Del Gaizo, Laura di Pietto, Marina De Marco, Ludovica Spinelli Barrile and Federica De Fazio
Pediatric Cardiology Unit—Luigi Vanvitelli—Campania University Hospital, Monaldi Hospital, Naples, Italy

*Address all correspondence to: giovannella.russo@ospedaledeicolli.it

## References

[1] Hoffman JI, Kaplan S. The incidence of congenital heart disease. Journal of the American College of Cardiology. 2002;**39**:1890-1900

[2] Pierpont ME, Brueckner M, Chung WK, et al. Genetic basis for congenital heart disease: Revisited: A scientific statement from the american heart association circulation. 2018;**138**:e653-e711

[3] Cowan JR, Ware SM. Genetics and genetic testing in congenital heart disease. Clinics in Perinatology. 2015;**42**:373-393

[4] Jin SC, Homsy J, Zaidi S, Lu Q, Morton S, DePalma SR, et al. Contribution of rare inherited and de novo variants in 2,871 congenital heart disease probands. Nature Genetics. 2017;**49**:1593-1601

[5] Huhta JC. Uses and abuses of fetal echocardiography: A pediatric cardiologist's view. Journal of the American College of Cardiology. 1986;**8**:451-458

[6] Khoshnood B, De Vigan C, Vodovar V, Goujard J, Lhomme A, Bonnet D, et al. Trends in prenatal diagnosis, pregnancy termination, and perinatal mortality of newborns with congenital heart disease in France, 1983-2000: A population-basedevaluation. Pediatrics. 2005;**115**:95-101

[7] Levey A, Glickstein JS, Kleinman C, Levasseur S, Chen J, Gersony W. The impact of prenatal diagnosis of complex congenital heart disease on neonatal outcomes pediatric cardiology. 2010;**31**:587-597

[8] Gupta N, Leven L, Stewart M, Cheung M, Patel N. Transport in infants with congenital heart disease: Benefits of antenatal diagnosis. European Journal of Pediatrics. 2014;**173**:655-660

[9] Bonnet D, Coltri A, Butera G, Fermont L, Bidois J, Kachaner J, et al. Detection of transposition of the great arteries in fetuses reduces neonatal morbidity and mortality. Circulation. 1999;**99**:916-918

[10] Chew C, Halliday JL, Riley MM, Penny DJ. Population-based study of antenatal detection of congenital heart disease by ultrasound examination. Ultrasound in Obstetrics & Gynecology. 2007;**29**:619-624

[11] Israel SW, Roofe LR, Saville BR, Walsh WF. Improvement in antenatal diagnosis of critical congenital heart disease implications for postnatal care and screening. Fetal Diagnostic Therapy. 2011;**30**:180-183

[12] Allan LD. Development of congenital lesions in mid or late gestation. International Journal of Cardiology. 1988;**19**:361e2

[13] Hutha J, Quintero RA, Suh E, Bader RS. Advances in fetal cardiac intervention. Current Opinion in Pediatrics. 2004;**16**:487-493

[14] Tworetzky W, Wilkins-Haug L, Jennings R, Van der Velde M, Marshall A, Marx G, et al. Balloon dilation of severe aortic stenosis in the fetus. Potential for prevention of hypoplastic left heart syndrome: Candidate selection, technique, and results of successful intervention. Circulation. 2004;**110**:2125-2131

[15] Friedman KG, Tworetzky W. Fetal cardiac interventions: Where do we stand?

Archives of Cardiovascular Disease. 2020;**113**:121-128

[16] Tulzer A, Arzt W, Tulzer G. Fetal aortic valvuloplasty may rescue fetuses with critical aortic stenosis and hydrops. Ultrasound in Obstetrics & Gynecology. 2021

[17] Pickard SS, Wong JB, Bucholz E, Newburger JW, Tworetzky W, Lafranchi T, et al. Fetal aortic valvuloplasty for evolving hypoplastic left heart syndrome: A decision analysis. Circulation: Cardiovascular Quality and Outcomes. 2020;**13**:e006127

[18] Rychiket J, Rome J, Collins MH, DeCampli WM, Spray TL. The hypoplastic left heart syndrome with intactatrial septum: Atrial morphology, pulmonary vascular histopathology and outcome. Journal of American College of Cardiology. 1999;**34**(2):554-560

[19] Vlahos AP, Lock J, McElhinney DB, Van der Velde M. Hypoplastic left heart syndrome with intact or highly restrictive atrial septum: Outcome after neonatale transcatheter atrial septostomy. Circulation. 2004;**109**:2326-2330

[20] Jantzen DW. Hypoplastic left heart syndrome with intact or restrictive atrial septum: A report from the international fetal cardiac intervention registry. Circulation. 2017;**136**:1346-1349

[21] Strainic J. Fetal cardiac intervention for right sided heart disease: Pulmonary atresia with intact ventricular septum. Birth Defects Research. 2019

[22] Moon-Grady AJ, Morris SA, Belfort M, et al. International fetal cardiac Intervention Registry: A Worldwide Collaborative Description a Preliminary Outcomes. Journal of American College of Cardiology. 2015;**66**:388-399

[23] Tulzer A, Artz W, Tulzer G. Immediate effects and outcome of *in-utero* pulmonary valvuloplasty in fetuses with pulmonary atresia with intact ventricular septum or critical pulmonary stenosis. Ultrasound in Obstetrics & Gynecology. 2018;**52**:230-237

[24] Tworetzky W, McElhinney DB, Marx G, Benson C, Brusseau R, Morash D, et al. In utero valvuloplasty for pulmonary atresia with hypoplastic right ventricle: Techniques and outcomes. Pediatrics. 2009;**124**:e510-e518

[25] Bravo-Valenzuela N, Alves Rocha L, Marcondes Machado Nardozza L, Araujo JL. Fetal cardiac arrhythmias: Current evidence. Annals of Pediatric Cardiology. 2018;**11**:148-163

[26] Kovacevic A, Elsässer M, Fluhr H, Müller A, Starystach S, Bär S, et al. Counseling for fetal heart disease—Current standards and best practice. Translational Pediatric. 2021;**10**:2225-2234

[27] Rossier MC, Mivelaz Y, Addor MC, Sekarski N, JanMeijboom E, Vial Y. Evaluation of prenataldiagnosis of congenitalheartdisease in a regionalcontrolled case study. Swiss Medical Weekly. 2014;**144**:w14068

[28] Dolk E, Loane M, Garne E. Congenital heart defects in Europe prevalence and perinatal mortality, 2000 to 2005 European Surveillance of Congenital Anomalies (EUROCAT) working group. Circulation. 2011;**123**: 841-849

[29] Bonnet D. Impacts of prenatal diagnosis of congenital heart diseases on outcomes. Translational Pediatrics. 2021;**10**:2241-2249

[30] Perolo A, Prandstraller D, Ghi T, Gargiulo G, Leone O, Bovicelli L, et al.

Diagnosis and management of fetal cardiac anomalies: 10 years of experience at a single institution. Ultrasound in Obstetrics & Gynecology. 2001;**18**:615-618

[31] Montaguti E, Balducci A, Perolo A, Livi A, Contro E, Casadio P, et al. Prenatal diagnosis of congenital heart defects and voluntary termination of pregnancy. American Journal of Obstetrics & Gynecology MFM. 2020;**2**:100207

[32] Evans W, Acherman R, Restrepo H. Prenatal diagnosis of significant congenital heart disease and elective termination of pregnancy in Nevada. The Journal of Maternal-Fetal & Neonatal Medicine. 2021;**23**:1-6

[33] Gowda M, Thiagarajan M, Satheesh S, Mondal N, Gochhait D, Godipelli L. Prenatal grading of fetalcongenitalheartdisease and itsinfluence on decision making during pregnancy and postata period: A prospective study. The Journal of Maternal-Fetal & Neonatal Medicine. 2020;**3**:1-9

[34] Hilton-Kamm D, Sklansky M, Chang R. How not to tell parentsabouttheirchild's new diagnosis of congenitalheartdisease: An Internet survey of 841 parents. Pediatric Cardiology. 2014;**35**:239-252

[35] Allan L, Huggon IC. Counselling following a diagnosis of congenital Heart disease. Prenatal Diagnostic. 2004;**24**:1136-1143

[36] Fouron JC. The changing and complex relationship between paediatric cardiologists and life. Cardiology in the Young. 2000;**10**:551-556

[37] Hutha JC. Uses and abuses of fetal echocardiography:apediatriccardiolog ist'sview. Journal of American College Cardiology. 1986;**8**:451-458

[38] Squarcia U. Fetaldiagnosis of congenital cardiac malformations—a challenge for physicians as well as parents. Cardiology in the Young. 1996;**6**:256-257

[39] Caniano A, Baylis F. Ethical considerations in prenatal surgical consultation. Pediatric Surgery International. 1999;*15:303*-309

[40] Flake AW. Prenatal intervention: Ethical considerations for life-threatening and non-life threatening anomalies. Seminars in Pediatric Surgery. 2001;**10**:212-221

[41] Aite L, Trucchi A, Nahom A, Zaccara A, La Sala E, Bagolan P. Antenatal diagnosis of surgically correctable anomalies: Effects of repeated consultations on parental anxiety. Journal of Perinatology. 2003;**23**:*652-654*

[42] Di Giusto M, Lazzari R, Giorgetti T, Paesano R, Pachi A. Psychological aspects of therapeutic abortion after early prenatal diagnosis. Clinical and Experimental Obstetrics & Gynecology. 1991;**18**:169-173

[43] Lorenz R, Kuhn M. Multidisciplinary team counselling for fetal anomalies. American Journal of Obstetrics and Gynecology. 1989;**161**:263-266

[44] Dallaire L, Lortie G, Des Rochers M, Clermont R, Vachon C. Parental reaction and adaptability to the prenatal diagnosis of fetal defect or genetic disease leading to pregnancy interruption. Prenatal Diagnosis. 1995;**15**:249-259

[45] Menahem S, Grimwade J. Pregnancy termination following prenatal diagnosis of serious heart disease in the fetus. Early Human Development. 2003;**73**:71-78

[46] Arya B, Glickstein J, Levasseur S, Williams I. Parents of children with

congenital heart disease prefer more information than cardiologists. Congenital Heart Diseases. 2013

[47] Boughman J, Berg KA, Astemborsky J, Clark E, Mc Carter R, Rubin JD, et al. Familial risks of congenital heart defect assessed in a population-based epidemiologic study. American Journal of Medical Genetetics. 1987;**26**:839

[48] Lin AE, Garver KL. Genetic counseling for congenital heart defects. The Journal of Pediatrics. 1988;**113**:1105

[49] Strauss AW, Johnson MC. The genetic basis of pediatric cardiovascular disease. Semina Perinatology. 1996;**20**(564)

[50] Lewin MB, Glass IA, Power P. Genotype-phenotype correlation in congenital heart disease. Current Opinion in Cardiology. 2004;**19**:221

Section 3

# Echocardiography

Chapter 3

# Clinical Benefits of New Echocardiographic Methods

*Teja Senekovič Kojc and Nataša Marčun Varda*

## Abstract

The main goals of a good echocardiographic examination are an accurate assessment of myocardial function and precise presentation of cardiac morphology. Therefore, some new echocardiographic methods, such as functional echocardiography, cardiac deformation imaging, and 3D echocardiography, are becoming increasingly useful. The main advantages of each method, the possibilities for clinical use, and the most important limitations are presented in this paper. Functional echocardiography enables real-time evaluation of cardiac performance, identifying the nature of cardiovascular compromise, guiding therapeutic decisions, and monitoring response to treatment. A better understanding of the cardiac function and hemodynamic changes in critically ill patients is a crucial clinical benefit of the method. Myocardial deformation imaging could be beneficial for the detection of early ventricular dysfunction, especially where classical methods are unreliable. The new methods do not rely on geometric assumptions and can quantify regional as well as global ventricular function. 3D echocardiography allows understanding of complex spatial cardiac relationships; furthermore, it can be valuable in understanding functional anatomy and help planning interventions.

**Keywords:** echocardiography, congenital heart disease, functional echocardiography, myocardial deformation imaging, speckle-tracking imaging, three-dimensional echocardiography, four-dimensional echocardiography

## 1. Introduction

Congenital heart diseases (CHD) are highly variable, ranging from simple to complex lesions. Therefore, pediatric echocardiography faces different challenges, especially in demonstrating complex anatomy and assessing myocardial function in ventricles with variable morphology [1]. At the same time, there is a desire to detect early changes in ventricular function in cardiac patients as well as in patients with systemic diseases potentially affecting the heart. Furthermore, bedside techniques are increasingly used in clinical medicine, which is also seen in pediatric echocardiography. Consequently, the development of new methods or the upgrade of existing ultrasound techniques is urgently needed.

Recent advances in pediatric echocardiography include functional imaging, myocardial deformation imaging, and 3D echocardiography. Advances in ultrasound techniques, especially in pediatric probes, allow imaging with high temporal and spatial resolution, which opens a new perspective on the mechanics and function of the myocardium. 3D echocardiography can help understand complex anatomy with associated functional changes, which is valuable for appropriate intervention planning. For pediatric cardiac patients, a highly variable ventricular morphology is typical, therefore, assessment of myocardial function may be challenging, especially assessment of right ventricular function and function of a single ventricle. Deformation imaging with strain and strain-rate quantification enables quantitative assessment of myocardial function independent of underlying morphology [1, 2]. Strain imaging also enables detecting minimal changes in the global and regional systolic function of the ventricles and allows recognition of the preclinical stage of different diseases affecting the heart [3].

Functional echocardiography has become increasingly useful in everyday clinical practice; nowadays it plays a central role in understanding and managing hemodynamics in critically ill patients [4]. Functional echocardiography facilitates real-time evaluation of cardiac performance, identifying the nature of cardiovascular compromise, guiding therapeutic decisions, and monitoring response to treatment [5]. Namely, early detection of cardiac dysfunction may help to choose an appropriate inotropic or vasopressor support. Good collaboration with pediatric cardiologists taking care of the patient is essential in the performance and interpretation of functional echocardiography [6].

## 2. Functional echocardiography

Bedside functional echocardiography provides physiological information and is a useful real-time noninvasive method among other monitoring tools for critically ill children. It is being increasingly used in making therapeutic clinical decisions and assessing response to treatment in unstable patients in the intensive and emergency units [7].

Functional echocardiography allows bedside use of cardiac ultrasound that brings fast and efficient investigation and recognition of the key hemodynamic changes, an assessment of cardiac function, pulmonary hypertension, pericardial effusion, and evaluation of the shunts. It provides insights into pathophysiology that leads to significant hemodynamic instability, and in addition, therapeutic interventions could be better planned and targeted. It also enables monitoring responses to treatment, which allows rapid therapeutic adjustments [7–10].

Functional echocardiography is also called targeted echocardiography, point-of-care cardiac ultrasound, or clinician performed ultrasound. It is being used to assess preload, afterload, and cardiac contractility while choosing inotropic or fluid therapy [4, 7].

Functional echocardiography performed in the newborn differs significantly from that performed in older children, because of the increased risk of critical or significant CHD. Therefore, the first echocardiography performed on a newborn should be accurate and structured with sequential segmental analysis of the heart. The subsequent scans can be functional, focused, or targeted to address specific clinical questions [7, 11–13].

**Table 1** summarizes the recommendations for the practice of functional echocardiography including neonatologist-performed echocardiography.

Clinical benefits of functional echocardiography are well seen in patients with hypotension and shock, which are common conditions in critically ill children, both likely to have high mortality. Furthermore, echocardiography is crucial in identifying

| Parameter | Recommendations |
|---|---|
| Left ventricular systolic function | • Qualitative assessment (eye-balling)<br>• Quantitative assessment (M-mode measurements of LVEDD and LVESD with a thickness of the septal and posterior wall)<br>• Shortening fraction can be measured by M-mode if there is no regional wall motion abnormality or abnormal septal motion<br>• Ejection fraction should be calculated using biplane volumetric Simpson's measurements |
| Left ventricular diastolic function | • Doppler mitral or tricuspid inflow flow and pulmonary venous flow<br>• TDI velocities at the mitral or tricuspid annulus |
| Right ventricular systolic function | • Qualitative visual assessment<br>• Quantitative assessment (TAPSE and FAC) |
| Volume status | • IVC size and collapsibility<br>• Measurement of LVEDD |
| Pulmonary artery pressure | • Estimation of RVSP and SPAP, MPAP and DPAP (Doppler measurement of tricuspid regurgitation and pulmonary regurgitation jets)<br>• Pressure gradient across the PDA |
| Cardiac output | • Left ventricular output method with pulsed Doppler tracing of TVI in the left ventricular outflow tract and measurement of the cross-sectional area of the left ventricular outflow tract (in the presence of a PDA, the left ventricular output method does not reflect systemic blood flow) |
| Pericardial effusion | • Measurements of effusion at the end of diastole<br>• Assessment of the hemodynamic significance |
| PDA | • The presence of a PDA<br>• Direction of the shunt and pressure gradient between the aorta and pulmonary arteries<br>• Hemodynamic significance in the case of left-to-right shunt by studying the degree of volume overload and left ventricular dimensions |
| PFO | • The presence of a PFO<br>• Shunt direction and the pressure gradient between the right and the left atrium |

*DPAP, diastolic pulmonary artery pressure; FAC, fractional area change; LVEDD, left ventricular end-diastolic dimension; LVESD, left ventricular end-systolic dimension; MPAP, mean pulmonary artery pressure; PAP, pulmonary artery pressure; PDA, patent ductus arteriosus; PFO, patent foramen ovale; RVSP, right ventricular systolic pressure; SPAP, systolic pulmonary artery pressure; SVC, superior vena cava; TAPSE, tricuspid annular plane systolic excursion; TDI, tissue Doppler imaging; TVI, time velocity integral.*

**Table 1.**
*Recommendations for functional echocardiography.*

the underlying pathophysiology, evaluating hemodynamics, and managing the response to treatment in patients with shock [7, 14].

Information from functional echocardiography in conjunction with other clinical parameters and monitoring tools can be used in choosing fluid resuscitation therapy and appropriate inotropic, vasopressor, or vasodilator therapy [15–17]. Early recognition of increased pulmonary pressure may help in the early institution of pulmonary vasodilators, especially in neonates with pulmonary hypertension [7, 9, 11, 17].

Functional echocardiography offers the potential for novel insights into cardiovascular impairment. Specifically, whether the concern relates to preload, afterload, or myocardial contractility. Serial echocardiography evaluation to monitor treatment response may provide a better understanding of physiology and guide the duration of treatment, which minimizes drug exposure [11].

Assessment of volume status is usually made with inferior vena cava (IVC) size and collapsibility, which is also the method of choice to evaluate right heart filling pressure. This can be done easily in spontaneously breathing children, but some limitations exist in ventilated patients. In the presence of cardiogenic shock and increased right heart filling pressure, the IVC will appear dilated with no respiratory variation [15].

Qualitative estimation of the severity of pulmonary hypertension can be made by assessing the shape of the left ventricle and interventricular septum (IVS) motion, which is obtained from the parasternal short-axis view. With rising pulmonary artery pressure (PAP), the left ventricle begins to lose its circular shape and IVS starts to flatten, furthermore, paradoxical septal movement may occur in severe pulmonary hypertension [7, 9]. The shunt across the patent foramen ovale (PFO) is generally bidirectional in the presence of pulmonary hypertension but can sometimes be left-to-right even in the presence of severe pulmonary hypertension. An exclusively right-to-left shunt across the PFO is always abnormal and suggests elevated right heart filling pressure [6]. Direct assessment of the pulmonary artery pressures can be done by a peak velocity of the tricuspid insufficiency jet using the modified Bernoulli equation. The pulmonary artery systolic pressure (PASP) may be estimated by adding right atrial pressure to the peak systolic pressure gradient between the right ventricle and right atrium. The mean pulmonary artery pressure (MPAP) is assessed by using the peak diastolic velocity of the pulmonary regurgitation jet. The end-diastolic velocity of the pulmonary regurgitation jet is used to estimate diastolic pulmonary artery pressure (DPAP) [6, 7]. Functional echocardiography is useful in the initiation of vasodilator treatment (such as inhaled nitric oxide) and monitoring the response to treatment [6].

Pericardial effusion is a common condition in intensive care units; functional echocardiography allows easy diagnosis and timely echo-guided pericardiocentesis [18]. The hemodynamic effect of pericardial effusion does not depend solely on the amount of pericardial fluid. A large amount of pericardial fluid can be well tolerated when the fluid accumulates slowly. However, rapidly increasing pericardial effusion is more dangerous and may lead to cardiac tamponade. The main echocardiographic signs of cardiac tamponade are distended IVC with no respiratory variation, right atrial collapse at the end of diastole, right ventricular free wall collapse during diastole, and respiratory variation of Doppler mitral inflow for more than 10% and tricuspid inflow for more than 25% [7].

Patent ductus arteriosus (PDA) is an independent risk factor for intraventricular hemorrhage, necrotizing enterocolitis, bronchopulmonary dysplasia (BPD), and acute pulmonary hemorrhage [19, 20]. The hemodynamic significance of a PDA may not be directly related to the size of the PDA but depends upon the magnitude of the shunt and the ability of the myocardium to adapt to a left-to-right shunt [7, 20–22]. PDA causes pulmonary hyperperfusion and systemic hypoperfusion, which could be assessed with functional echocardiography. The duration of the shunt and the level of diastolic flow reversal in the descending aorta are good indicators of the significance of PDA and can be used for follow-up. An additional factor in assessing the PDA is pulmonary artery pressure, which can be monitored based on PDA Doppler velocity magnitudes. A low-pressure gradient between the aorta and pulmonary artery may be associated with pulmonary hypertension. Non-restrictive PDA has a low peak systolic velocity with a high systolic to diastolic velocity gradient, while restrictive shunt is characterized by a high peak systolic velocity and a low systolic to diastolic velocity gradient [21]. Functional echocardiography has also been reported to improve the outcomes in infants being treated for PDA, the impact of this echocardiographic method is still the subject of ongoing research [23, 24]. Furthermore, it has been found that the performance of bedside echocardiography reduces the number of indomethacin doses used for treating PDA [25, 26]. The introduction of a functional echocardiography screening program for hemodynamically significant PDA on day 3 of life with the targeted intervention was associated with a reduction of severe intraventricular hemorrhage and ventilation duration [25, 27]. Serial echocardiography was associated with earlier identification and treatment of PDA, lower rates of severe intraventricular hemorrhage, and reduced ventilator days [11, 25].

## 3. Myocardial deformation imaging

Conventional methods for assessment of regional and global ventricular function, such as fractional shortening and ejection fraction, are largely dependent on loading conditions and geometric assumptions [28, 29]. Myocardial deformation imaging has introduced a new global parameter of left ventricular longitudinal deformation GLS (global longitudinal strain), which has turned out to be more sensitive for early detection of myocardial impairment compared to conventional echocardiographic systolic function parameters. Myocardial deformation parameters have diagnostic as well as prognostic values in several cardiac diseases [3].

Recent developments in the assessment of ventricular function are the measurement of myocardial tissue Doppler velocities (tissue Doppler imaging, TDI) and deformation imaging (strain and strain-rate quantification). TDI has some advantages over traditional echocardiographic techniques in providing measurements of cardiac tissue movements [7, 30]. Myocardial deformation analysis is a quantitative technique that helps define a global and regional function of both ventricles. Tissue deformation is measured by cardiac strain, and there is an additional parameter called strain rate that defines the rate of myocardial deformation in time [7].

Compared to traditional methods that measure cardiac function mainly in the radial direction, strain imaging does not rely on geometric assumptions and can quantify function in the longitudinal, radial, and circumferential direction of motion. Therefore, regional as well as global ventricular function may be better estimated. Strain rate measures the extent of shortening of the myocardium in the longitudinal and circumferential directions and thickening in the radial direction. These newer methods of myocardial function assessment have already shown great promise in several areas of pediatric echocardiography, but their use in clinical practice is still limited by the lack of data from large patient cohorts [1].

Recently, two-dimensional (2D) and three-dimensional (3D) speckle-tracking echocardiography (STE) has been introduced as a new method to quantify myocardial strain [29]. STE tracks the motion of speckles within the scan volume, allowing a more complete and accurate assessment of myocardial deformation in all three spatial dimensions [29, 31]. Strain imaging is a promising method for assessing left ventricular function for diagnosis, prognosis, and risk stratification of various congenital and acquired heart diseases; it is also useful for monitoring treatment outcomes before and after medical, percutaneous, and surgical interventions [29].

Strain and strain rate can be measured either from tissue Doppler velocities or with speckle-tracking techniques together with final analysis at the workstation. It

| Vendor | Software | Average value of GLS (%) | Lower limit of normal GLS (%) | Average value of GCS (%) | Average value of GRS (%) |
|---|---|---|---|---|---|
| GE | EchoPAC BT12 | −19.40 (−20.06 to −18.74) | −18 | −19.47 (−20.49 to −18.45) | 50.41 (47.96 to 52.87) |
| Philips | QLAB 7.1 | −19.67 (−21.27 to −18.08) | −14 | −22.13 (−26.73 to −17.52) | 59.24 (41.91 to 76.56) |
| Toshiba | UltraExtend | −17.04 (−17.91 to −16.17) | −15 | −28.79 (−32.90 to −24.68) | 33.17 (24.38 to 41.97) |

*Data are mean (95% CI—confidence interval); GLS, global longitudinal strain; GCS, global circumferential strain; GRS, global radial strain.*

**Table 2.**
*Normal left ventricular global longitudinal strain (GLS), global circumferential strain (GRS), and global radial strain (GRS) values for specific vendors' equipment based on data from the literature (adapted from Truong et al., Lang et al.).*

is necessary to be aware of the wide variability of the strain and strain rate measurements that depend on vendors, software packages, and echocardiographic laboratories, as shown in **Table 2** [32, 33]. Broad clinical use of the strain is still limited due to the intervendor differences and related difficult comparison of the results, thus, standardization is urgently needed [1, 34]. Higher heart rates, especially in younger children, require higher frame rates, particularly for strain rate imaging; therefore, this aspect of use requires further development. Another challenge for the implementation of strain imaging in everyday clinical practice is the availability of reference values for different age groups of children [1, 35].

3D speckle-tracking provides a more comprehensive evaluation of ventricular mechanics from pyramidal 3D datasets. Furthermore, it enables also more precise mechanical activation mapping compared to 2D strain, by being maximum opposing wall delay and SD (standard deviation) still significantly correlated with similar 2D strain measurements. 3D loops of regional strain are color-coded and divided into 16 or 18 segments for time-strain curves. The results are presented in a 16- or 18-segment polar map with segmental systolic strain values displayed in the bull's eye. GLS value is defined as the average peak longitudinal strain of the left ventricle [36, 37]. Future development and expansion of applications for 3D speckle tracking are anticipated.

Strain imaging has also been used to gain a greater understanding of the pathophysiology of cardiac ischemia and infarction, primary diseases of the myocardium, the effects of valvular disease on myocardial function, and understanding of diastolic function, as seen in **Table 3**. Strain imaging has also been used for heart failure patients undergoing cardiac resynchronization pacing therapy providing important quantitative information on the timing of mechanical activation. Strain imaging has become increasingly used for research purposes, in addition, it shows great potential for routine clinical practice in the light of the improved treatment of cardiovascular patients [37]. Therefore, deformation imaging also plays a role in the risk stratification of young individuals with a potentially increased risk for heart failure and sudden cardiac death [1, 38]. Strain imaging has also been used to help to differentiate between athlete's heart and individuals with potential cardiomyopathy [1, 39]. While multiple studies have shown the usefulness of strain quantification for risk stratification in various diseases, such as arterial hypertension, diabetes mellitus, metabolic

| Area of use | Clinical applications |
|---|---|
| CHD | • The effects of valvular disease on myocardial function<br>• Understanding of the diastolic function<br>• Timely treatment decisions |
| Primary diseases of the myocardium (cardiomyopathies) | • Early detection of ventricular dysfunction<br>• Potential need for additional diagnostics<br>• Timely treatment decisions |
| Cardiac ischemia and infarction | • Extent of the ischemic myocardium<br>• Assessing ventricular function, especially in patients with preserved LVEF |
| Cardiac resynchronization therapy | • Quantify abnormalities in the timing of mechanical activation of the left ventricle |
| Myocarditis | • Evaluation of ventricular function in patients with preserved LVEF<br>• Evaluation of regional myocardial dysfunction |
| Cardiotoxicity | • Recognition of subclinical myocardial dysfunction<br>• Adjustment of therapy |
| Risk stratification for heart failure and sudden cardiac death in children with a systemic disease | • Early detection of ventricular dysfunction in patients with arterial hypertension, diabetes mellitus, metabolic syndrome, chronic kidney disease, neuromuscular diseases<br>• Potential need for additional diagnostics<br>• Timely treatment decisions |

*CHD, congenital heart disease; LVEF, left ventricular ejection fraction.*

**Table 3.**
*Main clinical applications of myocardial deformation imaging.*

syndrome, chronic kidney disease, neuromuscular diseases, and others, the main limitation remains that strain values vary among methods, modalities, and software versions [40–42].

Ventricular morphology can be highly variable in CHD, and therefore traditional methods of assessment of ventricular function that rely on geometry are unreliable. Assessment of right ventricular function and evaluation of functional changes in patients with a single ventricle are particularly challenging. Assessment of regional function is also important in pediatric patients with coronary artery abnormalities [1]. Subtle impairment in myocardial function, detectable with strain imaging, can be used to identify asymptomatic patients who progress to require valve surgery, which improves timely planning of the appropriate treatment [43].

Due to geometric factors, strain imaging better reflects systolic function in patients with preserved ejection fraction (EF), which is also common in cardiomyopathies. Particularly, longitudinal shortening may vary in patients with cardiomyopathies significantly, as it has less effect on EF than circumferential shortening. Therefore, longitudinal shortening might potentially be a more sensitive marker of systolic dysfunction, which typically affects the subendocardial region first, and could be assessed with longitudinal strain [44]. Deformation parameters, especially global longitudinal strain, have better accuracy in detecting cardiac amyloidosis in patients with thickened hearts [45].

Strain imaging is a beneficial additional echocardiographic method in assessing the extent of the ischemic myocardium and ventricular function. Postsystolic shortening is an important feature of the ischemic myocardium as a marker of tissue viability, and when associated with systolic hypokinesis or akinesis, it indicates actively contracting myocardium. When combined with dyskinesis, however, postsystolic shortening seems to be a nonspecific marker of severe ischemia [46]. Semiautomated calculation of GLS is significantly related to all-cause mortality or heart failure in patients with myocardial infarction and left ventricular ejection fraction (LVEF) > 40% [47].

Strain imaging is effective in monitoring cardiac function in patients with the multisystem inflammatory syndrome in children (MIS-C), which occurs after COVID-19 infection. Patients with preserved LVEF in myocarditis within MIS-C had significantly lower GLS; furthermore, regional myocardial dysfunction may also be presented, as seen in **Figure 1**. Hence, even preserved EF patients show subtle changes in myocardial deformation, suggesting subclinical myocardial injury. During a follow-up of the patients with MIS-C, there was a good recovery of systolic function but the persistence of diastolic dysfunction [48, 49]. Speckle-tracking imaging can help in the diagnosis of acute myocarditis when cardiovascular magnetic resonance (CMR) is not readily available or cannot be performed. There is a good correlation between speckle-tracking imaging-based LVEF, global strain and magnetic resonance imaging (MRI) calculated LVEF [50].

Segmental strain curves in a four-chamber view (top left), two-chamber view (top right), three-chamber view/APLAX—apical long-axis view (bottom left), and

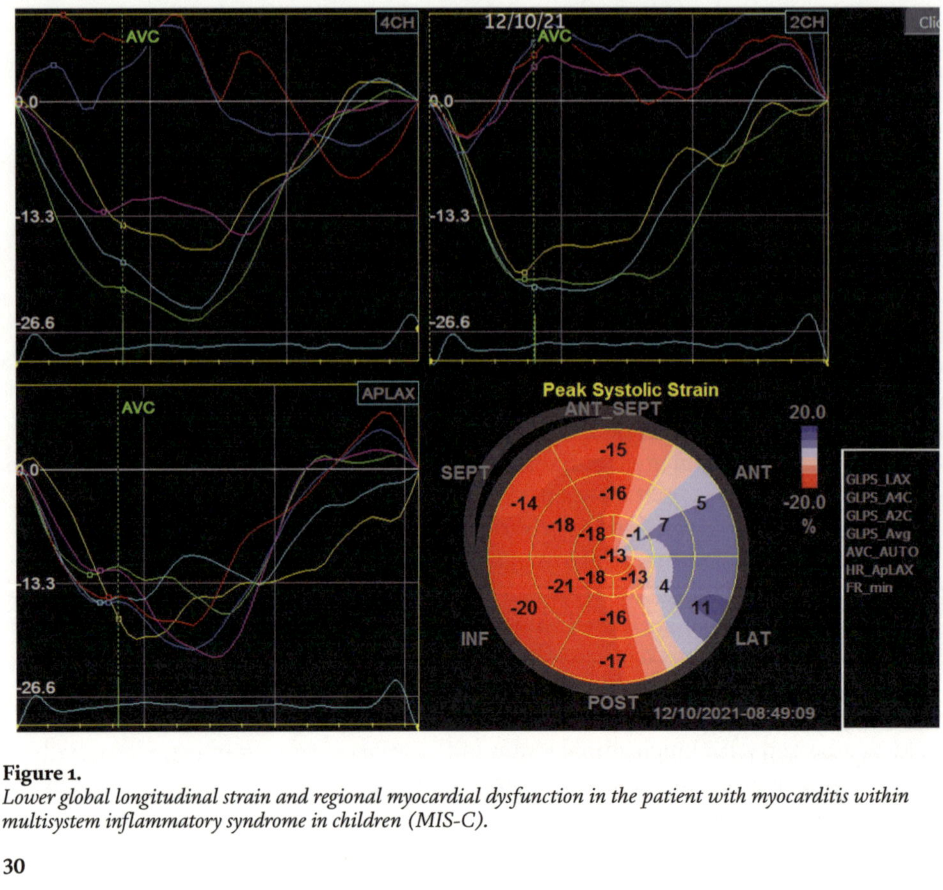


**Figure 1.**
*Lower global longitudinal strain and regional myocardial dysfunction in the patient with myocarditis within multisystem inflammatory syndrome in children (MIS-C).*

18-segment model or bull's eye (bottom right). The numbers in segments in the bull's eye are the peak longitudinal strain values in systole. The calculated value of global longitudinal strain (GLS) is −13.3%. Systolic values of the longitudinal strain are reduced in basal and mid-cavity segments of the anterior and lateral wall (blue color).

The recognition of early left ventricular dysfunction in cancer patients after cardiotoxic therapy may allow the identification of individuals at risk of future heart failure, allowing targeted monitoring and possibly institution of potential therapies such as angiotensin-converting enzyme inhibitors. The potential of strain imaging to prevent future cardiac toxicity by modulating cancer therapy and the institution of cardiac protective therapy is promising [51, 52].

GLS is the preferred indicator of left ventricular global systolic function. Strain measurements have proven to be more reproducible than LVEF due to minor dependency on segmental variability than LVEF calculations. Additionally, strain measurements should be obtained with the same analysis system and software version [42, 53–55].

Strain imaging is designed for the echocardiographic assessment of regional and global myocardial function, and has been well studied in the adult population, however, its use in pediatrics appears to be limited [56–58]. The duration of the investigation and the need to perform post-processing are major barriers to the more widespread implementation of the strain. Fully automated analysis with algorithms validated in the pediatric population may remove this problem [58].

## 4. 3D echocardiography

3D echocardiography (3DE) allows imaging and analysis of cardiovascular structures as they move in time and space, which enables the creation of 4D datasets (3D in real-time). Real-time 3DE is a major innovation in the history of cardiovascular ultrasound [59].

3DE is increasingly used in patients with congenital heart disease, as it allows the visualization of lesions in three dimensions, with opportunities for increased appreciation of complex spatial relationships. Alternative imaging modalities such as CMR or computed tomography (CT) have, compared to 3DE, some disadvantages, such as expense, general anesthesia (CMR), or exposure to radiation (CT) [1].

Clinical benefits of 3DE are evident in three main areas: better visualization and understanding of the spatial relationships and 3D morphology of congenital heart defects; quantification of cardiac mass and volumes; planning and guiding therapeutic interventions, as seen in **Table 4** [1, 60].

However, 3DE scanning modalities that use the ECG for gating, and then collect the data acquired over several heartbeats are often problematic in younger patients, as there is a large potential for movement artifact, especially with higher respiratory rates. The main shortcomings of 3D imaging have been the lower spatial and temporal resolution compared with 2D imaging, and the requirement for offline analysis [1, 60].

Compared to cross-sectional imaging methods 3DE does not use the same geometric assumptions, which allows a more accurate assessment of the cardiac function. At the same time, with better visualization also comes a better understanding of the anatomy of CHD, such as atrial and ventricular septal defects, atrioventricular (AV) septal defects, and atrioventricular valve or outflow tract abnormalities. In addition, 3DE enables better volumetric assessment of cardiac chambers in patients with borderline sized ventricles, it can also work as an important diagnostic tool for cardiac mass. 3DE findings correlate well with surgical findings, and can significantly improve the planning of therapeutic interventions, sometimes may also reduce the operative time [1].

| Area of use | Clinical applications |
|---|---|
| Morphology of CHD | • Atrial septal defects<br>• Ventricular septal defect<br>• Atrioventricular septal defects<br>• Atrioventricular valve abnormalities<br>• Outflow tract abnormalities |
| Quantification of cardiac mass and volumes | • Ventricular volume and mass quantification (borderline left ventricle, right ventricle)<br>• Atrial volume and mass quantification<br>• Dyssynchrony assessment (regional LV volumes) |
| Planning and guiding therapeutic interventions | • Presurgical imaging (including 3D printing of atrioventricular valves)<br>• Intraprocedural imaging (intraoperative epicardial and transesophageal 3DE, transcatheter procedures, endomyocardial biopsy) |
| Fetal echocardiography | • Spatial relationship of the cardiac structures and great vessels<br>• Quantification of cardiac volumes |

*CHD, congenital heart disease; LV, left ventricle.*

**Table 4.**
*Main clinical applications of 3D echocardiography.*

3DE offers the additional advantage to estimate the AV valve regurgitant volume, the mechanism, and the origin of regurgitation with clear visualization of the valves, which makes 3DE an ideal imaging modality to evaluate these structures and plan interventions [61–64]. 3DE is also a promising modality for 3D printing of AV valves, structures that are largely missing from cardiac models using exclusively MRI or CT data [64–66].

The 3DE and 4DE with spatiotemporal image correlation allow obtaining fetal cardiac volumes and their static and real-time analysis [67], and multiple two-dimensional images are stacked one behind the other to create a volume dataset [68–70]. 4DE is used mainly in the field of fetal echocardiography for the dynamic assessment of fetal cardiac structures and large vessels. The main challenge of fetal echocardiography is still a profound understanding of the spatial relationships and connections of the cardiac structures and great vessels, which 4DE overcomes with more accurate anatomic information. Although traditional 2D echocardiography is the basic modality for prenatal diagnosis of CHD, 3DE and 4DE should be considered as very useful additions [71].

## 5. Conclusions

Recently, the focus of the development of pediatric echocardiography has shifted toward accurate assessment of myocardial function and precise presentation of cardiac morphology. As in other areas of ultrasound examinations, there is an increasing need for bedside targeted echocardiography that provides fast answers to major clinical challenges. Therefore, some echocardiographic methods becoming increasingly useful, such as functional echocardiography, cardiac deformation imaging, and 3D echocardiography.

Functional echocardiography enables real-time evaluation of cardiac performance, identifying the nature of cardiovascular compromise, guiding therapeutic decisions, and monitoring response to treatment. An additional advantage of functional echocardiography is the noninvasiveness of the method. The decision-making process is easier with further information provided by targeted echocardiography, which also reduces a substantial proportion of interventions. Standardized training and close collaboration with pediatric cardiologists are essential for ensuring patients' safety and quality of examination, especially in neonatal units where the risk of a critical or major CHD is higher compared to older children. Future research should address short-term cardiovascular effects and long-term outcomes of functional echocardiography.

Myocardial deformation imaging may be beneficial for the detection of early ventricular dysfunction, especially where classical methods are unreliable. A better understanding of patterns of dysfunction may help clinicians to identify causative factors for global and regional ventricular dysfunction. Patients with progressive heart disease or systemic disease affecting the heart may be identified and treated timely. Furthermore, closer monitoring of the effects of therapy is also an important advantage of myocardial deformation. New methods of myocardial function assessment have already shown great promise in several areas of pediatric echocardiography, but the main limitation remains that strain values vary among methods, modalities, and software versions. Further investigation is warranted for the potential clinical applications in a pediatric population, especially in defining the normal range and maturational changes in strain.

3DE is a very promising and topical new echocardiographic method; recently, it has become more popular in patients with CHD, as it allows the visualization of defects in three dimensions, with opportunities for increased appreciation of complex spatial relationships. A current limitation of 3DE is a restriction of spatial and temporal resolution. Based on 3D modeling, virtual surgery may even be possible, to optimize device design for individual patients, or to determine the optimal surgical technique. In a near future, we are likely to see increased use of 3DE during transcatheter interventions and heart surgeries.

## Conflict of interest

The authors declare no conflict of interest.

## Author details

Teja Senekovič Kojc* and Nataša Marčun Varda
University Medical Centre Maribor, Maribor, Slovenia

*Address all correspondence to: teja.senekovic@gmail.com

## References

[1] Bharucha T, Mertens L. Recent advances in pediatric echocardiography. Expert Review of Cardiovascular Therapy. 2013;**11**:31-47. DOI: 10.1586/erc.12.168

[2] Smiseth OA, Torp H, Opdahl A, Haugaa KH, Urheim S. Myocardial strain imaging: How useful is it in clinical decision making? European Heart Journal. 2016;**37**:1196-1207. DOI: 10.1093/eurheartj/ehv529

[3] Kalam K, Otahal P, Marwick TH. Prognostic implications of global LV dysfunction: A systematic review and meta-analysis of global longitudinal strain and ejection fraction. Heart. 2014;**100**:1673-1680. DOI: 10.1136/heartjnl-2014-305538

[4] Harabor A, Soraisham AS. Utility of targeted neonatal echocardiography in the management of neonatal illness. Journal of Ultrasound in Medicine. 2015;**34**:1259-1263. DOI: 10.7863/ultra.34.7.1259

[5] Lavie-Nevo K, Dinur G, Almagor Y, Barzilay B, Rotschild A, Gover A. Functional echo in preterm infants—Past, present and future. Harefuah. 2020;**159**:759-763

[6] de Waal K, Kluckow M. Functional echocardiography; from physiology to treatment. Early Human Development. 2010;**86**:149-154. DOI: 10.1016/j.earlhumdev.2010.01.030

[7] Tissot C, Singh Y. Neonatal functional echocardiography. Current Opinion in Pediatrics. 2020;**32**:235-244. DOI: 10.1097/MOP.0000000000000887

[8] Groves AM, Singh Y, Dempsey E, Molnar Z, Austin T, El-Khuffash A, et al. Introduction to neonatologist-performed echocardiography. Pediatric Research. 2018;**84**:1-12. DOI: 10.1038/s41390-018-0076-y

[9] Singh Y. Echocardiographic evaluation of hemodynamics in neonates and children. Frontiers in Pediatrics. 2017;**5**:201. DOI: 10.3389/fped.2017.00201

[10] Beaulieu Y. Bedside echocardiography in the assessment of the critically ill. Critical Care Medicine. 2007;**35**:S235-S249. DOI: 10.1097/01.CCM.0000260673.66681.AF

[11] El-Khuffash AF, McNamara PJ. Neonatologist-performed functional echocardiography in the neonatal intensive care unit. Seminars in Fetal and Neonatal Medicine. 2011;**16**:50-60. DOI: 10.1016/j.siny.2010.05.001

[12] Mertens L, Seri I, Marek J, Arlettaz R, Barker P, McNamara P, et al. Targeted neonatal echocardiography in the neonatal intensive care unit: Practice guidelines and recommendations for training. Journal of the American Society of Echocardiography. 2011;**24**:1057-1078. DOI: 10.1016/j.echo.2011.07.014

[13] Singh Y, Gupta S, Groves AM, Gandhi A, Thomson J, Qureshi S, et al. Expert consensus statement 'Neonatologist-performed Echocardiography (NoPE)'—Training and accreditation in UK. European Journal of Pediatrics. 2016;**175**:281-287. DOI: 10.1007/s00431-015-2633-2

[14] Brierley J, Carcillo JA, Choong K, Cornell T, DeCaen A, Deymann A, et al. Clinical practice parameters for hemodynamic support of pediatric and neonatal septic shock: 2007 update from the American College of Critical

Care Medicine. Critical Care Medicine. 2009;**37**:666-688. DOI: 10.1097/CCM.0b013e31819323c6

[15] de Boode WP, van der Lee R, Horsberg Eriksen B, Nestaas E, Dempsey E, Singh Y, et al. The role of Neonatologist Performed Echocardiography in the assessment and management of neonatal shock. Pediatric Research. 2018;**84**:57-67. DOI: 10.1038/s41390-018-0081-1

[16] Landry DW, Oliver JA. The pathogenesis of vasodilatory shock. New England Journal of Medicine. 2001;**345**:588-595. DOI: 10.1056/NEJMra002709

[17] Wynn JL, Wong HR. Pathophysiology and treatment of septic shock in neonates. Clinics in Perinatology. 2010;**37**:439-479. DOI: 10.1016/j.clp.2010.04.002

[18] Pérez-Casares A, Cesar S, Brunet-Garcia L, Sanchez-de-Toledo J. Echocardiographic evaluation of pericardial effusion and cardiac tamponade. Frontiers in Pediatrics. 2017;**5**:79. DOI: 10.3389/fped.2017.00079

[19] Noori S, McCoy M, Friedlich P, Bright B, Gottipati V, Seri I, et al. Failure of ductus arteriosus closure is associated with increased mortality in preterm infants. Pediatrics. 2009;**123**:e138-e144. DOI: 10.1542/peds.2008-2418

[20] Noori S. Patent ductus arteriosus in the preterm infant: To treat or not to treat? Journal of Perinatology. 2010;**30**:S31-S37. DOI: 10.1038/jp.2010.97

[21] van Laere D, van Overmeire B, Gupta S, El-Khuffash A, Savoia M, McNamara PJ, et al. Application of Neonatologist Performed Echocardiography in the assessment of a patent ductus arteriosus. Pediatric Research. 2018;**84**:46-56. DOI: 10.1038/s41390-018-0077-x

[22] Arlettaz R. Echocardiographic evaluation of patent ductus arteriosus in preterm infants. Frontiers in Pediatrics. 2017;**5**:147. DOI: 10.3389/fped.2017.00147

[23] Sehgal A, McNemara PJ. Does point-of-care functional echocardiography enhance cardiovascular care in the NICU? Journal of Perinatology. 2008;**28**(11):729-735. DOI: 10.1038/jp.2008.100

[24] Sehgal A, Francis JV, James A, McNemara PJ. Patent ductus arteriosus ligation and post-operative hemodynamic instability: Case report and framework for enhanced neonatal care. Indian Journal of Pediatrics. 2010;**77**(8):905-907. DOI: 10.1007/s12098-010-0137-7

[25] O'Rourke D, El-Khuffash A, Moody C, Walsh K, Molloy E. Patent ductus arteriosus evaluation by serial echocardiography in preterm infants. Acta Paediatrica. 2008;**97**:574-578. DOI: 10.1111/j.1651-2227.2008.00745.x

[26] Carmo KB, Evans N, Paradisis M. Duration of indomethacin treatment of the preterm patent ductus arteriosus as directed by echocardiography. The Journal of Pediatrics. 2009;**155**:819-822.e1. DOI: 10.1016/j.jpeds.2009.06.013

[27] Poon W, Wong K. Neonatologist-performed point-of-care functional echocardiography in the neonatal intensive care unit. Singapore Medical Journal. 2017;**58**:230-233. DOI: 10.11622/smedj.2017036

[28] Dragulescu A, Mertens LL. Developments in echocardiographic techniques for the evaluation of ventricular function in children. Archives of Cardiovascular Diseases. 2010;**103**:603-614. DOI: 10.1016/j.acvd.2010.09.004

[29] Zhang L, Gao J, Xie M, Yin P, Liu W, Li Y, et al. Left ventricular

three-dimensional global systolic strain by real-time three-dimensional speckle-tracking in children: Feasibility, reproducibility, maturational changes, and normal ranges. Journal of the American Society of Echocardiography. 2013;**26**:853-859. DOI: 10.1016/j.echo.2013.05.002

[30] Nestaas E, Schubert U, de Boode WP, El-Khuffash A. Tissue Doppler velocity imaging and event timings in neonates: A guide to image acquisition, measurement, interpretation, and reference values. Pediatric Research. 2018;**84**:18-29. DOI: 10.1038/s41390-018-0079-8

[31] Gayat E, Ahmad H, Weinert L, Lang RM, Mor-Avi V. Reproducibility and inter-vendor variability of left ventricular deformation measurements by three-dimensional speckle-tracking echocardiography. Journal of the American Society of Echocardiography. 2011;**24**:878-885. DOI: 10.1016/j.echo.2011.04.016

[32] Truong VT, Phan HT, Pham KNP, Duong HNH, Ngo TNM, et al. Normal ranges of left ventricular strain by three-dimensional speckle-tracking echocardiography in adults: A systematic review and meta-analysis. Journal of the American Society of Echocardiography. 2019;**32**(12):1586-1597.e5. DOI: 10.1016/j.echo.2019.07.012

[33] Lang RM, Badano LP, Mor-Avi V, Afilalo J, Armstrong A, Ernande L, et al. Recommendations for cardiac chamber quantification by echocardiography in adults: An update from the American Society of Echocardiography and the European Association of Cardiovascular Imaging. European Heart Journal Cardiovascular Imaging. 2016;**17**(4):412. DOI: 10.1093/ehjci/jew041

[34] Lorch SM, Ludomirsky A, Singh GK. Maturational and growth-related changes in left ventricular longitudinal strain and strain rate measured by two-dimensional speckle tracking echocardiography in healthy pediatric population. Journal of the American Society of Echocardiography. 2008;**21**:1207-1215. DOI: 10.1016/j.echo.2008.08.011

[35] Marcus KA, Mavinkurve-Groothuis AMC, Barends M, van Dijk A, Feuth T, de Korte C, et al. Reference values for myocardial two-dimensional strain echocardiography in a healthy pediatric and young adult cohort. Journal of the American Society of Echocardiography. 2011;**24**:625-636. DOI: 10.1016/j.echo.2011.01.021

[36] Tanaka H, Hara H, Saba S, Gorcsan J. Usefulness of three-dimensional speckle tracking strain to quantify dyssynchrony and the site of latest mechanical activation. The American Journal of Cardiology. 2010;**105**:235-242. DOI: 10.1016/j.amjcard.2009.09.010

[37] Gorcsan J, Tanaka H. Echocardiographic assessment of myocardial strain. Journal of the American College of Cardiology. 2011;**58**:1401-1413. DOI: 10.1016/j.jacc.2011.06.038

[38] Printz BF. Noninvasive imaging modalities and sudden cardiac arrest in the young: Can they help distinguish subjects with a potentially life-threatening abnormality from normals? Pediatric Cardiology. 2012;**33**:439-451. DOI: 10.1007/s00246-012-0169-z

[39] Butz T, van Buuren F, Mellwig KP, Langer C, Plehn G, Meissner A, et al. Two-dimensional strain analysis of the global and regional myocardial function for the differentiation of pathologic and physiologic left ventricular hypertrophy: A study in athletes and in patients with hypertrophic cardiomyopathy. The

International Journal of Cardiovascular Imaging. 2011;**27**:91-100. DOI: 10.1007/s10554-010-9665-5

[40] Reichek N. Myocardial strain: Still a long way to go. Circulation. Cardiovascular Imaging. 2017;**10**(11): e007145. DOI: 10.1161/CIRCIMAGING.117.007145

[41] Collier P, Phelan D, Klein A. A test in context: Myocardial strain measured by speckle-tracking echocardiography. Journal of the American College of Cardiology. 2017;**69**:1043-1056. DOI: 10.1016/j.jacc.2016.12.012

[42] Amzulescu MS, de Craene M, Langet H, Pasquet A, Vancraeynest D, Pouleur AC, et al. Myocardial strain imaging: Review of general principles, validation, and sources of discrepancies. European Heart Journal Cardiovascular Imaging. 2019;**20**:605-619. DOI: 10.1093/ehjci/jez041

[43] Baumgartner H, Falk V, Bax JJ, de Bonis M, Hamm C, Holm PJ, et al. 2017 ESC/EACTS Guidelines for the management of valvular heart disease. European Heart Journal. 2017;**38**:2739-2791. DOI: 10.1093/eurheartj/ehx391

[44] Stokke TM, Hasselberg NE, Smedsrud MK, Sarvari SI, Haugaa KH, Smiseth OA, et al. Geometry as a confounder when assessing ventricular systolic function. Journal of the American College of Cardiology. 2017;**70**:942-954. DOI: 10.1016/j.jacc.2017.06.046

[45] Pagourelias ED, Mirea O, Duchenne J, van Cleemput J, Delforge M, Bogaert J, et al. Echo parameters for differential diagnosis in cardiac amyloidosis. Circulation. Cardiovascular Imaging. 2017;**10**:e005588. DOI: 10.1161/CIRCIMAGING.116.005588

[46] Skulstad H, Edvardsen T, Urheim S, Rabben SI, Stugaard M, Lyseggen E, et al. Postsystolic shortening in ischemic myocardium. Circulation. 2002;**106**:718-724. DOI: 10.1161/01.CIR.0000024102.55150.B6

[47] Ersbøll M, Valeur N, Mogensen UM, Andersen MJ, Møller JE, Velazquez EJ, et al. Prediction of all-cause mortality and heart failure admissions from global left ventricular longitudinal strain in patients with acute myocardial infarction and preserved left ventricular ejection fraction. Journal of the American College of Cardiology. 2013;**61**:2365-2373. DOI: 10.1016/j.jacc.2013.02.061

[48] Niaz T, Hope K, Fremed M, Misra N, Altman C, Glickstein J, et al. Role of a pediatric cardiologist in the COVID-19 pandemic. Pediatric Cardiology. 2021;**42**:19-35. DOI: 10.1007/s00246-020-02476-y

[49] Matsubara D, Kauffman HL, Wang Y, Calderon-Anyosa R, Nadaraj S, Elias MD, et al. Echocardiographic findings in pediatric multisystem inflammatory syndrome associated with COVID-19 in the United States. Journal of the American College of Cardiology. 2020;**76**:1947-1961. DOI: 10.1016/j.jacc.2020.08.056

[50] Leitman M, Vered Z, Tyomkin V, Macogon B, Moravsky G, Peleg E, et al. Speckle tracking imaging in inflammatory heart diseases. International Journal of Cardiovascular Imaging. 2018;**34**(5):787-792. DOI: 10.1007/s10554-017-1284-y

[51] Zamorano JL, Lancellotti P, Rodriguez Muñoz D, Aboyans V, Asteggiano R, Galderisi M, et al. 2016 ESC Position Paper on cancer treatments and cardiovascular toxicity developed under the auspices of the ESC Committee for Practice Guidelines. European Heart Journal. 2016;**37**:2768-2801. DOI: 10.1093/eurheartj/ehw211

[52] Hare JL, Brown JK, Leano R, Jenkins C, Woodward N, Marwick TH. Use of myocardial deformation imaging to detect preclinical myocardial dysfunction before conventional measures in patients undergoing breast cancer treatment with trastuzumab. American Heart Journal. 2009;**158**:294-301. DOI: 10.1016/j.ahj.2009.05.031

[53] Barbier P, Mirea O, Cefalù C, Maltagliati A, Savioli G, Guglielmo M. Reliability and feasibility of longitudinal AFI global and segmental strain compared with 2D left ventricular volumes and ejection fraction: Intra- and inter-operator, test–retest, and inter-cycle reproducibility. European Heart Journal Cardiovascular Imaging. 2015;**16**:642-652. DOI: 10.1093/ehjci/jeu274

[54] Medvedofsky D, Kebed K, Laffin L, Stone J, Addetia K, Lang RM, et al. Reproducibility and experience dependence of echocardiographic indices of left ventricular function: Side-by-side comparison of global longitudinal strain and ejection fraction. Echocardiography. 2017;**34**:365-370. DOI: 10.1111/echo.13446

[55] Knackstedt C, Bekkers SCAM, Schummers G, Schreckenberg M, Muraru D, Badano LP, et al. Fully automated versus standard tracking of left ventricular ejection fraction and longitudinal strain. Journal of the American College of Cardiology. 2015;**66**:1456-1466. DOI: 10.1016/j.jacc.2015.07.052

[56] Camarda JA, Patel A, Carr MR, Young LT. Practice variations in pediatric echocardiography laboratories. Pediatric Cardiology. 2019;**40**:537-545. DOI: 10.1007/s00246-018-2012-7

[57] Yingchoncharoen T, Agarwal S, Popović ZB, Marwick TH. Normal ranges of left ventricular strain: A meta-analysis. Journal of the American Society of Echocardiography. 2013;**26**:185-191. DOI: 10.1016/j.echo.2012.10.008

[58] Ziebell D, Bettermann E, Lipinski J, Border WL, Sachdeva R. Current practice and barriers to implementation of strain imaging in pediatric echocardiography labs: A national survey. Journal of the American Society of Echocardiography. 2021;**34**:316-318. DOI: 10.1016/j.echo.2020.11.011

[59] Correale M, Ieva R, Manuppelli V, Rinaldi A, di Biase M. Controversies in echocardiography: 2D vs 3D vs 4D. Minerva Cardioangiologica. 2009;**57**:443-455

[60] Shirali GS. Three-Dimensional echocardiography in congenital heart disease. Echocardiography. 2012;**29**:242-248. DOI: 10.1111/j.1540-8175.2011.01612.x

[61] Muraru D, Veronesi F, Maddalozzo A, Dequal D, Frajhof L, Rabischoffsky A, et al. 3D printing of normal and pathologic tricuspid valves from transthoracic 3D echocardiography data sets. European Heart Journal Cardiovascular Imaging. 2017;**18**:802-808. DOI: 10.1093/ehjci/jew215

[62] Mahmood F, Owais K, Taylor C, Montealegre-Gallegos M, Manning W, Matyal R, et al. Three-dimensional printing of mitral valve using echocardiographic data. JACC: Cardiovascular Imaging. 2015;**8**:227-229. DOI: 10.1016/j.jcmg.2014.06.020

[63] Mashari A, Montealegre-Gallegos M, Knio Z, Yeh L, Jeganathan J, Matyal R, et al. Making three-dimensional echocardiography more tangible: A workflow for three-dimensional printing with echocardiographic data. Echo Research and Practice. 2016;**3**:R57-R64. DOI: 10.1530/ERP-16-0036

[64] Mowers KL, Fullerton JB, Hicks D, Singh GK, Johnson MC, Anwar S. 3D Echocardiography Provides highly accurate 3D printed models in congenital heart disease. Pediatric Cardiology. 2021;**42**:131-141. DOI: 10.1007/s00246-020-02462-4

[65] Anwar S, Singh GK, Miller J, Sharma M, Manning P, Billadello JJ, et al. 3D Printing is a transformative technology in congenital heart disease. JACC: Basic to Translational Science. 2018;**3**:294-312. DOI: 10.1016/j.jacbts.2017.10.003

[66] Vukicevic M, Mosadegh B, Min JK, Little SH. Cardiac 3D printing and its future directions. JACC: Cardiovascular Imaging. 2017;**10**:171-184. DOI: 10.1016/j.jcmg.2016.12.001

[67] Jeanne Bravo-Valenzuela N, Borges Peixoto A, Carvalho Carrilho M, Letícia Siqueira Pontes A, Cevante Chagas C, Simioni C, et al. Fetal cardiac function by three-dimensional ultrasound using 4D-STIC and VOCAL—An update. Journal of Ultrasonography. 2019;**19**:287-294. DOI: 10.15557/JoU.2019.0043

[68] Gonçalves LF, Lee W, Chaiworapongsa T, Espinoza J, Schoen M, Falkensammer P, et al. Four-dimensional ultrasonography of the fetal heart with spatiotemporal image correlation. American Journal of Obstetrics and Gynecology. 2003;**189**:1792-1802. DOI: 10.1016/S0002-9378(03)00913-X

[69] DeVore GR, Falkensammer P, Sklansky MS, Platt LD. Spatio-temporal image correlation (STIC): New technology for evaluation of the fetal heart. Ultrasound in Obstetrics and Gynecology. 2003;**22**:380-387. DOI: 10.1002/uog.217

[70] DeVore GR, Satou G, Sklansky M. 4D fetal echocardiography—An update. Echocardiography. 2017;**34**:1788-1798. DOI: 10.1111/echo.13708

[71] Qin Y, Zhang Y, Zhou X, Wang Y, Sun W, Chen L, et al. Four-dimensional echocardiography with spatiotemporal image correlation and inversion mode for detection of congenital heart disease. Ultrasound in Medicine & Biology. 2014;**40**:1434-1441. DOI: 10.1016/j.ultrasmedbio.2014.02.008

Section 4

# Prevention of Sudden Cardiac Death in the Athlete

Chapter 4

# Pre-Sports Participation Cardiac Screening Evaluation – A Review

*P. Syamasundar Rao*


## Abstract

Sudden death is associated with sports, while rare is a disastrous event. Sudden death in athletes often has a cardiac etiology. Hypertrophic cardiomyopathy and congenital coronary artery anomalies are the two most frequent causes. The existing recommendations are to perform a pre-spots participation screening consisting of full personal and family history and detailed physical examination. If abnormal findings in history or physical examination are found, additional investigations should be performed to define the nature of abnormalities. Employing an electrocardiogram, echocardiogram, or magnetic resonance imaging as a routine screening technique is not recommended in the US. The rationale of pre-participation screening is to allow as many athletes as feasible to take part in the sports.


**Keywords:** sudden cardiac death, athlete, pre-participation screening, electrocardiogram, echocardiogram, hypertrophic cardiomyopathy, aberrant coronary artery, Marfan's syndrome

## 1. Introduction

Sudden cardiac death (SCD) is defined as any death secondary to a cardiac cause within minutes to 24 h of the exercise activity [1–3]. The SCD may be associated with a rhythm disturbance or circulatory collapse. The prevalence of SCD in children is approximately 600 per annum in the USA [3]. By contrast, sudden infant death syndrome (SIDS) occurs in 7000–10,000 infants per year, and SCD in adults is seen in 300,000–400,000 subjects per year [3]. Consequently, the prevalence of SCD in childhood (and young adult) athletes is a lot less frequent than SIDS in babies and SCD in adults. The objectives of this presentation are to list the most frequent cardiac causes of sudden death in athletes, describe clinical features of more common cardiac disease entities causing SCD, and discuss methods of pre-sports participation screening. The discussion will not include SIDS and SCD without an antecedent exercise activity.

## 2. Causes of sudden death in athletes

Disease processes causing SCD have changed remarkably over the years. In the 1970s, aortic valve stenosis, un-palliated cyanotic congenital heart defects (CHDs), and Eisenmenger's syndrome were the major culprits. In the 1990s, hypertrophic cardiomyopathy (HCM), congenital anomalies of the coronary arteries (CAs), premature atherosclerosis, rupture of the aorta in Marfan's syndrome, and arrhythmias were identified as major diseases entities causing SCD in athletes [2]. At the present time, HCM; congenital anomalies of the CAs; Marfan's syndrome; structural cardiac defects, namely, repaired tetralogy of Fallot, repaired transposition of the great arteries by Mustard or Senning procedures, single ventricle lesions addressed by Fontan operation; CHD without prior surgery, including aortic is responsible for SCD [2–4]. Less common causes namely, acute or chronic myocarditis; complex forms of mitral prolapse, arrhythmogenic right ventricular cardiomyopathy (ARVC), Eisenmenger's syndrome; long QT syndrome; other abnormalities of the coronary artery such as Kawasaki disease and familial hyperbeta hyperlipoproteinemia; commotio cordis; catecholaminergenic polymorphic ventricular tachycardia; and Brugada syndrome were also found to be responsible for SCD [4–7]. Some of these entities will be reviewed in the ensuing paragraphs. In the US, SCD is seen more frequently following basketball and football than with other sports; this is likely to be related to the requirement for high level of physical activity in these sports [5, 6].

## 3. Hypertrophic cardiomyopathy

### 3.1 Introduction

This condition has been called asymmetric septal hypertrophy (ASH), hypertrophic obstructive cardiomyopathy (HOCM), dynamic muscular subaortic stenosis, idiopathic hypertrophic subaortic stenosis (IHSS), diffuse muscular subaortic stenosis, Brock's Disease, Teare's Disease, and others, but is now best described as hypertrophic cardiomyopathy. HCM is a primary, often inherited, disease of the myocardium affecting the sarcomeric proteins. This results in hypertrophy and disorganization of myofibrils and fibrosis of interstitia. Autosomal dominant inheritance with a high degree of penetrance is noted. Matrilineal, X-linked, and autosomal-recessive inheritance patterns have also been described. One hundred or more different mutations in 10 genes have been discovered (chromosomes 1, 14 & 15). Troponin-T, beta myosin heavy chain, and alpha tropomyosin may also be involved.

### 3.2 Pathology and pathophysiology

HCM is characterized by hypertrophy of the left ventricle (more often) and/or right ventricle (RV). Concentric left ventricular (LV) hypertrophy is present without an identifiable hemodynamic reason. Frequently, there is asymmetric interventricular septal hypertrophy. Diastolic dysfunction including, delayed relaxation and increased muscle stiffness are present. LV outflow obstruction, which is dynamic is seen in 25% of cases. Systolic anterior motion (SAM) of the mitral valve may contribute to the LV outflow tract narrowing. RV outflow obstruction is rare but is more frequent in infants with HCM. There appear to be areas of localized hypertrophy in the LV muscle in addition to those in the septum and serve as potential arrhythmogenic foci.

### 3.3 Symptoms

There are usually no symptoms in infants and children; they are most often detected because of a cardiac murmur or family history of HCM. Symptoms in infancy usually indicate a poor prognosis. In early adulthood, the presenting symptoms are exertional dyspnea, lightheadedness, chest pain, syncope, or palpitations.

### 3.4 Physical examination

In the non-obstructive HCM, the findings are subtle with minimal or no increase in LV impulse. A third or fourth heart sound may be auscultated at the apex. There may either be a soft systolic murmur or no murmur. In the obstructive HCM, increased LV impulse, double or triple impulse may be felt. Pulses bisfiriens may be felt in some subjects. An ejection systolic murmur is heard at the left mid and right upper sternal borders. The murmur changes with postural maneuvers: decreases in intensity on squatting which may increase in a standing position. The murmur of HCM is usually auscultated at the left mid sternal border and increases in intensity with the Valsalva maneuver.

### 3.5 Chest X-ray and electrocardiogram (ECG)

Chest X-ray is of limited value; the size of the heart may be normal or cardiomegaly may be present. The size of the heart may be normal even with marked LV hypertrophy. ECG is abnormal in 90% of patients; bizarre patterns are seen, but none are characteristic of HCM. Most commonly, increased LV voltages (deep S waves in V1 and V2 and tall R wave in V5 and V6) are detected. T wave inversion, deep q waves, and enlargement of the left atrium may be identified on the ECG in some patients. Unfortunately, the ECG pattern does not discriminate between obstructive and non-obstructive types or those at risk for sudden death. However, Holter monitoring is likely to detect arrhythmia [8, 9] and may help prognosticate [9].

### 3.6 Echo-doppler studies

Echocardiogram is the most useful test in the diagnosis of this condition. It demonstrates LV hypertrophy (**Figure 1**), asymmetric septal hypertrophy (**Figures 1** and 2),

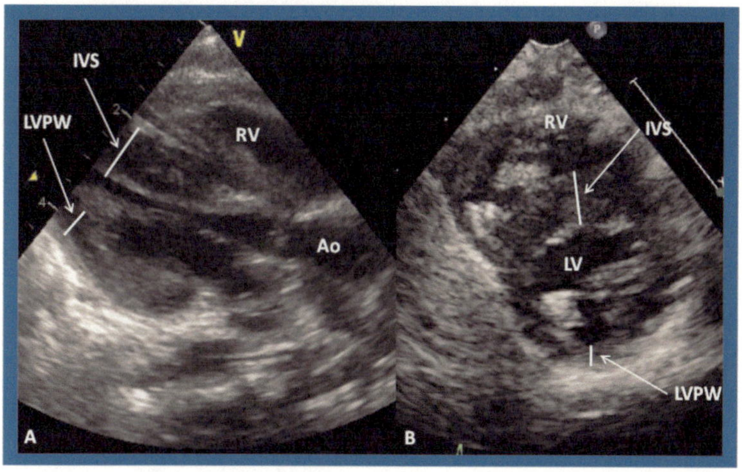


**Figure 1.**
*A. Parasternal long (A) and short (B) axis views of the left ventricle (LV) illustrating LV hypertrophy and strikingly thickened inter-ventricular septum (IVS). Ao, aorta; LVPW, LV posterior wall; RV, right ventricle. (reproduced from reference [10]).*

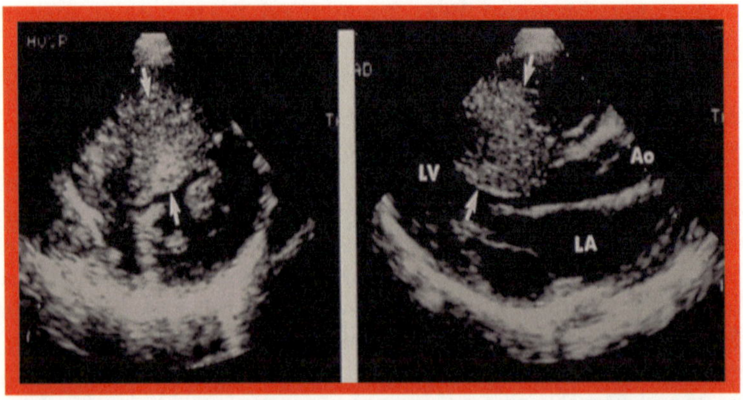


**Figure 2.**
*Parasternal short (left) and long (right) axis views of the left ventricle (LV) illustrating distinctly thickened inter-ventricular septum (arrows in both images). Ao, aorta; LA, left atrium.*

and SAM of the mitral valve (**Figure 3**). The LV cavity is completely obliterated in systole (**Figure 4**). Doppler studies will detect abnormal mitral inflow Doppler patterns and mitral insufficiency and help to quantify LV outflow tract obstruction (**Figures** 5 and **6**).

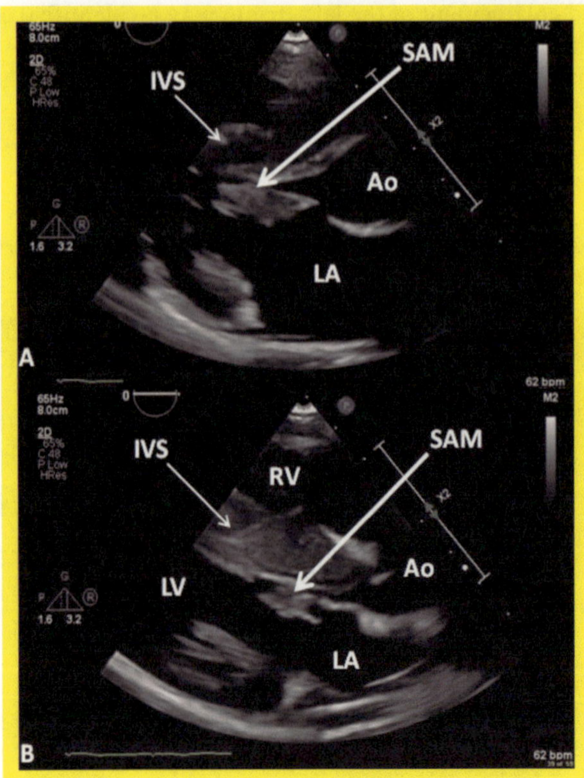


**Figure 3.**
*Parasternal echocardiographic long axis views of the left ventricle (LV) and mitral valve illustrating systolic anterior motion (SAM) of the mitral valve (thick arrows in both 'A' and 'B'). Note thickened inter-ventricular septum (thin arrows), particularly noticeable in 'B'. Ao, aorta; LA, left atrium; RV, right ventricle.*

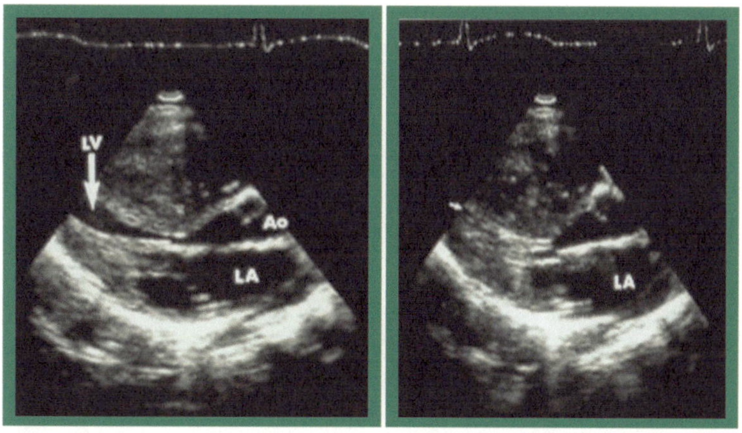


**Figure 4.**
*Parasternal long-axis views of the left ventricle (LV) of a child with hypertrophic cardiomyopathy demonstrating total obliteration of the cavity of the LV (right image) in systole (arrows).*

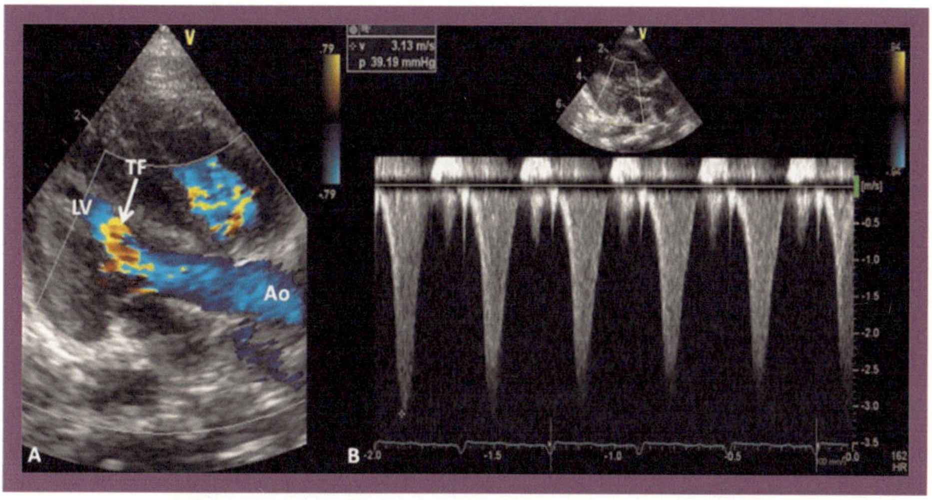


**Figure 5.**
*A. Parasternal long axis 2D and color doppler recording showing turbulent flow (TF) in the left ventricular (LV) outflow tract. B. Continuous-wave doppler indicates a gradient of 39 mmHg (the insert in B). The triangular pattern of the doppler recording is suggestive of subaortic narrowing. Ao, aorta. (reproduced from reference [10]).*

Localized, atypical hypertrophy patterns as demonstrated in **Figures 7–9** may also be detected.

### 3.7 Differentiation from athlete's heart

Some athletes develop LV hypertrophy and differentiation of this LV hypertrophy from that seen with HCM maybe not easy. Criteria that help differentiate these conditions [7] are listed in **Table 1**.

### 3.8 Sudden cardiac death in HCM

Yearly mortality rate in subjects with HCM is in the order of 2 to 4% of the HCM cases; this is largely based on patients cared for in large tertiary care centers.

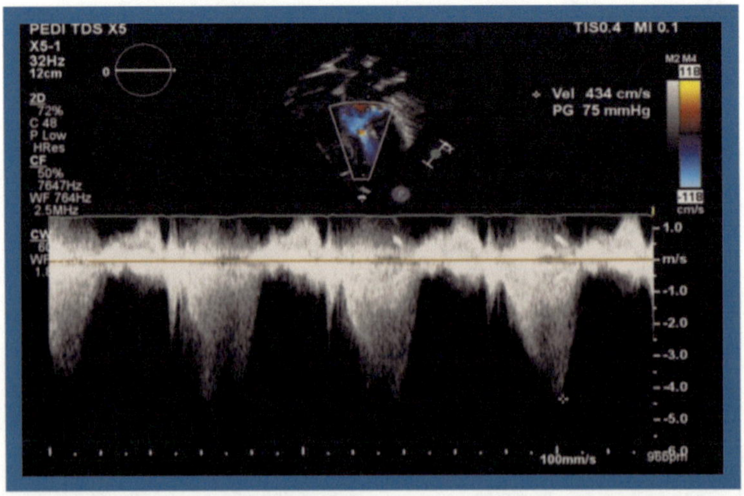


**Figure 6.**
*Apical five-chamber view with continuous-wave doppler across the left ventricular outflow tract demonstrating a peak gradient of 75 mmHg. The triangular pattern of the doppler recording is suggestive of subaortic narrowing.*

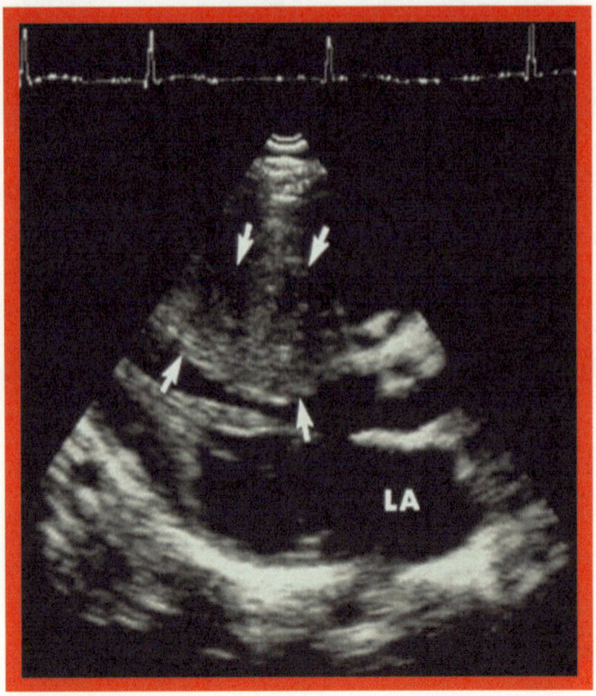


**Figure 7.**
*Parasternal long-axis views of the left ventricle of a patient with hypertrophic cardiomyopathy showing marked inter-ventricular septal thickening (arrows). LA, left atrium.*

Consequently, the true population prevalence is unknown. Examination of SCD in competitive athletes revealed that HCM is the most frequent reason for SCD and accounted for 36% of deaths [5–7]. The mortality is largely confined to the 12-to-35-year age patient group. Most of these patients are asymptomatic or mildly

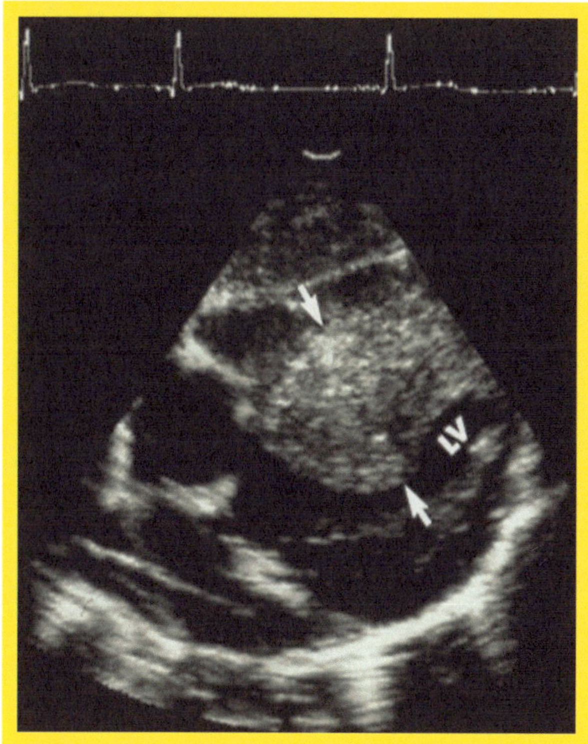


**Figure 8.**
*Subcostal view of the left ventricle (LV) of a patient with hypertrophic cardiomyopathy showing marked inter-ventricular septal thickening (arrows).*

symptomatic and therefore, risk stratification of HCM is difficult. In some investigations, risk factors for SCD in HCM patients have been identified and these include, a family history of sudden death related to HCM, history of syncope or pre-syncope, history of having survived sudden death episode, massive LV hypertrophy (> 30 mm), non-sustained ventricular tachycardia, unusual blood pressure (BP) response to exercise, and high LV outflow tract gradient [1–4, 11–13].

### 3.9 Sudden cardiac death prevention in HCM

The mechanism by which HCM results in SCD following exercise is not clearly understood, but the development of ventricular arrhythmia, leading to ventricular fibrillation is thought to be responsible for SCD [2]. Even at the present time, we have limited knowledge as to how to prevent SCD in HCM. We continue to lack sound criteria of individual severity and relative prognostic risk, in general, and especially in athletes. Early studies showed the usefulness of beta-blockers in reducing mortality, but recent studies did not corroborate the usefulness of beta-blocker usage in the prevention of mortality. Exercise limitation may be helpful in decreasing the probability of sudden death. Indeed, the athlete with HCM should not be permitted to take part in the strenuous sports activity. If non-sustained ventricular tachycardia is present, Amiodarone has been shown to be beneficial. Intra-cardiac defibrillators (ICDs) for high-risk patients with ventricular tachycardia induced by programmed ventricular stimulation may be helpful.

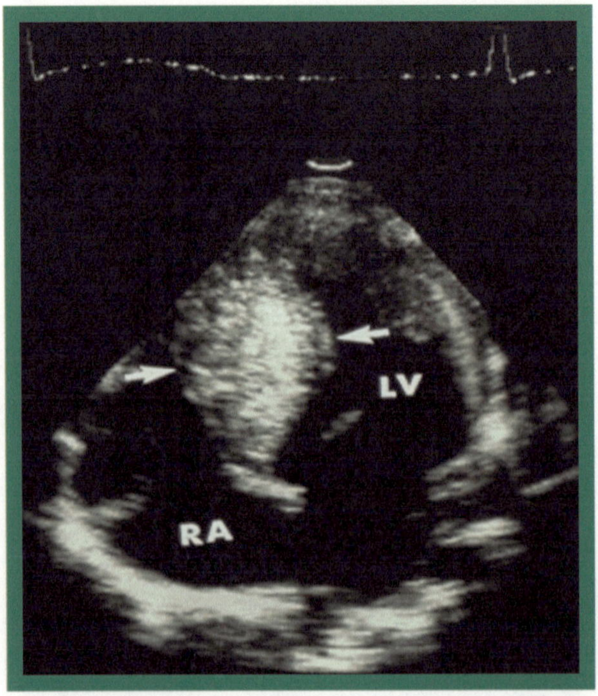


**Figure 9.**
*Apical four-chamber view of the left ventricle (LV) of a patient with hypertrophic cardiomyopathy showing marked inter-ventricular septal thickening (arrows). RA, right atrium.*

| Parameter | Hypertrophic cardiomyopathy | Athlete's heart |
|---|---|---|
| Unusual patterns of LVH on echo | Positive | Negative |
| LV Cavity <45 mm | Positive | Negative |
| LV Cavity >55 mm | Negative | Positive |
| Left atrial enlargement | Positive | Negative |
| Bizarre ECG patterns | Positive | Negative |
| Abnormal LV filling | Positive | Negative |
| Female gender | Positive | Negative |
| Decreased LV muscle thickness with de-conditioning | Negative | Positive |
| Family history of hypertrophic cardiomyopathy | Positive | Negative |

*ECG, electrocardiogram; LV, left ventricle; LVH, left ventricular hypertrophy.*

**Table 1.**
*Criteria to distinguish athlete's heart from HCM.*

## 4. Congenital coronary artery anomalies

### 4.1 Normal coronary arteries

In normal subjects, the left and right coronary arteries (CAs) originate from left and right sinuses of Valsalva, respectively. The left main CA is short and divides into two branches, namely the left anterior descending (LAD) and circumflex. The LAD continues in the same course as the left main CA and traverses in the interventricular groove. The circumflex traverses perpendicular to the axis of the left main CA and keeps on going in the posterior atrioventricular groove. The left CA perfuses the LV and interventricular septum [14, 15]. The right CA originates from the right sinus of Valsalva and continues in the right atrioventricular sulcus and does not branch out similar to the left CA. The right CA supplies the RV [14, 15]. The site of origin and the course of the CAs proximally can easily be demonstrated in echocardiographic studies (**Figures 10** and **11**). Color flow mapping of the CAs (**Figures 11** and **12**) should also be undertaken concurrently to ensure that the parallel lines of the transverse sinus of the pericardium are not mistaken for CAs [16].

### 4.2 Aberrant coronary arteries

The aberrant origin of the CA is a rare abnormality with its origin from the contralateral aortic sinus of Valsalva [16]. In aberrant left CA, the left CA originates from the right sinus of Valsalva (rarely from the right CA) with a short intramural (within the aortic wall) course and continues between the pulmonary trunk anteriorly and the aorta posteriorly. The ostium of the left CA is often Slit-like forming a potential site for obstruction to coronary blood flow. In aberrant right CA, the right coronary artery arises from the left sinus of Valsalva (less commonly from the left main CA). This is the counterpart of aberrant left CA. The right CA then traverses rightward with a short intramural course within the aortic wall and then traverses between the pulmonary artery and aorta to get to its usual course. There is adequate coronary flow at rest, but during exercise, ischemia may develop secondary to either

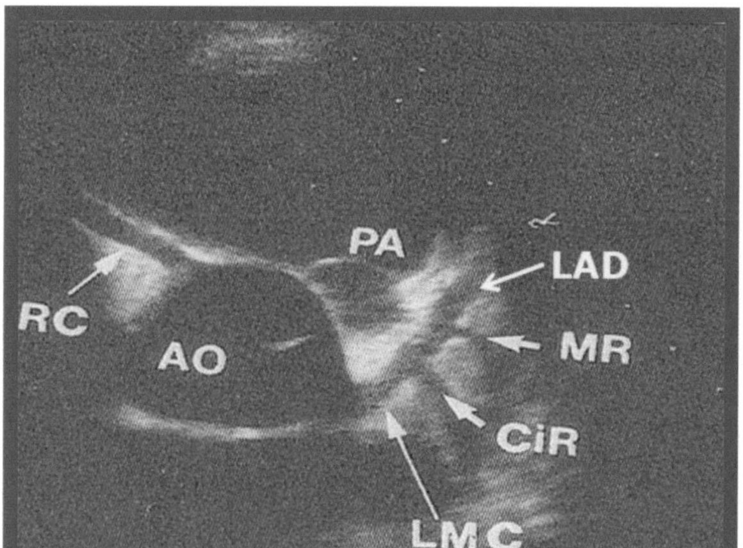


**Figure 10.**
*A short-axis view at the level of aortic sinuses demonstrating normal left and right (RC) coronary arteries and their branches. The left main coronary artery (LMC) continues in the same direction to become the left anterior descending (LAD) artery. The circumflex (CiR) and marginal (MR) branches traverse perpendicular to the axis of LMC. The aorta (AO) and pulmonary artery (PA) are also shown. Demonstration of color flow within the coronary arteries is required to ensure that these indeed are coronary arteries. (modified from reference [16]).*

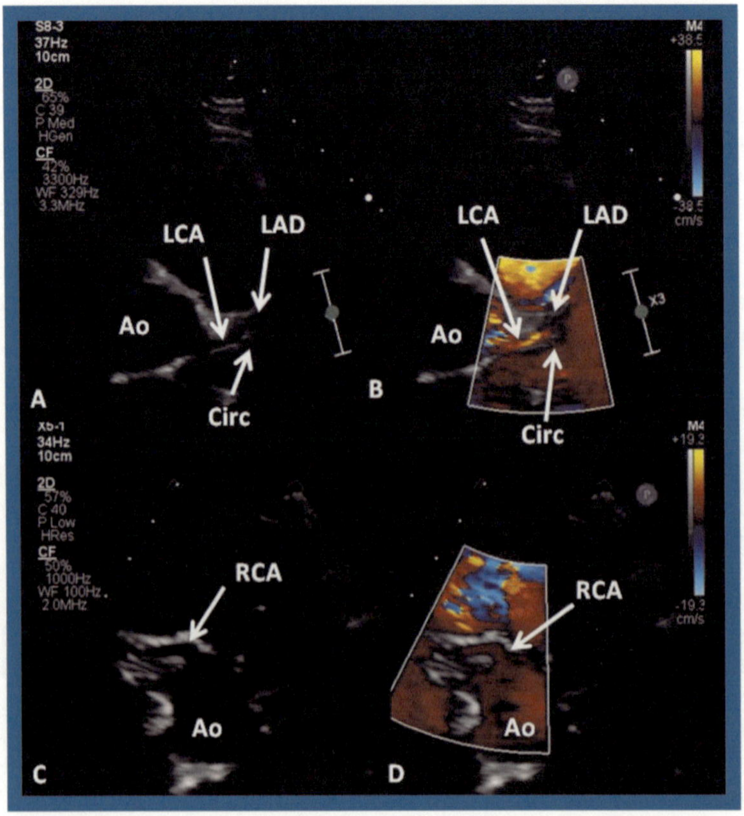


**Figure 11.**
*The short-axis views at the level of aortic sinuses demonstrate the origin and course of the left (LCA) (A and B) and right (RCA) (C and D) coronary arteries. The LCA continues in the same direction to become the left anterior descending artery (LAD). The circumflex (CIRC) traverses perpendicular to the axis of LCA. Color flow within the coronary arteries is demonstrated in 'B' and 'D' and is required to ensure that these indeed are coronary arteries and not parallel lines of the transverse sinus of the pericardium. Ao, aorta.*

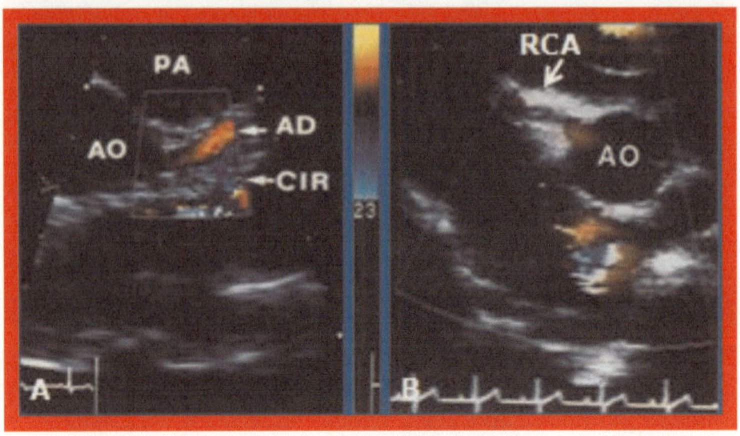


**Figure 12.**
*A. a short-axis view at the level of aortic sinuses, similar to* ***Figures 10*** *and* ***11****, focusing on the left main coronary artery showing its division into left anterior descending (AD) and circumflex (CIR) coronary arteries. Note the red flow in the AD and the blue flow in the CIR. B. a short-axis view at the level of aortic sinuses, similar to figure a, but focusing on to the right coronary artery (RCA) showing its origin from the right sinus with the color flow within it. AO, aorta.*

partial or total occlusion of the CA [17, 18]. Several hypotheses have been proposed to elucidate the reason(s) for inadequate CA blood flow. One such hypothesis is compression of the CA (left or right) between the great arteries by the expansion of the aorta and pulmonary artery against each other during the exercise. Another hypothesis suggests that an angle is created between ostium of the CA and its main axis creating additional tension, during aortic expansion [19–21]. The intramural course of the coronary artery also contributes to the risk of SCD during exertion. Echocardiographic examples of aberrant left CA arising from the right sinus of Valsalva (**Figure 13**) and of aberrant right CA arising from the left sinus of Valsalva (**Figures 14–16**) are shown in **Figures 13–16**.

### 4.3 Aberrant coronary arteries and SCD

The aberrant origin of the left CA is strongly associated with SCD [19, 20]. While not as common, aberrant right CA is also seen with SCD associated with exercise [21]. Aberrant CAs constitute 17% of all SCDs following exercise [5–7] and are next only to HCM with regard to frequency.

### 4.4 Clinical and laboratory features of aberrant coronary arteries

Often, the first presentation of most patients with aberrant coronary arteries is SCD with exercise. A few patients may present with symptoms of angina or syncope following exercise [22]. Some patients may be detected during echocardiograms performed for some other reason. Routine physical examination is completely normal. Patients with complaints of angina or syncope following exercise should be evaluated

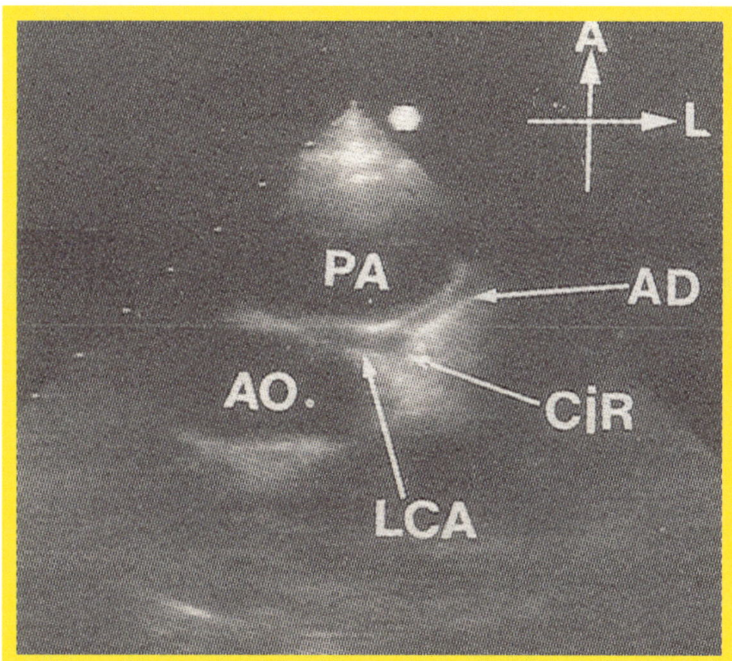


**Figure 13.**
*A short-axis view of the aorta demonstrating aberrant left coronary artery from the right sinus of Valsalva, traversing between the aorta (AO) and pulmonary artery (PA). (reproduced from reference [16]).*

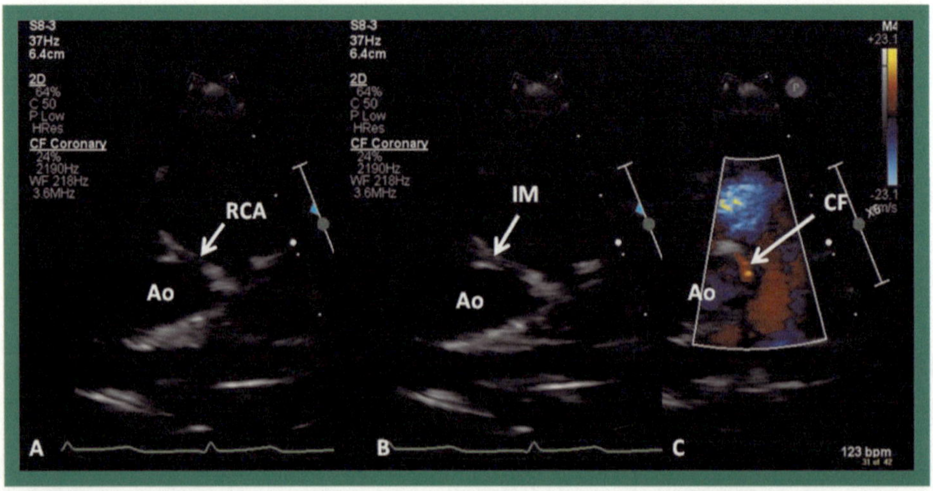


**Figure 14.**
*The short-axis views of the aorta (Ao) demonstrate aberrant right coronary artery (RCA) from the left sinus of Valsalva by two-dimensional (A and B) and color flow (CF) (C) imaging. The intramural (IM) course of the right coronary artery is shown in 'B'.*

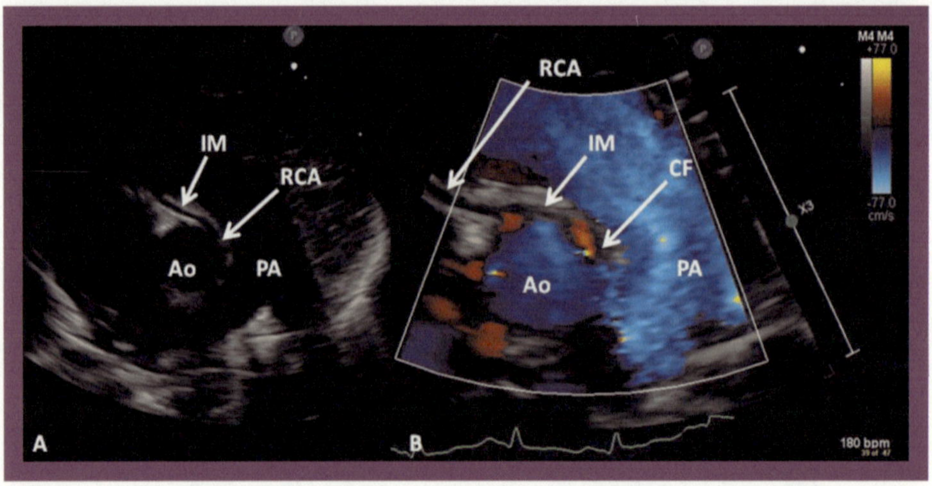


**Figure 15.**
*The short-axis views of the aorta (Ao) demonstrate aberrant right coronary artery (RCA) from the left sinus of Valsalva by two-dimensional (A) and color flow (B) imaging. Color flow (CF) at the origin of RCA (B) and intramural (IM) course of the RCA (A and B) are shown. PA. Pulmonary artery.*

by a cardiologist. Stress testing, while routinely used for complaints of this nature, a regular stress test may not yield abnormal results in subjects with aberrant CAs particularly if the stress test is sub-maximal [16, 17]. If the stress test with maximal activity is performed, it may precipitate a coronary event or even sudden death. Instead, the author recommends echocardiographic studies, focusing on imaging of proximal CAs [16]. Reliable echocardiographic screening methods to identify aberrant CAs (**Figure 17**) have been described [23, 24] and may be used. However, normalcy (**Figures 10–12**) of the CAs or aberrancy (**Figures 13–16**) should be documented by direct visualization of the CAs by transthoracic echocardiographic studies. With the

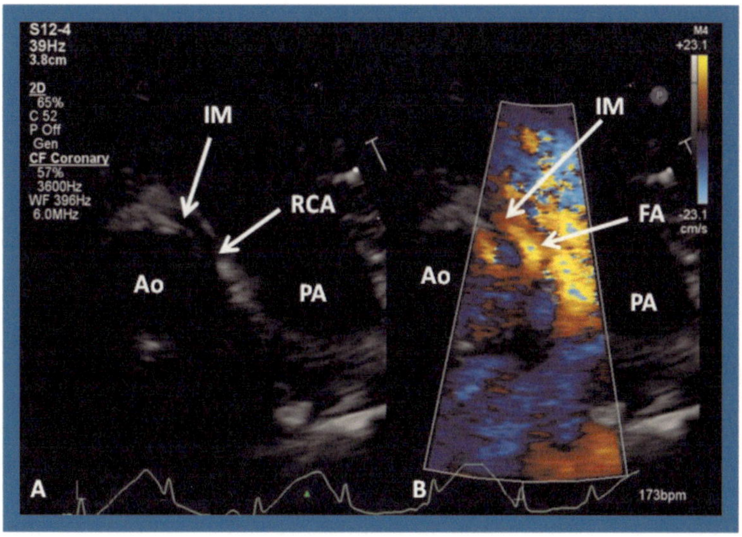


**Figure 16.**
*The short-axis views of the aorta (Ao) demonstrate aberrant right coronary artery (RCA) from the left sinus of Valsalva by two-dimensional (A) and color flow (B) imaging. Color flow acceleration (FA) at the origin of RCA (B) may suggest stenosis at the origin of RCA. The intramural (IM) course of the RCA (A and B) is seen. PA. Pulmonary artery.*

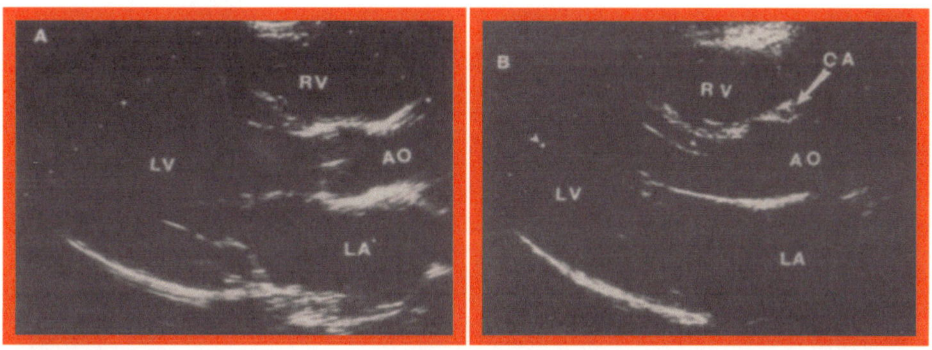


**Figure 17.**
*Parasternal long-axis two-dimensional echo images of the left atrium (LA), left ventricle (LV) and aorta (AO) in a normal child are shown in A. A similar view of the heart in a child with an aberrant coronary artery (CA) is shown in B which demonstrated a cross-sectional image of the CA in the anterior wall of the AO (arrow in B). RV, right ventricle. Modified from Jureidini SB, Marino CJ, Singh GK, Balfour IC, Rao PS. J Am Society of Echocard 2003; 16: 756–763 [23].*

current state-of-the-art echocardiographic equipment, echo studies are the primary tools of investigation. If transthoracic echocardiographic images are not clear, especially in adolescents and adults with poor acoustic windows, other studies such as transesophageal echocardiography (TEE), computed tomography (CT) scan, or angiography may have to be performed to demonstrate the CA anatomy. Surgical re-implantation of the aberrant CAs along with enlarging the coronary ostium and un-roofing the intramural portion of the CA, as deemed appropriate, can be safely performed, and subsequent to recovery from surgery, participation in the full athletic activity is feasible.

## 5. Marfan's syndrome

Marfan's syndrome is a disorder of the connective tissue with multisystem involvement, particularly of the musculoskeletal, ocular, and cardiovascular systems [25, 26]. Mutations of the fibrillin-1 gene are believed to be responsible for this syndrome. The overall prevalence is one in 10,000 to 20,000 individuals [27]. The inheritance pattern is autosomal dominant with variable expression. In approximately 15% of cases, it may manifest sporadically [25]. Several reviews of SCD in young athletes disclosed aortic rupture in Marfan's syndrome patients (2 to 3%) as a causative factor [1, 5–7, 26, 28].

Clinical manifestations of Marfan's syndrome are tall stature with arm span >105% of the height, scoliosis, arachnodactyly, pectus deformity, hyper-extensible joints, and dislocation of the lens. They may also have glaucoma and retinal detachment. Some of the clinical features are illustrated in **Figure 18**. Cardiovascular abnormalities include mitral valve prolapse (**Figure 19**) in almost 100% of patients, some with mitral regurgitation (**Figure 19**), and aortic root dilatation (**Figures 20** and **21**) in a high percentage of patients [26, 29]. The mitral prolapse and mitral regurgitation may be appreciated on careful auscultation and confirmed by echocardiography. However, echocardiography is necessary to detect aortic root dilatation [29]; the measurements are compared with normal subjects, and *Z* scores are determined. The diagnosis of Marfan's syndrome is largely on the basis of Ghent nosology criteria [27, 30] using a mixture of major and minor clinical features and the family history. In the absence of

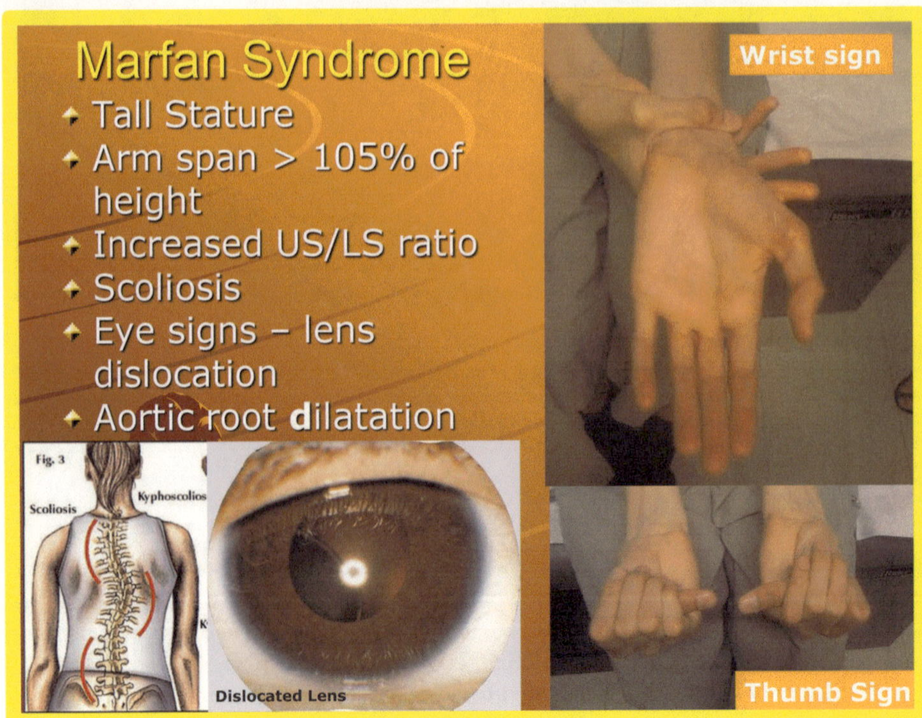


**Figure 18.**
*A summary of clinical features of Marfan's syndrome.*

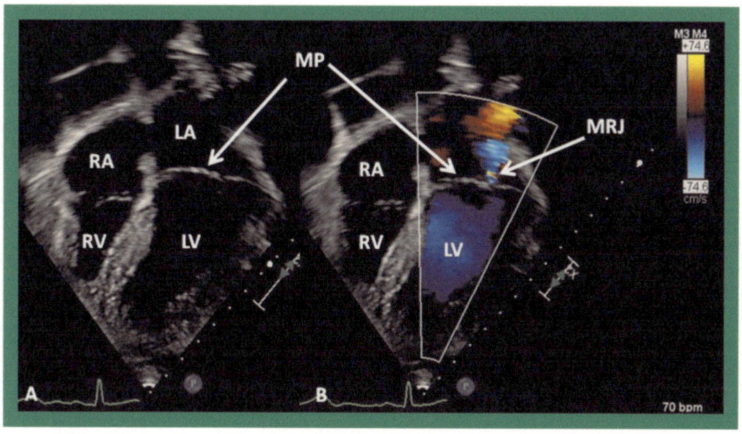


**Figure 19.**
*Selected video frames from apical four-chamber views demonstrating mitral valve prolapse (MP) and mitral regurgitation jet (MRJ) in a patient clinically diagnosed as Marfan's syndrome. LA, left atrium; LV, left ventricle; RA, right atrium; RV, right ventricle.*

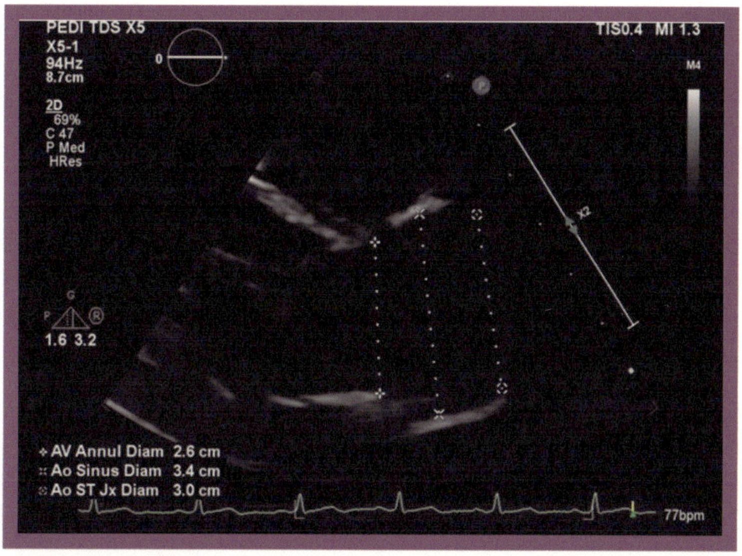


**Figure 20.**
*Selected video frame from parasternal long-axis view demonstrating measurements of the dilated aortic root in a patient clinically diagnosed as Marfan's syndrome. Note the measurements are listed at the left bottom. The Z scores of the dilated aortic root varied between 2.9 and 3.8.*

these criteria, a scoring system is utilized [31] for the diagnosis. Spontaneous aortic dissection has been observed. To prevent such catastrophes, surgery to replace the aortic root is suggested if the aortic diameter exceeds 5.0 cm or if the rate of growth of the aorta is more than 0.5–1.0 cm/year [30]. Beta-blocking drugs, angiotensin converting enzyme (ACE) inhibiting medications and more recently, losartan (to attenuate TGFß signaling) have been used to decrease the rate of growth of the aorta. In an attempt to prevent aortic dissection and SCD, restriction from participation from sports is generally recommended [31].

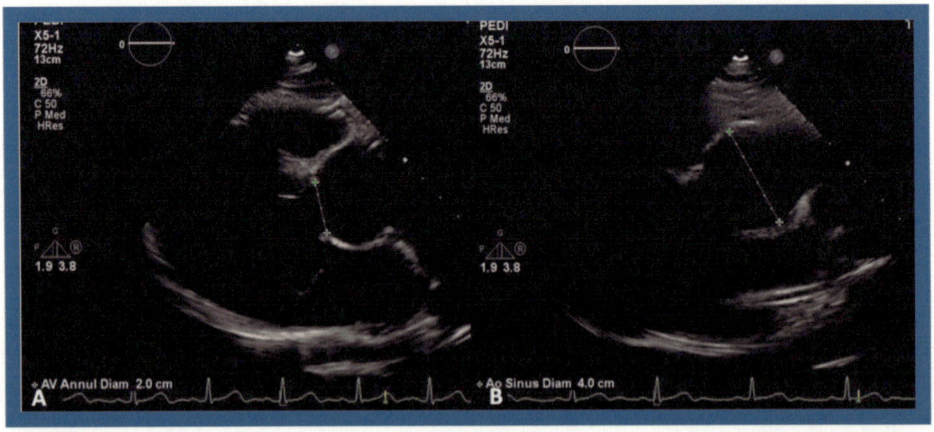


**Figure 21.**
*Selected video frames from parasternal long-axis view demonstrating measurements of the dilated aortic root in a patient clinically diagnosed as Marfan's syndrome. The measurements are listed at the left bottom in both 'A' and 'B'. while the Z score of the aortic valve (AV) annulus was within normal limits, the Z score of the dilated aortic sinus was +5.5.*

## 6. Structural heart defects

Congenital cardiac defects following repair (tetralogy of Fallot—total correction; transposition of the great arteries—Mustard or Senning operation, and single ventricle lesions—Fontan operation) in 2% and un-operated CHDs, including aortic stenosis in 3% have been reported as causative factors for SCD following exercise activity [4–7]. The clinical features of these disease entities [32–37] and their long-term squealae [38, 39] were reviewed elsewhere [32–39] for the interested reader and will not be reviewed here.

## 7. Arrhythmogenic right ventricular cardiomyopathy

Arrhythmogenic right ventricular cardiomyopathy (ARVC) is a rare myocardial disorder inherited in an autosomal dominant pattern with an estimated prevalence of 1:1000–1:5000 [40]. It has been identified as a cause of SCD following sports participation in approximately 4% of cases [5–7]. Cardiomyopathic changes most frequently involve the right ventricular myocardium; however, cases involving the LV have also been reported. Exercise may be important in eliciting ventricular arrhythmias. The usual presenting symptoms are palpitations, syncope, or aborted cardiac arrest. Congestive heart failure may occur in the late stages. T-wave inversion in the right chest leads, indicative of repolarization abnormalities are seen in the ECG. However, the ECG is not sensitive in detecting ARVC [41]. The diagnosis is largely based on major and minor criteria in the echocardiographic and MRI studies, reviewed elsewhere [40, 42]. The mechanism for SCD following exercise is the development of ventricular arrhythmia 40].

## 8. Other disease entities

There are number of other diseases/defects that have been known to have a causal relationship with SCD following exercise; the prevalence of each of these varied

| Disease entities | Percent prevalence | Comments |
|---|---|---|
| Myocarditis | 6% [5–7] | Early studies indicated a higher prevalence ranging from 18 to 29% [28, 43, 44] |
| Complex Forms of Mitral Prolapse | 4% [5–7] | Family history of SCD and exercise-induced arrhythmias in mitral prolapse cases are likely to be related to SCD [2] |
| Ion Channelopathies | 3 to 4% [5–7] | Long QT syndromes (Jervell and Lange-Nielson syndrome and Romano-Ward syndrome) and Brugada syndrome |
| Myocardial Bridging of the Left Anterior Descending Coronary Artery | 3% [5–7] | Has also been reported in other studies [16, 45, 46] |
| Atherosclerotic Coronary Artery Disease | 3% [5–7] | Premature atherosclerotic coronary artery disease secondary to hyperbeta hyperlipoprotenemia |
| Dilated Cardiomyopathy | 2% [5–7] | — |
| Wolf Parkinson White syndrome | 2% [7] | — |
| Pulmonary Hypertension (Eisenmenger's Syndrome), Sarcoidosis, Kawasaki Disease, Commotio Cordis | ~1% each [2, 5, 6, 28, 47] | Pulmonary Hypertension (Eisenmenger's Syndrome) [28], Sarcoidosis [5], Kawasaki Disease [2, 6], Commotio Cordis [6, 47] |

*ECG, electrocardiogram; SCD, sudden cardiac death.*

**Table 2.**
*Other disease entities associated with SCD following exercise.*

between 1 and 6% [5–7]. These are listed in **Table 2**. A detailed discussion of these entities is beyond the scope of this paper.

## 9. Pre-sports participation screening

Pre-sports participation screening is commonly suggested by most medical societies [5, 48–52] including the American Academy of Pediatrics (AAP), American Heart Association (AHA), and the American College of Cardiology (ACC). Yet, the heart conditions which predispose to SCD happen in 5 in 100,000 persons and SCD occurs in 1 in 200,000 subjects. This degree of low risk makes the appraisal hard and the cost-effectiveness of screening techniques is low. The aim of any program is to discover individuals at risk for SCD during tough exercise without invasive testing and in a cost-effective manner. However, no generally established standards for screening are available at the present time. This issue was tackled differently in different countries. In the US, the pre-participation screening [5, 48, 51, 52] includes securing sports person's personal and family history and complete physical examination (**Tables 3** and **4**) without an ECG or any other imaging studies and if abnormalities are detected in this initial screening process, further workup is pursued. In Italy [49, 53], Israel [54], and Japan [55], an ECG is also performed along with history and physical examination; this is mandated by the respective country's laws. Screening of the athletes in other European countries is limited to the individuals participating in international, Olympic, or other professional sports [56]. Denmark, on the other hand

| Personal history |
|---|
| 1. Chest pain or discomfort during exertional activities |
| 2. Unexplained syncope or near-syncope |
| 3. Excessive exertional and unexplained dyspnea/fatigue or palpitations associated with exercise |
| 4. Previously recognized heart murmur |
| 5. Elevated systemic blood pressure |
| 6. History of prior restriction from participation in sports |
| 7. Results of prior testing of the heart by another physician/healthcare giver |
| **Family history** |
| 8. History of premature death (sudden and unexpected, or otherwise) prior to age 50 years secondary to a cardiac issue in more than 1 relative. |
| 9. Disability from heart disease in close relatives less than 50 years of age |
| 10. History of hypertrophic or dilated cardiomyopathy, long-QT syndrome or other ion channelopathies, Marfan's syndrome, clinically significant arrhythmias, or genetic cardiac conditions in family members |

**Table 3.**
*Personal and family history [5, 48, 51, 52].*

| Physical examination |
|---|
| 11. Complete physical examination including blood pressure in a sitting position* |
| 12. Palpation of femoral pulses to exclude coarctation of the aorta |
| 13. Look for physical stigmata of Marfan's syndrome |
| 14. Careful auscultation to exclude left ventricular outflow tract obstruction** |

**The numbering continues from Table 3.*
***Auscultation should be undertaken with the athlete in both the supine and standing positions (and with Valsalva maneuver) particularly to discover murmurs associated with HCM (dynamic left ventricular outflow tract obstruction).*

**Table 4.**
*Pre-participation physical examination [5, 48, 51, 52].*

completely rejected systematic screening for the athletes; their stated justification was a low event rate [57].

Some investigators employed screening studies utilizing ECG [58–61], echocardiogram [61–64], or MRI [65], and these investigators demonstrated that the prevalence of high-risk cardiac condition that is likely to predispose to SCD following exercise is low: ECG—0.33 to 11.5%; echocardiogram—1.26 to 5.1%; and MRI—1.25% of the athletic population screened [58–65].

The current recommendations by the AHA and ACC [5, 48, 51, 52] are to examine the personal history and family history (**Table 3**) and to carry out an orderly and complete physical examination (**Table 4**), whether it is undertaken in primary care doctors' clinic or in mass pre-participation screening programs. The rationale of the pre-participation screening is not to exclude youths from participation in sports, but to enable as many of them as possible to participate in sports to their full potential.

As mentioned above, the present AHA/ACC suggestions are that screening assessments are executed by trained examiners. This appraisal should consist of the 14-key elements of personal and family history and physical examination (**Tables 3** and **4**). Such assessment should be carried out in a setting favorable for best auscultation of the heart. These all-inclusive screening assessments should be re-done in two years for high school athletes and in three years for the college student athletes. It is not realistic to presume that usual large-scale screening assessments are capable of excluding all clinically pertinent diseases. The writer of this chapter strongly believes that such appraisals should be undertaken by the primary care doctors (pediatricians, internists, family practitioners, and other primary care providers who care for children, adolescents and young adults) as a part of their annual regular physicals, but they should make sure that the AHA/ACC suggested 14-key elements of personal and family history and physical examination (**Tables 3** and **4**) are included.

If abnormalities are detected in the previously expressed, 14-Element AHA/ACC recommendations (**Tables 3** and **4**) for pre-participation cardiovascular screening, additional testing, as suitable, should be undertaken (**Table 5**).

### 9.1 Electrocardiogram

ECG is the first test that should be performed if any abnormalities are detected in the 14-element screening (Routine pre-participation screening ECG is not recommended in the US and the justification for such will be reviewed in the next section of this chapter). The ECG may identify patients with HCM because, as mentioned in the HCM section, many patients with HCM exhibit ECG abnormalities although the ECG abnormalities are not diagnostic of HCM. The value of ECG in identifying coronary abnormalities is limited. However, the ECG is useful in detecting long QT syndrome, Wolf-Parkinson-White (WPW) syndrome, atrioventricular block, and Brugada syndrome.

### 9.2 Echocardiogram

Echocardiogram should be performed to investigate abnormalities detected during history taking, performing a physical examination, or unexplained ECG findings. However, it is absolutely impracticable to use the echocardiogram as a screening tool for SCD [2 22]. Hypertrophic cardiomyopathy (**Figures 1–9**) and other types of cardiomyopathies can easily be diagnosed by echo-Doppler studies. Aberrant CAs should be specifically imaged in an attempt to document normalcy (**Figures 10–12**) or to establish aberrancy (**Figures 13** through **17**). Echo is also useful in quantifying dilatation of the aortic root (**Figures 20** and **21**) in Marfan's syndrome. The presence of prolapse of the mitral valve and mitral valve insufficiency (**Figure 19**) can be detected easily in echo-Doppler studies.

### 9.3 Other studies

A number of other studies may be useful in investigating these patients and they should focus on specific issues/concerns discovered during the screening process (**Table 5**). Exercise testing may help resolve the significance of exercise-induced symptoms. Holter or Event monitors may be used to document arrhythmias. An invasive electrophysiology study may be needed in some children. Genetic screening for HCM, Marfan's syndrome, and long QT syndrome is currently available and may be performed as indicated for a given clinical scenario. MRI and CT scans may be

| |
|---|
| 1. Secure careful personal and family history (**Table 3**) |
| 2. Perform methodical pre-participation physical examination (**Table 4**) |
| 3. Obtain a 12-lead electrocardiogram if any abnormalities are detected during history and/or physical examination (items 1 and 2) |
| 4. If abnormalities are detected during history taking and physical examination or if unexplained ECG findings are seen, an echocardiogram should be performed. Particular focus should be paid to address the type of abnormality detected during items 1, 2, and 3 |
| 5. If problems are detected during items 1 through 4, additional studies, specifically addressing the detected abnormalities, are in order:<br>• Exercise testing if exercise-induced symptoms were noted<br>• Holter or Event monitors may be used to document arrhythmias<br>• Genetic screening for HCM, Marfan's syndrome, and long QT syndrome, if indicated<br>• MRI and CT scans may be performed to address issues not resolved by an echo<br>• Cardiac catheterization and cineangiography are rarely needed |
| *CT, Computed tomography; HCM, Hypertrophic cardiomyopathy; MRI, magnetic resonance imaging.* |

**Table 5.**
*Stepwise approach to cardiac screening evaluation.*

employed in specific situations, not resolved by echocardiography. Cardiac catheterization and cineangiography are rarely needed.

Given the easy accessibility of echocardiography and its utility in the detection and quantification of causes of sudden death in athletes (as reviewed in Sections 2–8 of this chapter), echocardiography has become the primary mode of investigation to address issues identified during history, physical examination and ECG screening. However, in subjects with poor echo windows, noninvasive studies such as MRI and CT scans may be utilized. These studies are particularly useful in evaluating aortic arch and pulmonary artery anomalies. Another condition in which MRI is useful is arrhythmogenic right ventricular cardiomyopathy; indeed, MRI criteria forms the basis for diagnostic confirmation of ARVC. In patients with Marfan syndrome, aortic dilatation can be quantitated and aortic dissection detected by MRI. MRI and CT scans are also useful in evaluating anomalous origin and course of the coronary arteries as well in assessing other coronary artery abnormalities listed in **Table 2**.

## 10. Routine ECG as a screening tool

The Task Force on Preparticipation Screening for Cardiovascular Disease in Competitive Athletes of AHA/ACC [5, 48, 51, 52] does not recommend routine ECGs and echocardiograms for pre-participation screening. On the other hand, the International Olympic Committee [66] and the European Society of Cardiology [67] guidelines recommend routine screening with a 12-lead ECG along with history and physical examination. Pre-participation screening ECG does not increase the diagnostic accuracy, is not practical, is not sensitive, and is not specific. In addition, both false positives and false negatives (5–20%) exist with the ECG [68]. However, it may detect patients with hypertrophic cardiomyopathy, WPW syndrome, atrioventricular block, long QT syndrome, and Brugada syndrome.

The justification for AHA/ACC guidelines for not recommending routine recording of ECGs as a part of pre-participation screening may be summarized as follows: 1. ECG is not sensitive and is not specific with false-positive ECGs taking place way above true-positive ECGs, 2. The incidence of cardiac conditions leading to sports-related deaths is rather low (5 out of 100,000 subjects), 3. The athlete group to be screened is of the considerable size (10 million in the USA and much larger worldwide), 4. Routine ECG screening will impose a large price tag of roughly 2 Billion dollars/year, and 5. There is no adequate physician pool to do and interpret this large number of ECGs. Furthermore, the subjects with undiagnosed cardiac abnormality may present with symptoms, namely chest pain, exertional dyspnea, or syncope which may be uncovered by the screening questionnaire. Since some of the entities have a genetic and familial origin, they may be discovered by the screening protocol. Finally, studies comparing the strategies with and without ECG during screening did not demonstrate a mortality benefit in the group with routine ECGs [52, 54, 69]. Based on these and other considerations, the author is in support of not performing ECG during pre-participation screening [3] and recommends careful attention to implementing the 14-point AHA/ACC pre-participation screening protocol.

## 11. Summary and conclusions

Sudden death associated with sports participation often has a cardiovascular cause and the two most frequent etiologies are HCM and aberrant CAs. Clinical features of HCM, aberrant CAs, Marfan's syndrome, and ARVC were reviewed and other entities responsible for SCD were listed/tabulated. The existing recommendations are a pre-spots participation review of full personal and family history and systematic physical examination, preferably in the primary care doctors' office. Additional investigative studies should be undertaken if history or physical examination detect any abnormalities. Using ECG, echocardiogram, or MRI as routine screening techniques is contentious and is not currently recommended in the USA. The rationale of pre-sports participation evaluation is to allow as many athletes as feasible to partake instead of being excluded from sports participation.

## Conflict of interest

The author declares no conflict of interest.

## Author details

P. Syamasundar Rao
McGovern Medical School and Children's Memorial Hermann Hospital, University of Texas Health Sciences Center at Houston, Houston, Texas, USA

*Address all correspondence to: p.syamasundar.rao@uth.tmc.edu

## References

[1] Maron BJ, Epstein SE, Roberts WC. Causes of sudden death in competitive athletes. Journal of the American College of Cardiology. 1986;7:204-214

[2] McCaffrey FM, Braden DS, Strong WB. Sudden cardiac death in young athletes. A review. The American Journal of Diseases of Children. 1991; **145**:177-183

[3] Rao PS. Prevention of sudden death in athletes. Pediat Therapeut. 2015;**5**:e129. DOI: 10.4172/2161-0665.1000e129

[4] Maron BJ, Shirani J, Poliac LC, et al. Sudden death in young competitive athletes. Clinical, demographic, and pathological profiles. Journal of the American Medical Association. 1996;**276**: 199-204

[5] Maron BJ, Thompson PD, Ackerman MJ, Balady G, Berger S, Cohen D, et al. Recommendations and considerations related to preparticipation screening for cardiovascular abnormalities in competitive athletes: 2007 update: a scientific statement from the American Heart Association Council on Nutrition, Physical Activity, and Metabolism: endorsed by the American College of Cardiology Foundation. Circulation. 2007;**115**:1643-1655

[6] Maron BJ, Doerer JJ, Haas TS, Tierney DM, Mueller FO. Sudden deaths in young competitive athletes: Analysis of 1866 deaths in the United States, 1980-2006. Circulation. 2009;**119**: 1085-1092

[7] Maron BJ. Distinguishing hypertrophic cardiomyopathy from athlete's heart physiological remodeling: Clinical significance, diagnostic strategies and implications for preparticipation screening. British Journal of Sports Medicine. 2009;**43**: 649-656

[8] Canedo MI, Frank MJ, Abdulla AM. Rhythm disturbances in hypertrophic cardiomyopathy: Prevalence, relation to symptoms, and management. The American Journal of Cardiology. 1980; **45**:848-855

[9] Maron BJ, Savage DD, Wolfson JK, Epstein SE. Prognostic significance of 24-hour ambulatory electrocardiographic monitoring in patients with hypertrophic cardiomyopathy: A prospective study. The American Journal of Cardiology. 1981;**48**:252-257

[10] Rao PS. Echocardiographic evaluation of neonates with suspected heart disease. In: Rao PS, Vidyasagar D. editors. A Multidisciplinary Approach to Perinatal Cardiology. Vol. 1. New Castle upon Tyne, UK: Cambridge Scholars Publishing; 2021. pp. 314–408. ISBN-13: 978-1-5275-6722-1

[11] Maron BJ, Epstein SE, Roberts WC. Hypertrophic cardiomyopathy: A common cause of sudden death in the young competitive athlete. European Heart Journal. 1983; **4** Suppl F:135–144. DOI: 10.1093/eurheartj/4.suppl_f.135

[12] Maron BJ, Roberts WC, McAllister HA, Rosing DR, Epstein SE. Sudden death in young athletes. Circulation. 1980;**62**:218-229. DOI: 10.1161/01.cir.62.2.218

[13] Maron BJ, Haas TS, Ahluwalia A, Murphy CJ, Garberich RF. Demographics and epidemiology of sudden deaths in young competitive athletes: From the United States National Registry. The American Journal of

Medicine. 2016;**129**:1170-1177. DOI: 10.1016/j.amjmed.2016.02.031

[14] Smith JR, Henry MJ. Demonstration of the coronary arterial system with neoprene latex. The Journal of Laboratory and Clinical Medicine. 1945; **30**:462-466

[15] Kamban J, Rao PS. Anomalous origin of left coronary artery (bland-white-Garland syndrome). In: Kamban J, editor. Cardiac Anesthesia for Infants and Children. St. Louis, MO: Mosby-Year Book, Inc.; 1993. pp. 361-367

[16] Jureidini SB, Marino CJ, Rao PS. Congenital coronary artery anomalies. Indian Journal of Pediatrics. 1998;**65**: 217-229

[17] Barth CW, Robert WC. Left main coronary artery origin from the right sinus of Valsalva and coursing between the aorta and pulmonary trunk. Journal of the American College of Cardiology. 1986;**7**:36-73

[18] Krogel AH, Roberts WC. Anomalous origin of either the right or left main coronary artery from the aorta with subsequent coursing between aorta and pulmonary trunk: Analysis of 32 necropsy cases. The American Journal of Cardiology. 1988;**62**:771-777

[19] Cheitlin MD, DeCastro CM, McAllister HA. Sudden death as a complication of anomalous left coronary origin from the anterior sinus of Valsalva. Circulation. 1974;**50**:780-787

[20] Strong WB, Alpert BS. The child with heart disease: Play, recreation, and sports. Current Problems in Cardiology. 1981;**6**:1-37

[21] Roberts WC, Siegel RJ, Zipes DP. Origin of the right coronary artery from the left sinus of Valsalva and its functional consequences: Analysis of 10 necropsy patients. The American Journal of Cardiology. 1982;**49**:863-868

[22] Braden DS, Strong WB. Preparticipation screening for sudden cardiac death in high school and college athletes. The Physician and Sports Medicine. 1988;**16**:128-140

[23] Jureidini SB, Marino CJ, Singh GK, Balfour IC, Rao PS. Aberrant coronary arteries: A reliable echocardiographic screening method. The Journal of the American Society of Echocardiography. 2003;**16**:756-763

[24] Frommelt PC, Berger S, Pelech AN, Bergstrom S, Williamson JG. Prospective identification of anomalous origin of left coronary artery from the right sinus of Valsalva using transthoracic echocardiography: Importance of color Doppler flow mapping. Pediatric Cardiology. 2001;**22**:327-332

[25] Missri JC, Swett DD. Marfan syndrome: A review. Cardiovascular Reviews & Reports. 1982;**3**:1648-1653

[26] Cantwell JD. Marfan's syndrome: Detection and management. The Physician and Sports Medicine. 1986;**14**:51-55

[27] Yuan SM, Jing H. Marfan's syndrome: An overview. São Paulo Medical Journal. 2010;**128**:360-366

[28] Lambert EC, Vijayan AM, Wagner HR, Vlad P. Sudden unexpected death from cardiovascular disease in children, a cooperative international study. The American Journal of Cardiology. 1974;**34**:89-96

[29] Geva T, Hegesh J, Frand M. The clinical course and echocardiographic features of Marfan's syndrome in childhood. American Journal of Diseases of Children. 1987;**141**:1179-1182

[30] Loeys BL, Dietz HC, Braverman AC, Callewaert BL, De Backer J, Devereux RB, et al. The revised Ghent nosology for the Marfan syndrome. Journal of Medical Genetics. 2010;**47**:476-485

[31] Van Laer L, Loeys B. Connective tissue disorders. In: Moller JH, Hoffman JIE. editors. Pediatric Cardiovascular Medicine. 2nd ed. Oxford, UK: Wiley-Blackwell/A John Wiley & Sons Ltd; 2012. pp. 969–981

[32] Rao PS. Diagnosis and management of acyanotic heart disease: Part I - obstructive lesions. Indian Journal of Pediatrics. 2005;**72**:496-502

[33] Singh GK, Rao PS. Left heart outflow obstructions. In: Crawford MH, DiMarco JP, Paulus WJ. editors. Cardiology, 3rd ed. Edinburgh, UK: Mosby Elsevier; 2010. pp. 1507–1518. ISBN: 978–0–7234-3485-6

[34] Rao PS. Congenital heart defects—A review. In: Rao PS editor. Congenital Heart Disease—Selected Aspects. Rijeka, Croatia: InTech; 2012. pp. 3–44. ISBN: 978-953-307-472-6

[35] Rao PS. Diagnosis and management of cyanotic congenital heart disease: Part I. Indian Journal of Pediatrics 2009; **76**:57-70.

[36] Rao PS. Diagnosis and management of cyanotic congenital heart disease: Part II. Indian Journal of Pediatrics. 2009;**76**:297-308

[37] Rao PS. Tricuspid atresia. In: Rao PS, editor. Pediatric Cardiology: How it Has Evolved over the Last 50 Years. New Castle upon Tyne, UK: Cambridge Scholars Publishing; 2020. pp. 24-69. ISBN-13: 9781527548886

[38] Rao PS. What an adult cardiologist should know about cyanotic congenital heart disease? Journal of Cardiovascular Diseases & Diagnosis. 2013;**1**:104. DOI: 10.4172/2329- 9517.100010

[39] Rao PS. Fontan operation: Indications, short- and long-term outcomes. Indian Journal of Pediatrics. 2015;**82**:1147-1156

[40] Haugaa KH, Haland TF, Leren IS, Saberniak J, Edvardsen T. Arrhythmogenic right ventricular cardiomyopathy, clinical manifestations, and diagnosis. Europace. 2016;**18**: 965-972

[41] Landry CH, Fatah M, Connelly KA, Angaran P, Hamilton RM, Dorian P. Evaluating the 12-Lead electrocardiogram for diagnosing ARVC in young populations: Implications for preparticipation screening of athletes. CJC Open. 2020;**3**:498-503

[42] Marcus FI, McKenna WJ, Sherrill D, Basso C, Bauce B, Bluemke DA, et al. Diagnosis of arrhythmogenic right ventricular cardiomyopathy/dysplasia: Proposed modification of the task force criteria. Circulation. 2010;**121**:1533-1541

[43] Koskenvuo K. Sudden death among Finnish conscripts. BMJ. 1976;**2**: 1413-1415

[44] Kramer MR, Drori Y, Lev B. Sudden death in young soldiers, high incidence of syncope prior to death. Chest. 1988; **93**:345-347

[45] Angolini P, Trivollato M, Donis J, Leacman RD. Myocardial bridges: A review. Progress in Cardiovascular Diseases. 1983;**26**:75-88

[46] Furniss SS, Williams DO, McGregor CGA. Systolic coronary occlusion due to myocardial bridging: A rare cause of ischemia. International Journal of Cardiology. 1990;**26**:116-117

[47] Maron BJ, Poliac LC, Kaplan JA, Mueller FO. Blunt impact to the chest leading to sudden death from cardiac arrest during sports activities. The New England Journal of Medicine. 1995;**333**: 337-342

[48] Maron BJ, Thompson PD, Puffer JC, et al. Cardiovascular preparticipation screening of competitive athletes. A statement for health professionals from the sudden death committee (clinical cardiology) and congenital cardiac defects committee (cardiovascular disease in the young), American Heart Association. Circulation. 1996;**94**: 850-856

[49] Corrado D, Pelliccia A, Bjørnstad HH, Vanhees L, Biffi A, Borjesson M, et al. Study Group of Sport Cardiology of the Working Group of Cardiac Rehabilitation and Exercise Physiology and the Working Group of Myocardial and Pericardial Diseases of the European Society of Cardiology. Cardiovascular pre-participation screening of young competitive athletes for prevention of sudden death: proposal for a common European protocol. Consensus Statement of the Study Group of Sport Cardiology of the Working Group of Cardiac Rehabilitation and Exercise Physiology and the Working Group of Myocardial and Pericardial Diseases of the European Society of Cardiology. European Heart Journal. 2005; **26**:516–524

[50] Maron BJ, Friedman RA, Kligfield P, et al. Assessment of the 12-Lead electrocardiogram as a screening test for detection of cardiovascular disease in healthy general populations of young people (12–25 years of age): A scientific statement from the American Heart Association and the American College of Cardiology. Journal of the American College of Cardiology. 2014;**64**:1476-1516. DOI: 10.1016/j.jacc.2014.05.006

[51] Maron BJ, Levine BD, Washington RL, Baggish AL, Kovacs RJ, Maron MS. American Heart Association Electrocardiography and Arrhythmias Committee of Council on Clinical Cardiology, Council on Cardiovascular Disease in Young, Council on Cardiovascular and Stroke Nursing, Council on Functional Genomics and Translational Biology, and American College of Cardiology. Eligibility and Disqualification Recommendations for Competitive Athletes With Cardiovascular Abnormalities: Task Force 2: Preparticipation Screening for Cardiovascular Disease in Competitive Athletes: A Scientific Statement From the American Heart Association and American College of Cardiology. Circulation. 2015;**132**:e267–272

[52] Maron BJ, Levine BD, Washington RL, Baggish AL, Kovacs RJ, Maron MS. Eligibility and disqualification recommendations for competitive athletes with cardiovascular abnormalities: Task force 2: Preparticipation screening for cardiovascular disease in competitive athletes: A scientific statement from the American Heart Association and American College of Cardiology. Journal of the American College of Cardiology. 2015;**66**:2356-2361

[53] Corrado D, Basso C, Pavei A, Michieli P, Schiavon M, Thiene G. Trends in sudden cardiovascular death in young competitive athletes after implementation of a preparticipation screening program. Journal of the American Medical Association. 2006; **296**:1593-1601

[54] Steinvil A, Chundadze T, Zeltser D, Rogowski O, Halkin A, Galily Y, et al. Mandatory electrocardiographic screening of athletes to reduce their risk for sudden death: Proven fact or wishful thinking? Journal of the American College of Cardiology. 2011;**57**:1291-1296

[55] Haneda N, Mori C, Nishio T, Saito M, Kajino Y, Watanabe K, et al. Heart diseases discovered by mass screening in the schools of Shimane prefecture over a period of 5 years. Japanese Circulation Journal. 1986;**50**: 1325-1329

[56] Corrado D, Schmied C, Basso C, Borjesson M, Schiavon M, Pelliccia A, et al. Risk of sports: Do we need a pre-participation screening for competitive and leisure athletes? European Heart Journal. 2011;**32**:934-944

[57] Holst AG, Winkel BG, Theilade J, Kristensen IB, Thomsen JL, Ottesen GL, et al. Incidence and etiology of sports-related sudden cardiac death in Denmark: Implications for preparticipation screening. Heart Rhythm. 2010;**7**:1365-1371

[58] Pelliccia A, Culasso F, Di Paolo FM, Accettura D, Cantore R, Castagna W, et al. Prevalence of abnormal electrocardiograms in a large, unselected population undergoing pre-participation cardiovascular screening. European Heart Journal. 2007;**28**:2006-2010

[59] Wilson MG, Basavarajaiah S, Whyte GP, Cox S, Loosemore M, Sharma S. Efficacy of personal symptom and family history questionnaires when screening for inherited cardiac pathologies: The role of electrocardiography. British Journal of Sports Medicine. 2008;**42**:207-211

[60] Le VV, Wheeler MT, Mandic S, Dewey F, Fonda H, Perez M, et al. Addition of the electrocardiogram to the preparticipation examination of college athletes. Clinical Journal of Sport Medicine. 2010;**20**:98-105

[61] Anderson JB, Grenier M, Edwards NM, Madsen NL, Czosek RJ, Spar DS, et al. Usefulness of combined history, physical examination, electrocardiogram, and limited echocardiogram in screening adolescent athletes for risk for sudden cardiac death. The American Journal of Cardiology. 2014;**114**:1763-1767

[62] Wyman RA, Chiu RY, Rahko PS. The 5-minute screening echocardiogram for athletes. Journal of the American Society of Echocardiography. 2008;**7**:786-788

[63] Grazioli G, Merino B, Montserrat S, et al. Usefulness of echocardiography in preparticipation screening of competitive athletes. Revista Española de Cardiología (English Edition). 2014;**67**: 701-705

[64] Yim ES, Basilico F, Corrado G. Early screening for cardiovascular abnormalities with preparticipation echocardiography: Utility of focused physician-operated echocardiography in preparticipation screening of athletes. Journal of Ultrasound in Medicine. 2014; **33**:307-313

[65] Angelini P, Cheong BY, Lenge De Rosen VV, Lopez JA, Uribe C et al. Magnetic resonance imaging-based screening study in a general population of adolescents. Journal of the American College of Cardiology. 2018;**71**:579–580

[66] IOC Medical Commission, International Olympic Committee. Journal of the American College of Cardiology. 2004. http://multimedia.olympic.org/pdf/en_report_886.pdf

[67] Pelliccia A, Fagard R, Bjørnstad HH, et al. Recommendations for competitive sports participation in athletes with cardiovascular disease: A consensus document from the study Group of Sports Cardiology of the working Group of Cardiac Rehabilitation and Exercise Physiology, and the working Group of Myocardial and Pericardial diseases of

the European Society of Cardiology. European Heart Journal. 2005;**26**: 1422-1445

[68] Rowin EJ, Maron BJ, Appelbaum E, Link MS, Gibson CM, Lesser JR, et al. Significance of false negative electrocardiograms in preparticipation screening of athletes for hypertrophic cardiomyopathy. The American Journal of Cardiology. 2012;**110**:1027-1032

[69] Maron BJ, Haas TS, Doerer JJ, Thompson PD, Hodges JS. Comparison of U.S. and Italian experiences with sudden cardiac deaths in young competitive athletes and implications for preparticipation screening strategies. The American Journal of Cardiology. 2009;**104**:276-280

Section 5

# Individual Heart Defects

Chapter 5

# Ventricular Septal Defects: A Review

*Unnati Doshi and Elizabeth Wang-Giuffre*

## Abstract

Ventricular septal defects (VSDs) account for up to 30% of all congenital cardiac anomalies and are one of the most common lesions encountered in day-to-day practice. The etiology is thought to be multifactorial inheritance but it is sometimes associated with chromosomal abnormalities such as aneuploidies and microdeletions. Most of these defects, close spontaneously and do not require treatment. Symptoms are primarily dependent upon the degree of shunt across the ventricles. Echocardiography remains the main modality of definitive diagnosis for isolated defects. Surgical repair is recommended in hemodynamically significant shunts or if there is aortic prolapse and regurgitation. Prognosis after surgical repair remains excellent especially with isolated defects but complete atrioventricular block or worsening valve regurgitation may occur in some patients. Newer techniques involving catheter based or hybrid device closures are being used in select cases such as muscular defects. Large unrepaired shunts, although uncommon in the developed world, may cause irreversible changes in pulmonary vasculature leading to Eisenmenger's syndrome.

**Keywords:** ventricular septal defect, congenital heart defects, heart disease, pediatrics, Acyanotic heart defects

## 1. Introduction

The incidence of congenital heart disease varies from 6/1000 live births for moderate to severe forms and increases to ~75/1000 if trivial forms are included [1]. Ventricular septal defect (VSD) is a defect in the interventricular septum and one of the most common congenital cardiac anomalies accounting for up to 30% of all congenital heart defects [2]. Many trivial defects are unaccounted for as they close before one year of age or in fetal life and therefore, a precise prevalence is difficult to obtain. Prevalence is reported up to 5% in newborn babies [3]. They can occur in isolation or as a part of several other complex cardiac anomalies including tetralogy of Fallot, truncus arteriosus and atrioventricular septal defect. In this paper, we will primarily discuss isolated VSDs.

## 2. Embryology/genetics

The interventricular septum (IVS) is composed of the mesenchymal and muscular portions. The ventricular septal growth starts around the fifth week of embryonic



IntechOpen

development and involves fusion of different septal components. The atrioventricular endocardial cushions form part of the interventricular septum [4]. The muscular interventricular septum arises from the primary fold or ring and grows upward from the floor of the ventricles towards the already fused endocardial cushions [5]. The outflow tract cushions composed of mesenchymal cells as well as neural crest cells contribute to the septation of the common outflow tract, the semilunar valves and also move downward into the ventricles forming the aortopulmonary septum. By the eighth week of gestation, when the endocardial cushions, muscular septum and aortopulmonary septum fuse, the membranous septum is formed and the ventricular septation is complete [6].

Several theories are currently postulated to determine factors affecting normal cardiac septation. The etiology of ventricular septal defect is heterogenous and may involve environmental and genetic factors, commonly referred to as multifactorial inheritance. Known chromosomal abnormalities such as aneuploidies (e.g. trisomy 21 or trisomy 18) and microdeletions such as DiGeorge syndrome are known to be associated with ventricular septal defects [7]. Single gene defects involving TBX-5 causes Holt Oram syndrome and is characterized by a constellation of birth defects, including ventricular septal defects. Transcription factor encoding genes such as TBX, NKX2–5,GATA4 play an important role in the ventricular septum positioning during cardiogenesis. Other genes that may play a possible role in cardiac septation include GATA6, HOMEX and PLG1 [8].

## 3. Anatomy

Even though VSDs are encountered on a day to day basis by cardiologists and cardiovascular surgeons alike, its classification and nomenclature continues to remain variable among different groups. Two famous schools of thought come from descriptions by Soto et al. [9] and Van Praagh et al. [10].

Soto et al., broadly divided the ventricular septum into the membranous and muscular portions. The membranous septum is separated by the septal leaflet of

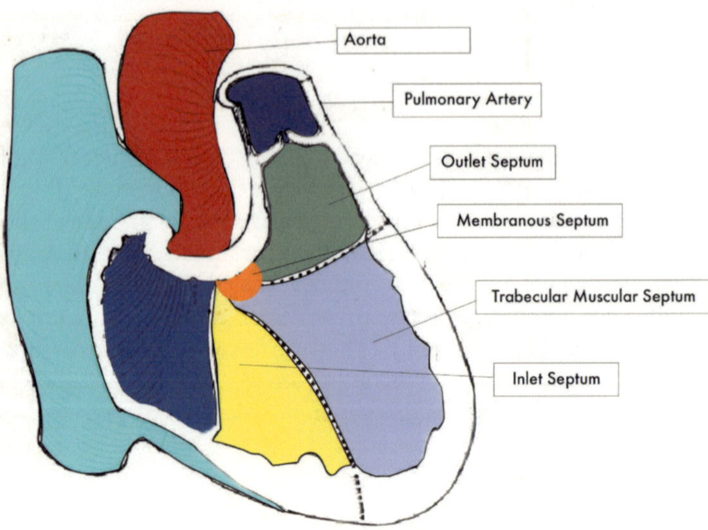


**Figure 1.**
*Anatomy of the ventricular septum from the right ventricular aspect.*

tricuspid valve tissue into atrioventricular and interventricular components. The muscular septum in turn is described as having three different components, (**Figure 1**): The inlet muscular septum is small and divides the mitral and tricuspid valves. The trabecular septum is the largest portion of the ventricular septum extending to the ventricular apex. The infundibular septum is the portion above the crista supraventricularis that separates the aortic and pulmonary valves. The other part of the crista is between the tricuspid and pulmonary valves [11].

Van Praagh and associates have described these defects as atrioventricular canal, muscular, conoventricular, and conal septal type ventricular septal defects.

Accordingly, the ventricular septal defects may be classified as follows: (**Figure 2**).

A. Perimembranous defects: These are defects in the membranous septum and may further extend into inlet, trabecular or outlet muscular septum. On the left ventricular side, these defects typically lie in the outflow tract below the aortic valve. On the right ventricular side, the defects appear beneath the crista supraventricularis and posterior to the medial papillary muscle. All defects have a rim which is formed by the tricuspid, mitral and aortic fibrous continuity. Approximately 80% of ventricular septal defects occur in this area [2].

B. Muscular defects are further divided into the inlet, trabecular and outlet septal defects. These account for ~5–20% of all VSDs.

C. Subarterial infundibular defects are located in the area of the septum, adjacent to the arterial valves which are contiguous. These are also called doubly committed juxtaarterial/subarterial defects. They account for ~5–7% of all VSDs. Of note,

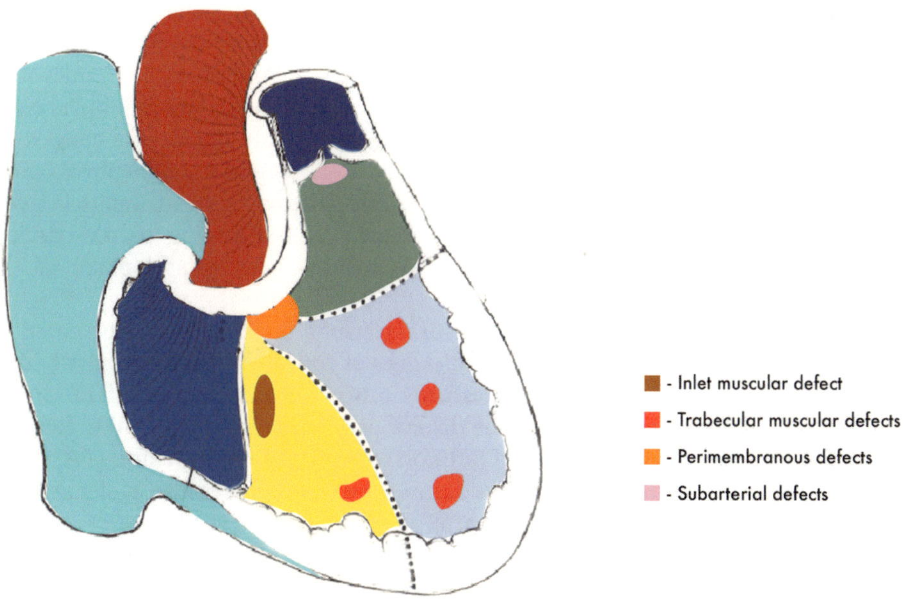


**Figure 2.**
*Types of ventricular septal defects by location.*

it is more common among Asians with reported incidence up to 30% in Japanese population.

D. Atrioventricular septal defects are located in the inlet septum and will not be reviewed in this chapter.

VSDs are also classified based on their size: those less than one-third (~33%) the size of the aortic valve annulus are considered as small; more than half (50%) as large and moderate being in between.

## 4. Pathophysiology

The degree of shunting across the VSD is primarily dependent on the size of the defect. In large non-restrictive defects, the difference in the pulmonary vascular resistance (PVR) and systemic vascular resistance (SVR) determines the magnitude of the shunt. The degree of shunt is frequently described as the ratio of pulmonary blood flow (Qp) to systemic blood flow (Qs) and shunts with Qp:Qs ≥1.5 are typically considered hemodynamically significant.

In neonates, right after birth, there is significant drop in PVR as the gas exchange changes from placental circulation to the lung. Thereafter there is progressive rise in SVR, and decline of PVR, with consequent increase in pulmonary blood flow which continues over a period of the first 6–8 weeks of life. It is this rate of decline in PVR that determines the amount of left to right shunting in patients with VSDs.

In patients with small VSDs, the decrease in PVR does not influence pulmonary over circulation as the size of the defect intrinsically restricts flow. In comparison, in patients with large VSDs, the drop in PVR primarily determines the amount of pulmonary blood flow and direction of flow across the two ventricles. Once the pulmonary resistance decreases, blood flow from the left to the right ventricle causes over circulation to the lungs and increases preload to the left atrium and ventricle. Pulmonary mechanics are altered due to increased pulmonary blood flow including decreased lung compliance and tidal volume [12]. Another mechanism contributing to clinical symptoms of congestive heart failure is neurohormonal activation with increased levels of norepinephrine and renin – angiotensin seen in these infants [13]. In some patients, the medial muscle layer in the small pulmonary vessels does not regress as rapidly, in turn leading to slower decline of the PVR [14]. In such patients, there may be subsequent delay in development of symptoms.

Chronic exposure of volume and pressure overload due to large uncorrected VSDs leads to structural and functional changes of the pulmonary vascular bed. There is development of endothelial dysfunction, smooth muscle proliferation, vascular remodeling, and intravascular thrombosis. These changes lead to increase in pulmonary vascular resistance and pulmonary arterial hypertension (PAH) [15]. The definition of PAH includes a mean pulmonary arterial pressure ≥ 25 mmHg at rest, a left atrial pressure ≤ 15 mmHg, and normal resting cardiac output, suggesting a resting pulmonary vascular resistance of ≥3 Woods units (WU). Eisenmenger's syndrome (ES) is the most advanced stage of pulmonary arterial hypertension in patients with unrepaired shunts of congenital heart disease and often irreversible.

## 5. Natural history of ventricular septal defects

Conventional descriptions of natural history of VSDs include spontaneous closure, progression to pulmonary vascular obstructive disease (PVOD), development of infundibular stenosis, and progression to aortic insufficiency. Each of these will be reviewed briefly.

### 5.1 Spontaneous closure

Approximately 70% of ventricular septal defects do not require any intervention either due to spontaneous closure or due to hemodynamically insignificant shunts. Trabecular muscular VSDs tend to close more often than membranous defects. Most defects close by 2 years of age but in some cases, closure may take place through 8 years of age. However, the process of spontaneous closure continues through adolescence and adulthood. Membranous defects close due to apposition of tricuspid valve leaflets against the VSD; also described as "aneurysmal" formation [16].

### 5.2 Progression to pulmonary vascular obstructive disease

PVOD may develop in 10% of untreated VSDs. This is likely to be due to the exposure of the pulmonary vascular bed to high flow and high pressure. Speedy diagnosis and closure of the VSD at least prior to 18 months of age is expected to decrease the incidence of development of PVOD.

With the advent of better echocardiographic imaging as well as its availability, the incidence of Eisenmenger's syndrome and irreversible PVOD has decreased but still exists in less than 10% of patients. Such patients are often are diagnosed in adulthood, particularly in developing countries. In many of these patients, prognosis maybe worse after surgical repair. In a subset of patients with VSD and PAH, newer treatment modalities such as pulmonary vasodilators have made some patients amenable to repair. However, immediate post-operative survival does not necessarily assure good long-term outcomes [17].

### 5.3 Development of infundibular stenosis

Development of infundibular stenosis, originally described by Gasul, occurs in 8% of VSDs. Some specific signs, namely, right aortic arch and increased angle of the right ventricular outflow tract that may influence the VSDs to undergo Gasul's transformation. Although the onset of infundibular stenosis ultimately needs surgery, it truly protects the pulmonary circulation and prevents development of PVOD.

### 5.4 Progression to aortic insufficiency

While most spontaneous VSD closures are due apposition of tricuspid valve tissue against the VSD, sometimes aortic valve cusps prolapse down towards the VSD to produce partial or complete closure. This may either be due to prolapse of an aortic valve cusp into the VSD or lack of support to the aortic root. This complication appears to occur more commonly with doubly committed subarterial VSDs than with other types.

Combination of VSD and aortic regurgitation (AR) due to prolapse of right coronary or, less frequently, non-coronary cusp is known as Laubry-Pezzi syndrome. Aortic valve prolapse can be seen in some patients with perimembranous defects and more commonly those with the subarterial defects where the tissue supporting aortic cusp is lacking. It is commonly seen in those with smaller defects due to venturi effect on the leaflets. The lifetime risk of developing aortic valve prolapse in patients with VSD is ~6.3% [18]. Long term follow up is recommended in these patients and surgery is indicated in patients with more than trivial AR. Based on a recent study of 261 pediatric and adult patients with VSD and AR, it was found that AR tends to be detected between the ages of 3–8 years [19]. Only the patients with aortic valve abnormalities or delayed operation had AR progression or persistence of more than mild degree of AR. The study authors concluded that surgical closure of subarterial VSD is indicated in patients with significant leaflet deformity as well as those with subarterial VSDs with moderate to severe AR.

### 5.5 Other natural history events

#### *5.5.1 Double chambered right ventricle*

First described in 1858 by TB Peacock, double chambered right ventricle may evolve as a complication in some patients with VSD. It is characterized by a mid-cavitary obstruction either due to hypertrophy of the crista supraventricularis or of septoparietal trabeculations causing the right ventricle to divide into a high-pressure proximal portion and a low-pressure distal portion. It can occur in up to 8–10% of patients with VSDs [20].

#### *5.5.2 Development of infective endocarditis*

VSDs even when not hemodynamically significant carry a lifetime risk of developing infective endocarditis (IE). The incidence of IE in unrepaired VSDs is 1.5 to 2.4 per 1000 patient-years, especially if associated with aortic insufficiency or with left ventricle-to-right atrial shunt [21]. Based on a Swedish registry study, risk of IE in adult VSD patients without previous intervention is 20–30 times higher than the general population [22]. The second natural history study reported risk of IE is twice as likely in unrepaired defects as compared to after surgical repair. However, the incidence of IE after closure of VSD was still higher than normal risk curve [23, 24]. Based on the 2007, AHA guidelines, prophylaxis for IE is not recommended on patients with isolated VSDs. The exceptions are VSDs within 6 months of surgical or intervention closure, with ES, with residual defects after surgery or patients with previous history of IE [25].

## 6. Clinical presentation

Small VSDs: Patients with small VSDs are usually asymptomatic and are detected incidentally on routine physical examination. A holosystolic murmur with or without a thrill is best heard at the left lower sternal border in muscular and membranous defects while the holosystolic murmur is heard at the left upper sternal border in sub-arterial defects due to direction of VSD jet towards the pulmonary outflow tract. In very small defects, the murmur is shorter and does not last through the entire systole.

Moderate to large VSDs: Subjects with hemodynamically significant, moderate to large VSDs usually present with signs of congestive heart failure due to pulmonary over-circulation and left ventricular volume overload. Due to equalization of pressures in both right and left ventricles, the right ventricular impulse in the lower left sternal border or subxiphoid region is prominent. In patients with chronic left ventricular overload, the left ventricular impulse is hyperdynamic and shifts laterally. A mid diastolic flow rumble may be heard at the apex due to relative mitral stenosis from increased left to right shunt. This usually indicates a Qp:Qs >2:1.

Eisenmenger syndrome: Patients with ES may present with central cyanosis, clubbing, peripheral edema, abdominal tenderness, right ventricular heave, a loud pulmonary ejection click and an accentuated pulmonary component of the second heart sound.

## 7. Diagnostic testing

### 7.1 Non-invasive imaging

In current times, transthoracic echocardiogram (TTE) is the main modality for definitive diagnosis of VSDs. It allows to delineate size and location of the defect as well as other details such as outflow tracts, associated lesions, evidence of chamber dilation and pressures (**Figures 3–6**). Transesophageal echocardiographic (TEE)

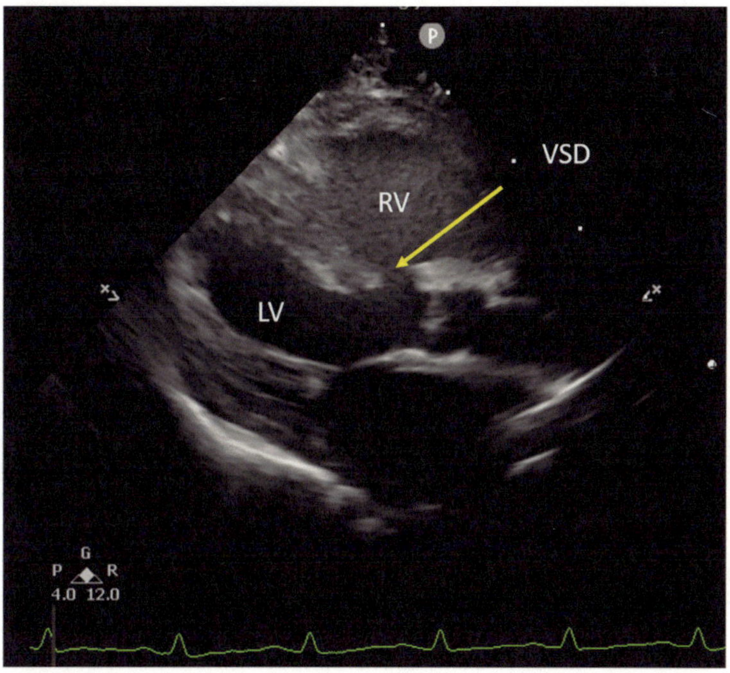


**Figure 3.**
*Echocardiographic parasternal long axis view showing perimembranous ventricular septal defect (VSD). RV = right ventricle; LV = left ventricle.*

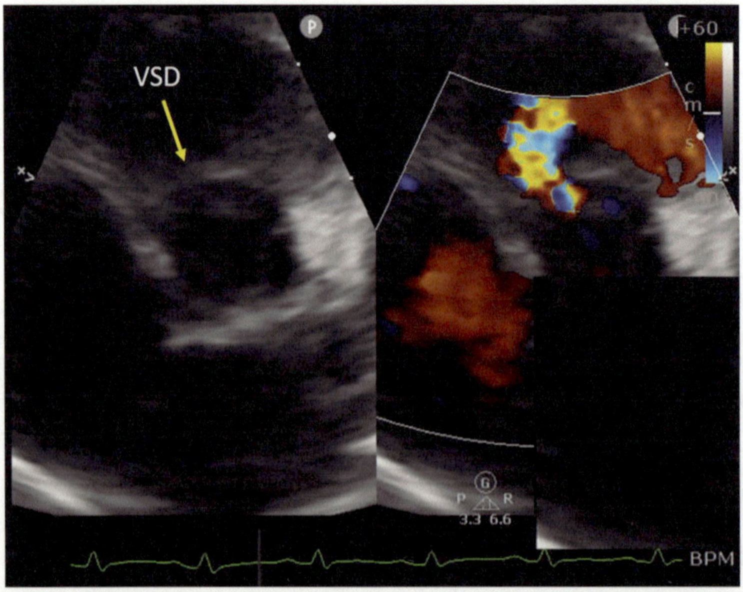


**Figure 4.**
*Echocardiographic parasternal short axis color compare view showing perimembranous ventricular septal defect (VSD) at ~110' clock position. The red flow represents indicates left to right shunt during systole across it.*

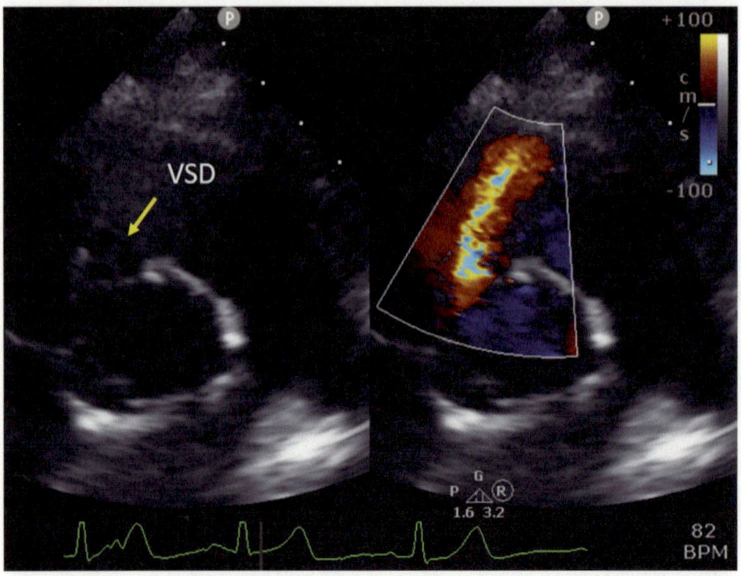


**Figure 5.**
*Echocardiographic image (parasternal short axis color compare view) showing subarterial ventricular septal defect (VSD) at ~12–1 o'clock position. The red flow represents indicates left to right shunt during systole across it.*

imaging is routinely used for evaluation of anatomy intraoperatively. It also helps to better delineate associated pathologies especially those involving valve abnormalities such as valve prolapse and regurgitation. Postoperatively, it is used to detect presence of residual defects as well as ventricular function assessment.

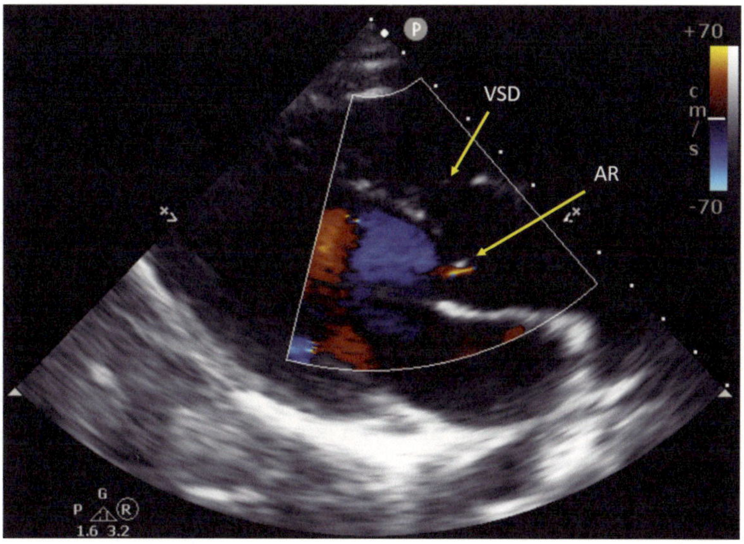


**Figure 6.**
*Echocardiographic parasternal long axis view showing trivial aortic regurgitation (AR) is seen by color flow in the presence of aortic cusp prolapse into the subarterial ventricular septal defect (VSD).*

Electrocardiographic changes such as left atrial enlargement as well as left ventricular hypertrophy is seen in hemodynamically significant defects. Right ventricular hypertrophy maybe seen in patients with significant pulmonary arterial hypertension. Chest X-rays serve as adjuncts to clinical assessment. Cardiomegaly, and increased pulmonary vascular markings are seen in patients with moderate to large VSDs. Left atrial dilation may cause superior deviation of the left main bronchus. In patients with Eisenmenger's, there is evidence of right heart enlargement with main pulmonary artery dilation without increased pulmonary vascular markings.

Advanced imaging such as cardiac magnetic resonance (CMR) imaging is not necessary in the routine evaluation of isolated VSDs. However, it is a helpful adjunct in the diagnosis of complex anatomical variants and in the evaluation of associated defects or complications such as double chambered right ventricle and pulmonary arterial hypertension (PAH). 3D phase contrast-CMR may help obtain additional information with regards to quantification of pulmonary blood flow.

### 7.2 Cardiac catheterization

Although a mainstay in diagnosis of all congenital heart defects in the past, cardiac catheterization is now reserved for cases requiring measurements of PVR. In the patients with PAH, cardiac catheterization may be undertaken to determine operability. Catheterization data indicating operability suggests the likelihood of a favorable versus an unfavorable outcome [17]. But, there is no validated consensus data accurate enough to define which patients will be free of major postoperative complications related to pulmonary vascular disease. However, a baseline ratio between indexed pulmonary vascular resistance (PVRi) and indexed systemic vascular resistance (SVRi) of <0.3 and PVRi of <6 indexed Woods units/m2 (iWU. m2) is indicative of favorable outcome. Pulmonary vasoreactivity study with $O_2$ and iNO has been used to determine operability in subjects with PVRi of 6–9 iWU m2 or resistance ratio (PVRi/SVRi) of 0.3–0.5. A positive test is defined as decrease of both PVRi and resistance ratio by 1/5th of initial value as well as final PVRi of 6 iWUm2 and resistance ratio of <0.3. All patients should meet all of these criteria before being considered operable with decreased risk of serious postoperative complications [26, 27]. In patients with PVRi >10 iWUm2 and resistance ratio of >0.7, surgical repair is not beneficial [28].

Other protocols have been proposed for the vasoreactivity studies to assess operability as well as to assess prognosis and indication for specific anti PAH therapies. Measurements of resistance and flow in systemic and pulmonary vascular beds are carried out in several conditions such as room air, nitric oxide, IV epoprostenol or inhaled iloprost and in some cases oral phosphodiesterase 5 inhibitors. Some recommend to avoid use of high oxygen concentrations in these patients if other agents are available due to high amounts of dissolved oxygen as a potential source of error causing overestimation of Qp [29].

## 8. Treatment

### 8.1 Medical management

Most small VSDs do not require intervention unless complications occur. In moderate to large defects, medical therapy is initiated if signs of pulmonary overcirculation and congestive heart failure develop. Standard medical therapy consists of diuretics, commonly furosemide. This helps to decrease preload and relieves symptoms such as tachypnea and tachycardia. Spironolactone is usually added to counter the hypokalemia related to the loop diuretic use. One other approach is afterload reduction, mostly with the use angiotensin converting enzyme (ACE) inhibitors such as captopril or enalapril to reduce the SVR which in turn decreases pulmonary blood flow and increases systemic flow. Digoxin, still preferred by some cardiologists, is not very commonly used anymore since the theoretical effect in the presence of normal systolic function is not well known. Medical therapy for congestive heart failure should be continued either until the defect size decreases, closes spontaneously, or until surgery as the case may be.

Medical management of patients with ES with anti – PAH drug therapy remains the main stay for treatment of Eisenmenger's syndrome. Three groups of pulmonary vasodilators have emerged since 1995. These include, prostacyclins such as epoprostenol, treprostinil, iloprost; endothelin receptor antagonists (bosentan, ambrisentan, macitentan); and phosphodiesterase-5 inhibitors, namely tadalafil and sildenafil [30]. One of the newer FDA approved therapy is a soluble guanylate cyclase stimulator, Riociguat. They are often used as mono, dual or triple therapy, as per the clinical scenario. Detailed discussion of the pulmonary vasodilators is beyond the scope of this chapter. Optimizing hemoglobin and iron levels is important, usually with oral and occasionally intravenous iron supplementation may become necessary. Phlebotomies and routine anticoagulation are not recommended. When polycythemia is found to be problematic (hematocrit >70%), erythropheresis instead phlebotomy is recommended. Oxygen supplementation is not shown to provide symptomatic relief or survival benefits in patients with ES. Definitive treatment is lung transplantation with VSD closure or heart–lung transplantation.

### 8.2 Surgical intervention

Hemodynamically significant VSDs are those with congestive heart failure and pulmonary artery hypertension, and those causing failure to thrive or repeated respiratory infections [24]. VSDs producing cardiomegaly beyond a year of age are also considered hemodynamically significant [24].

Surgical closure of VSD remains the mainstay of treatment for most VSDs. Indications for surgical closure include hemodynamically significant shunts causing left ventricular volume overload and failure of medical therapy. A Qp:Qs >2:1 although difficult to calculate by non-invasive imaging modalities, is an indication for surgery in older and adult patients if there is normal or reversible pulmonary vascular resistance. Other indications include aortic valve prolapse with regurgitation, double chambered right ventricle with significant obstruction, left ventricular systolic dysfunction, or patients with previous history of bacterial endocarditis.

Majority of perimembranous VSDs are closed using a Dacron patch via right atriotomy with or without detachment of the tricuspid valve leaflets. Tricuspid valve detachment adds to the cardiopulmonary bypass and cross clamp time but there is no significant difference in postoperative residual shunts or degree of tricuspid regurgitation [31]. A transpulmonary approach is used in sub arterial, doubly committed VSDs. Although not widespread, some surgeons have reported use of the right axillary approach for closure of selected VSDs. Use of such methods are limited to certain centers and in mostly older adolescents and adults. Most muscular defects are difficult to close by surgical approach.

Surgery is relatively safe and the surgical mortality is low. Long term prognosis after surgical closure is excellent. After closure, catch up growth may take ~6–12 months and the left ventricular volume and mass eventually return to normal. Complications, although rare, include residual lesions, sinus node dysfunction, pulmonary hypertension, and modest progression of aortic insufficiency [32]. The incidence of complete heart block after closure of perimembranous defects is between 0.7 and 1% [33].

Although commonly used few decades ago, main pulmonary artery banding is rarely used in the management of most isolated VSDs. In rare situations such as in a child with other comorbidities where a complete repair is not feasible or where the VSD is difficult to close by standard techniques such as muscular "swiss-cheese" type defects, a main pulmonary artery banding procedure may be considered. Later, the band is removed with repair of main pulmonary artery and patch closure of VSD. In some cases, the muscular defects close spontaneously or at least become hemodynamically insignificant to require closure [32].

### 8.3 Percutaneous device closure

Device closure of VSDs is an alternative for some residual defects, centrally located muscular defects and those not amenable to surgery such as apical muscular defects [34]. Various devices have been used to close VSDs, since its initial description by Rashkind in the 1970s [35]. Since then, several devices including the Amplatzer muscular and membranous VSD occluders, Nit-occlud, and duct occluders I and II are being used for different types of VSD [36]. At this time, only the Amplatzer muscular VSD occluder has received approval for clinical use by the Food and Drug Administration (FDA) and others devices are used on "off-label" basis. Within a year of device placement, up to 92% of patients achieve complete closure of the muscular VSDs. Complications, although rare, include device embolization or malposition, valve regurgitation, residual shunt, hemolysis, arrhythmias, tamponade, cardiac perforation, and death [32]. Nit-occlud devices are associated with residual shunt when compared to other devices. Transient and permanent atrioventricular block is the most serious complication reported with device closure, especially with closure of perimembranous defects [37]. However, more recent studies have reported success of device closure of VSD may depend on patient selection as well as the distance of VSD to aorta and tricuspid valve [36]. The newer ADO II devices are being used in younger patients with perimembranous or muscular VSDs. In a single center trial, lesser complication rates with good success were reported [38]. However, longer, multicenter, prospective data is needed to establish the safety and efficacy.

### 8.4 Hybrid approach

In rare cases, such as small infants with hemodynamically significant muscular VSDs a hybrid "perventricular" approach has been utilized without placing patient on cardiopulmonary bypass; this procedure is performed under TEE guidance. In these cases, access is obtained through a median sternotomy or subxiphoid incision. The device delivery sheath is inserted under TEE guidance from right to left ventricle. The success rate of closure with these devices is reported from 82 to 100% in different studies. Complications include arrythmias, device malposition or missing additional defects. Unsuccessful implantations are converted to conventional open-heart surgical repair [32]. These percutaneous perventricular approach has also been described for successful closure of subarterial VSDs in a small number of patients [39].

Detailed description of percutaneous and perventricular device closures of VSDs is beyond scope of this chapter; the interested is referred elsewhere [32].

## 9. Eisenmengers syndrome

An unrepaired large VSD with unrestricted left to right shunt over a period of time, if not corrected, will lead to increased PVR and irreversible PVOD due to vascular remodeling. There is a bidirectional shunt initially and eventually, right to left shunt develops, as pulmonary artery pressures and PVR exceed systemic pressures and SVR, causing central cyanosis. There is a secondary erythrocytosis, polycythemia and coagulation abnormalities develop. Maladaptation of the right ventricle (RV) as a result of pressure and volume overload with time causes progressive right heart failure. Other factors that may influence risk of developing ES is presence of complex anatomy and underlying genetic and environmental factors. Diagnosis of ES is made by clinical features and echocardiography is a common monitoring tool. The patients may develop dyspnea, decreased exercise tolerance and syncope. Parameters such as $O_2$ saturation, WHO functional class, level of exercise intolerance, reflected by six min walk distance, and NT proBNP are used for serial assessments as well as predictors of survival. Other models of risk stratification in these patients describe various clinical, laboratory and diagnostic markers to determine predictors of mortality [40]. Various other biomarkers reflecting RV dysfunction, endothelial dysfunction and some that may predict potential reversibility of pulmonary vascular lesions are being studied [17]. In a large adult study, older age, pre-tricuspid shunt (such as atrial septal defects and partial anomalous pulmonary venous return), $O_2$ saturations at rest, absence of sinus rhythm, and presence of pericardial effusion were determined as predictors of mortality [41]. Right heart catheterization remains gold standard to confirm diagnosis of ES. In ES patients with established reversed shunt and significant vascular remodeling and PVOD repair is not indicated [17]. Pregnancy is associated maternal and fetal mortality and is contraindicated. Management of patients with ES with drug therapy was reviewed in the section on 8.1. Medical Management and will not be repeated. Many other novel treatment trials and targeted PAH therapies have promising results with improvement in functional capacity and hemodynamic parameters; however, prospective randomized studies are needed to assess their effect on mortality.

## 10. Conclusions

Smaller VSDs may self-resolve and the majority of the patients do well without intervention. On the other hand, recognition of unrestrictive defects, and prompt medical and surgical intervention may prevent development of irreversible pulmonary vaso-occlusive disease. Newer therapeutic options such as a minimally invasive approach as well as catheter based closures are appealing and can dramatically improve cosmetic outcomes in many of these patients. Development of newer devices and ongoing trials provide promise in non-surgical approach for VSD closure. Adult patients with Eisenmenger's syndrome continue to present a challenge due to increased morbidity and mortality. Specialized targeted anti pulmonary arterial hypertension therapies with endothelin receptor antagonists, phosphodiesterase 5 inhibitors and prostacyclins show improved exercise capacity and hemodynamics in this patient population.

## Author details

Unnati Doshi and Elizabeth Wang-Giuffre
University of Texas at Houston, Children's Heart Institute, McGovern Medical School and Children's Memorial Hermann Hospital, Houston, Texas, USA

*Address all correspondence to: unnati.h.doshi@uth.tmc.edu

## References

[1] Hoffman JI, Kaplan S. The incidence of congenital heart disease. Journal of the American College of Cardiology. 2002;**39**(12):1890-1900. DOI: 10.1016/s0735-1097(02)01886-7

[2] Rubio A, Lewin M. Ventricular septal defects. In: Allen H, Shaddy R, Penny D, Feltes T, Cetta F, editors. Moss and Adams' Heart Disease in Infants, Children, and Adolescents: Including the Fetus and Young Adult. Eighth ed. Philadelphia: Wolters Kluwer/Lippincott Williams & Wilkins; 2013. pp. 713-721

[3] Penny DJ, Vick GW. Ventricular septal defect. Lancet. 2011;**377**(9771):1103-1112. DOI: 10.1016/S0140-6736(10)61339-6 Epub 2011 Feb 23

[4] Kloesel B, DiNardo JA, Body SC. Cardiac embryology and molecular mechanisms of congenital heart disease: A primer for anesthesiologists. Anesthesia and Analgesia. 2016;**123**(3):551-569. DOI: 10.1213/ANE.0000000000001451

[5] Rojas CA, Jaimes C, Abbara S. Ventricular septal defects: Embryology and imaging findings. Journal of Thoracic Imaging. 2013;**28**(2):W28-W34. DOI: 10.1097/RTI.0b013e31824b5b95

[6] Gittenberger-de Groot AC, Bartelings MM, Deruiter MC, Poelmann RE. Basics of cardiac development for the understanding of congenital heart malformations. Pediatric Research. 2005;**57**(2):169-176. DOI: 10.1203/01.PDR.0000148710.69159.61 Epub 2004 Dec 20

[7] Bellmann K, Perrot A, Rickert-Sperling S. Human genetics of ventricular septal defect. In: Rickert-Sperling S, Kelly R, Driscoll D, editors. Congenital Heart Diseases: The Broken Heart. Vienna: Springer; 2016. pp. 307-328

[8] Chen HX, Zhang X, Hou HT, Wang J, Yang Q, Wang XL, et al. Identification of a novel and functional mutation in the TBX5 gene in a patient by screening from 354 patients with isolated ventricular septal defect. European Journal of Medical Genetics. 2017;**60**(7):385-390. DOI: 10.1016/j.ejmg.2017.04.011 Epub 2017 Apr 18

[9] Soto B, Becker AE, Moulaert AJ, Lie JT, Anderson RH. Classification of ventricular septal defects. British Heart Journal. 1980;**43**(3):332-343. DOI: 10.1136/hrt.43.3.332

[10] Van Praagh R, Geva T, Kreutzer J. Ventricular septal defects: How shall we describe, name and classify them? Journal of the American College of Cardiology. 1989;**14**(5):1298-1299. DOI: 10.1016/0735-1097(89)90431-2

[11] Soto B, Ceballos R, Kirklin JW. Ventricular septal defects: a surgical viewpoint. Journal of the American College of Cardiology. 1989;**14**(5):1291-1297. DOI: 10.1016/0735-1097(89)90430-0

[12] Yau KI, Fang LJ, Wu MH. Lung mechanics in infants with left-to-right shunt congenital heart disease. Pediatric Pulmonology. 1996;**21**(1):42-47. DOI: 10.1002/(SICI)1099-0496(199601)21:1<42::AID-PPUL7>3.0.CO;2-S

[13] Buchhorn R, Hammersen A, Bartmus D, Bürsch J. The pathogenesis of heart failure in infants with congenital heart disease. Cardiology in the Young. 2001;**11**(5):498-504. DOI: 10.1017/s1047951101000725

[14] Rudolph AM. Circulatory adjustments after birth: Effects on ventricular septal defect. British Heart Journal. 1971;**33**(Suppl):32-34. DOI: 10.1136/hrt.33.suppl.32

[15] Beghetti M, Galiè N. Eisenmenger syndrome a clinical perspective in a new therapeutic era of pulmonary arterial hypertension. Journal of the American College of Cardiology. 2009;**53**(9):733-740. DOI: 10.1016/j.jacc.2008.11.025

[16] Minette MS, Sahn DJ. Ventricular septal defects. Circulation. 2006;**114**(20):2190-2197. DOI: 10.1161/CIRCULATIONAHA.106.618124 Erratum in: Circulation. 2007 Feb 20;115(7): e205

[17] Myers PO, Tissot C, Beghetti M. Assessment of operability of patients with pulmonary arterial hypertension associated with congenital heart disease. Circulation Journal. 2014;**78**(1):4-11. DOI: 10.1253/circj.cj-13-1263 Epub 2013 Nov 13. Erratum in: Circ J. 2014;78(7):1774

[18] Backer CL, Winters RC, Zales VR, Takami H, Muster AJ, Benson DW Jr, et al. Restrictive ventricular septal defect: How small is too small to close? The Annals of Thoracic Surgery. 1993;**56**(5):1014-1018; discussion 1018-9. DOI: 10.1016/0003-4975(95)90006-3

[19] Krishnasamy S, Sivalingam S, Dillon J, Mokhtar RAR, Yakub A, Singh R. Syndrome of ventricular septal defect and aortic regurgitation - a 22-year review of its management. Brazilian Journal of Cardiovascular Surgery. 2021;**36**(6):807-816. DOI: 10.21470/1678-9741-2020-0207

[20] Lascano ME, Schaad MS, Moodie DS, Murphy D Jr. Difficulty in diagnosing double-chambered right ventricle in adults. The American Journal of Cardiology. 2001;**88**(7):816-819. DOI: 10.1016/s0002-9149(01)01862-8

[21] Knirsch W, Nadal D. Infective endocarditis in congenital heart disease. European Journal of Pediatrics. 2011;**170**(9):1111-1127. DOI: 10.1007/s00431-011-1520-8 Epub 2011 Jul 20

[22] Berglund E, Johansson B, Dellborg M, Sörensson P, Christersson C, Nielsen NE, et al. High incidence of infective endocarditis in adults with congenital ventricular septal defect. Heart. 2016;**102**(22):1835-1839. DOI: 10.1136/heartjnl-2015-309133 Epub 2016 Jul 21

[23] Kidd L, Driscoll DJ, Gersony WM, Hayes CJ, Keane JF, O'Fallon WM, et al. Second natural history study of congenital heart defects. Results of treatment of patients with ventricular septal defects. Circulation. 1993;**87** (Suppl. 2):I38-I51

[24] Waldman JD. Why not close a small ventricular septal defect? The Annals of Thoracic Surgery. 1993;**56**(5):1011-1012. DOI: 10.1016/0003-4975(95)90004-7

[25] Wilson W, Taubert KA, Gewitz M, Lockhart PB, Baddour LM, Levison M, et al. Endocarditis, and Kawasaki disease committee; American Heart Association Council on cardiovascular disease in the young; American Heart Association Council on clinical cardiology; American Heart Association Council on cardiovascular surgery and anesthesia; quality of care and outcomes research interdisciplinary working group. Prevention of infective endocarditis: Guidelines from the American Heart Association: A guideline from the American Heart Association rheumatic fever, endocarditis, and Kawasaki disease committee, council on cardiovascular disease in the young, and the council on clinical cardiology, council on

cardiovascular surgery and anesthesia, and the quality of care and outcomes research interdisciplinary working group. Circulation. 2007;**116**(15):1736-1754. DOI: 10.1161/CIRCULATIONAHA.106.183095 Epub 2007 Apr 19. Erratum in: Circulation. 2007 Oct 9;116(15):e376-7

[26] Lopes AA, O'Leary PW. Measurement, interpretation and use of haemodynamic parameters in pulmonary hypertension associated with congenital cardiac disease. Cardiology in the Young. 2009;**19**(5):431-435. DOI: 10.1017/S1047951109990771 Epub 2009 Aug 27

[27] Talwar S, Keshri VK, Choudhary SK, Gupta SK, Ramakrishnan S, Juneja R, et al. Surgical strategies for patients with congenital heart disease and severe pulmonary hypertension in low/middle-income countries. Heart Asia. 2015;7(2):31-37. DOI: 10.1136/heartasia-2015-010645

[28] Kaemmerer H, Mebus S, Schulze-Neick I, Eicken A, Trindade PT, Hager A, et al. The adult patient with eisenmenger syndrome: A medical update after Dana point part I: Epidemiology, clinical aspects and diagnostic options. Current Cardiology Reviews. 2010;**6**(4):343-355. DOI: 10.2174/157340310793566154

[29] Apitz C, Hansmann G, Schranz D. Hemodynamic assessment and acute pulmonary vasoreactivity testing in the evaluation of children with pulmonary vascular disease. Expert consensus statement on the diagnosis and treatment of paediatric pulmonary hypertension. The European Paediatric pulmonary vascular disease network, endorsed by ISHLT and DGPK. Heart. 2016;**102**(Suppl. 2):ii23-ii29. DOI: 10.1136/heartjnl-2014-307340

[30] Liew N, Rashid Z, Tulloh R. Strategies for the management of pulmonary arterial hypertension in patients with congenital heart disease. Journal of Congenital Heart Diseases. 2020;**4**:21. DOI: 10.1186/s40949-020-00052-w

[31] Ling Y, Bian X, Wang Y, Qian Y. Does tricuspid valve detachment improve outcomes compared with the non-tricuspid valve detachment approach in ventricular septal defect closure? Interactive Cardiovascular and Thoracic Surgery. 2021;**32**(3):483-488. DOI: 10.1093/icvts/ivaa289

[32] Rao PS, Harris AD. Recent advances in managing septal defects: Ventricular septal defects and atrioventricular septal defects. F1000Res. 2018;7:F1000 Faculty Rev:498. DOI: 10.12688/f1000research.14102.1

[33] Jonas RA. Ventricular septal defect. In: Jonas RA, editor. Comprehensive Surgical Management of Congenital Heart Disease. 2nd ed. London: CRC Press; 2014. pp. 730-331

[34] Knauth AL, Lock JE, Perry SB, McElhinney DB, Gauvreau K, Landzberg MJ, et al. Transcatheter device closure of congenital and postoperative residual ventricular septal defects. Circulation. 2004;**110**(5):501-507. DOI: 10.1161/01.CIR.0000137116.12176.A6 Epub 2004 Jul 19

[35] Lock JE, Block PC, McKay RG, Baim DS, Keane JF. Transcatheter closure of ventricular septal defects. Circulation. 1988;**78**(2):361-368. DOI: 10.1161/01.cir.78.2.361

[36] Bergmann M, Germann CP, Nordmeyer J, Peters B, Berger F, Schubert S. Short- and long-term outcome after interventional VSD closure: A single-center experience in pediatric and adult patients. Pediatric Cardiology. 2021;**42**(1):78-88.

DOI: 10.1007/s00246-020-02456-2 Epub 2020 Oct 3

[37] Rao PS. Perimembraneous ventricular septal defect closure with the Amplatzer device. (editorial). The Journal of Invasive Cardiology. 2008;**20**:217-218

[38] Polat TB, Türkmen E. Transcatheter closure of ventricular septal defects using the Amplatzer duct Occluder II device: A single-center experience. Postepy Kardiol Interwencyjnej. 2016;**12**(4):340-347. DOI: 10.5114/aic.2016.63635 Epub 2016 Nov 17

[39] Wang L, Xie L, Ruan W, Li T, Gan C, Lin K. Percutaneous-perventricular device closure of ventricular septal defect: Mid-term follow-up. BMC Surgery. 2020;**20**(1):208. DOI: 10.1186/s12893-020-00854-0

[40] Arvanitaki A, Giannakoulas G, Baumgartner H, Lammers AE. Eisenmenger syndrome: Diagnosis, prognosis and clinical management. Heart. 2020;**106**(21):1638-1645. DOI: 10.1136/heartjnl-2020-316665 Epub 2020 Jul 20

[41] Kempny A, Hjortshøj CS, Gu H, Li W, Opotowsky AR, Landzberg MJ, et al. Predictors of death in contemporary adult patients with Eisenmenger syndrome: A multicenter study. Circulation. 2017;**135**(15):1432-1440. DOI: 10.1161/CIRCULATIONAHA.116.023033 Epub 2016 Dec 15

Chapter 6

# Atrioventricular Septal Defects

*Rakesh Donthula, Animisha Rudra and P. Syamasundar Rao*

## Abstract

Atrioventricular septal defects (AVSD) are a group of malformations involving the atrioventricular (AV) septum and common AV junction. They are divided into complete, partial, intermediate and transitional AVSD. It is most commonly associated with Down Syndrome. All of them share a few common features. Complete AVSDs are also classified as balanced and unbalanced. Echocardiography is the primary imaging tool to diagnose these defects. Patients with complete and intermediate forms clinically present early and require surgical correction during infancy, whereas partial, and transitional forms become symptomatic in early childhood. Patients who are ineligible for complete surgical repair initially undergo palliative pulmonary artery banding. The surgical management of unbalanced AVSDs is complex. Most of these patients fall into either single ventricle, one and a half or bi-ventricular repair. Overall surgical outcomes for AVSDs are excellent. Left atrioventricular valve regurgitation is the most common reason for reoperation.

**Keywords:** atrioventricular septal defects, atrioventricular canal, recent advances, complete atrioventricular septal defect partial atrioventricular septal defect, transitional atrioventricular septal defect, intermediate atrioventricular septal defect

## 1. Introduction

Atrioventricular septal defects are a group of malformations involving the atrioventricular (AV) septum and common atrioventricular junction (**Figure 1**). Previously, referred to as atrioventricular canal or endocardial cushion defects, is now called AV septal defect (AVSD). For the purpose of this chapter, we will use the term AV septal defects. They are divided into complete, partial and variations of both of them based on the orifices and septal communications which will be discussed in detail in this chapter.

## 2. Prevalence

Congenital heart disease (CHD) accounts for around 1–1.2% of live births both in the United States and globally [1, 2]. AVSDs account for around 4–5% of all CHDs, with 5.38 cases per 10,000 live births, an increase from prior reports [1, 3]. It is the most common fetal cardiac anomaly detected on prenatal screening (**Figure 2**). Around half of the patients with AVSD have Down syndrome. However, approximately 45% of CHD patients with Down syndrome have AVSD [4, 5]. Most of these

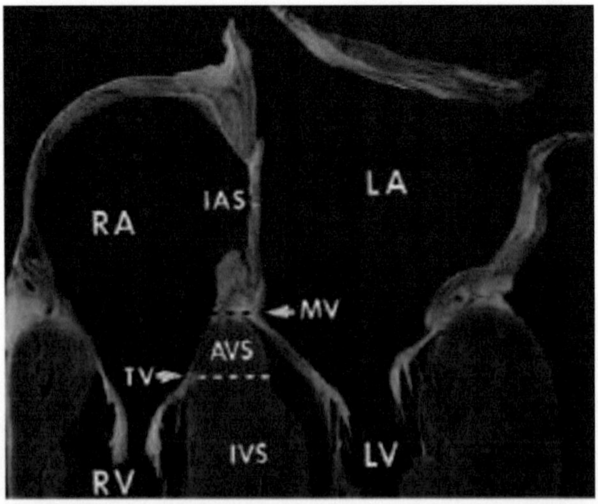


**Figure 1.**
*Atrioventricular septum in the normal heart. The atrioventricular septum (AVS) lies between the right atrium (RA) and the left ventricle (LV). LA, left atrium; RV, right ventricle; MV, mitral valve; TV, tricuspid valve. "From: Cetta F, Truong D, Minich LL, Maleszewski JJ, O'Leary PW, Dearani JA & Burkhart HM. Chapter 29: Atrioventricular Septal Defects. In: Allen HD, editor. Moss & Adams' Heart Disease in Infants, Children, and Adolescents, Including the Fetus and Young Adult, 9th Edition. Philadelphia: Lippincott Williams & Wilkins, 2016; used with permission of Mayo Foundation for Medical Education and Research, all rights reserved."*

cases are isolated, although some may have pulmonary stenosis or atresia. There is an association with other anomalies like heterotaxy and Ellis-Van Creveld syndrome [6].

## 3. Pathology

In a normal heart, tricuspid and mitral valve annuli are positioned at different levels because of the atrioventricular septum. In AV septal defects, tricuspid valve annulus is located more apically in relation to mitral valve. The portion of the offset between tricuspid and mitral valve is the location of atrioventricular septum. It has overlapping atrial and ventricular walls [7]. Aortic valve is located anterior and superior between tricuspid and mitral valve, what is referred to as wedged between these valves. This makes the subaortic outflow region placed in between tricuspid and mitral valves. The papillary muscles in the left ventricle are located antero-superior and postero-inferior region. Another feature of importance to this topic, the distance from mitral valve to apex of left ventricle is same as the distance from left ventricular apex to aortic valve (**Figure 3**).

In patients with AV septal defect, the fundamental abnormality is absence of the atrioventricular septum or having a common atrioventricular junction. This results in a cascade of features that are different from normal hearts. The common features shared by all forms of atrioventricular septal defects are:

a. Presence of common atrioventricular valve

b. Elongation of the left ventricular outflow tract

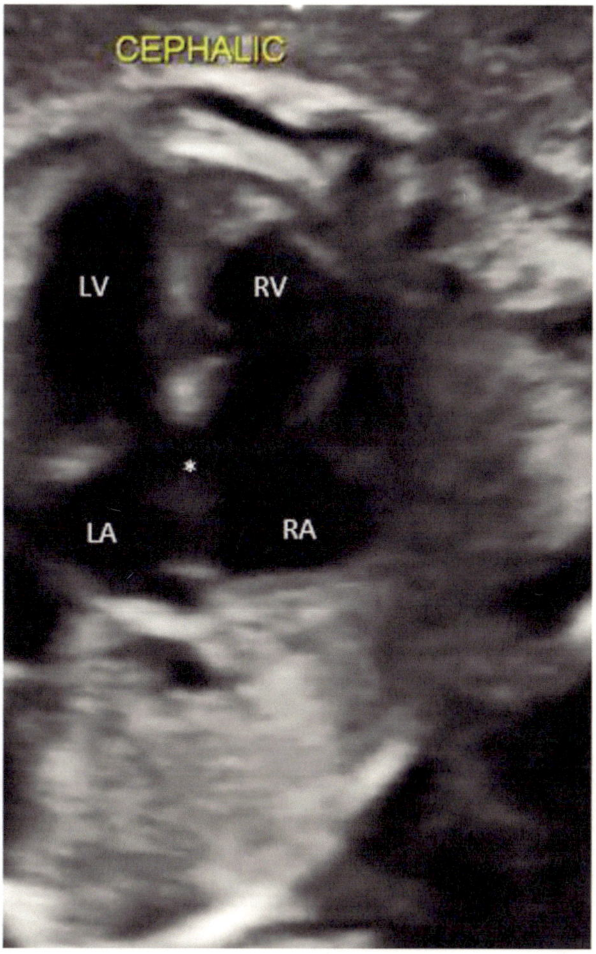


**Figure 2.**
*Fetal echocardiogram four-chamber view: Complete AVSD. RA, right atrium; LA, left atrium; RV, right ventricle; LV, left ventricle. *Primum atrial septal defect and inlet ventricular septal defect.*

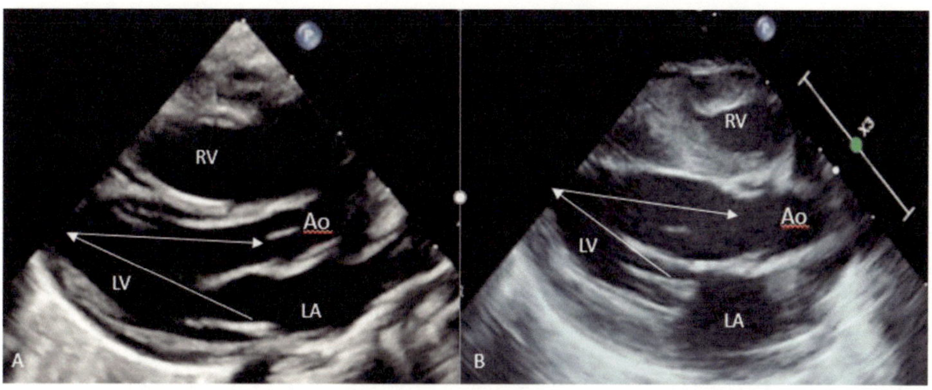


**Figure 3.**
*2D echocardiogram parasternal long axis view: A. In normal cardiac anatomy, distance from the mitral valve to left ventricular (LV) apex and from LV apex to aortic valve is same. B. In AVSD, LVOT is elongated and distance from LV apex to left AV valve annulus is shorter. LA, left atrium; RV, right ventricle; Ao, aorta.*

c. Clockwise rotation of papillary muscles

d. Cleft in the left AV valve

## 4. Classification

There are two major types of AV septal defects: complete and partial AVSDs. Two sub-types are described: intermediate and transitional, which are variations of complete and partial AV septal defects, respectively (**Figure 4**). It is preferable to describe the features of these subtypes rather than identifying them as an entity. Different combinations of shunting across atria and ventricles could happen based on the attachments and relationship of the bridging leaflets to septal structures. In general, we would see ostium primum defect and ventricular septal defect (VSD). If the bridging leaflets are attached to the atrial septum, there could be only a ventricular level shunt (**Figure 5**). When the bridging leaflets are attached to the crest of ventricular septum, it results in an atrial level shunt with an ostium primum defect. In rare instances, where the bridging leaflets close the septal defect(s), we will still see features of the

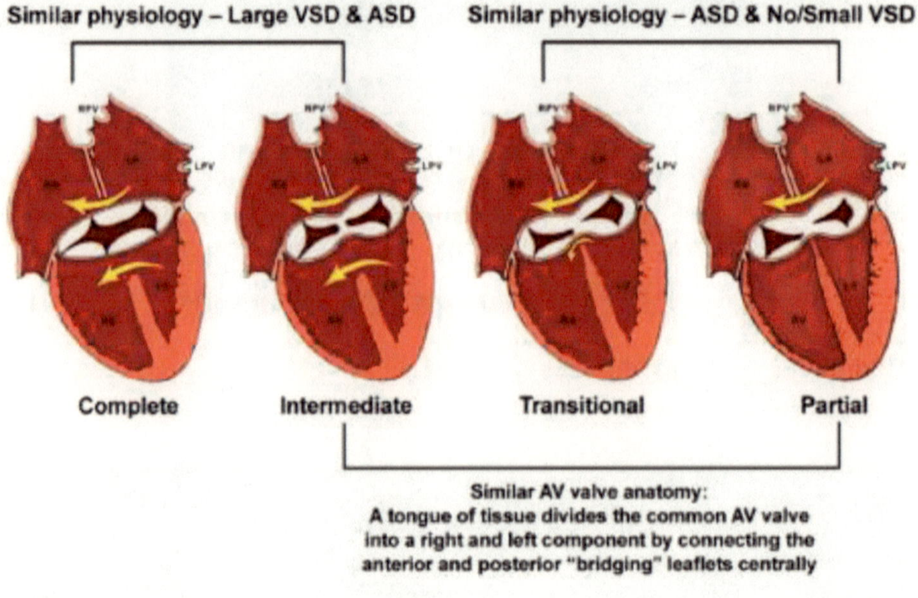


**Figure 4.**
*Summary of AVSD. Anatomic and physiologic similarities between the different forms of atrioventricular septal defect (AVSD) are illustrated. Complete AVSDs have one orifice with large interatrial and interventricular communications. Intermediate defects (two orifices) are a subtype of complete AVSD. Complete AVSDs have physiology of VSDs and atrial septal defects (ASDs). In contrast, partial AVSDs have physiology of ASDs. Transitional defects are a form of partial AVSD in which a small inlet VSD is present or the ventricular level shunt has been obliterated by chordal tissue. Partial AVSDs and the intermediate form of complete AVSD share a similar anatomic feature: A tongue of tissue divides the common atrioventricular valve into distinct right and left orifices. LA, left atrium; LPV, left pulmonary vein; LV, left ventricle; RA, right atrium; RPV, right pulmonary vein; RV, right ventricle. "From: Cetta F, Truong D, Minich LL, Maleszewski JJ, O'Leary PW, Dearani JA & Burkhart HM. Chapter 29: Atrioventricular Septal Defects. In: Allen HD, editor. Moss & Adams' Heart Disease in Infants, Children, and Adolescents, Including the Fetus and Young Adult, 9th Edition. Philadelphia: Lippincott Williams & Wilkins, 2016; used with permission of Mayo Foundation for Medical Education and Research, all rights reserved."*

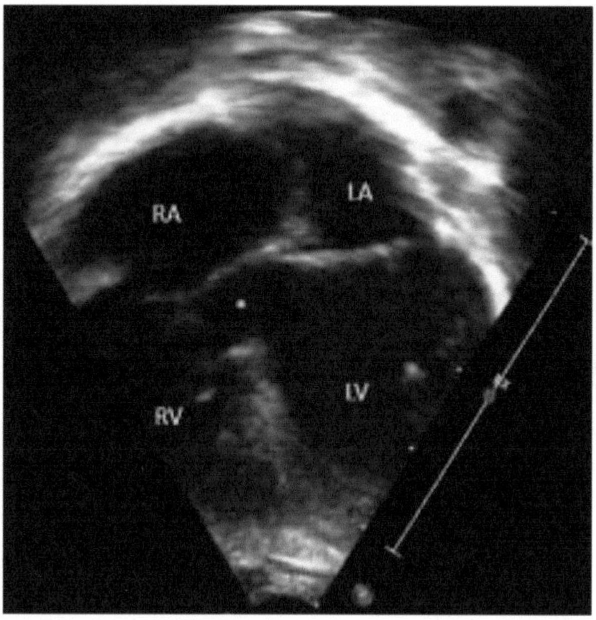


**Figure 5.**
*2D echocardiogram apical four-chamber view: A rare form of AVSD with large inlet ventricular septal defect (*) without a primum atrial septal defect. Note that AV valves are at same level. RA, right atrium; RV, right ventricle; LA, left atrium; LV, left ventricle.*

common atrioventricular valve [8–10]. Complete AVSDs are classified further into three types based on the morphology of anterior bridging leaflet and is named after Giancarlo Rastelli who made significant contributions in his short career and life span:

1. Type A: In this type, anterior bridging leaflet (ABL) is divided and attached to the crest of the interventricular septum. It is the most common defect and is associated with Down syndrome.

2. Type B: ABL is partly divided and is not attached to the crest of the septum. Chordae attach usually to papillary muscle in the right ventricle (RV), on the septal surface. It is the least common of all types.

3. Type C: ABL is not attached or divided and is termed "free-floating". There are chordal attachments to RV free wall. This type is seen in Down syndrome patients with Tetralogy of Fallot; double outlet right ventricle, complete transposition of the great arteries, and heterotaxy syndromes.

## 5. Other features

### 5.1 Left AV valve

In normal hearts, mitral valve has two leaflets, anterior and posterior with a zone of opposition in one plane. In hearts with AV septal defects, the left AV valve closes in tri-foliate fashion with zones of opposition between posterior, superior and inferior bridging leaflets. This characteristic feature of the left AV valve in AV septal defects will never achieve a mitral valve as in normal hearts. Usually, jet of LAVV cleft is directed to the ventricular septum when compared to isolated mitral valve clefts which are directed anteriorly towards the aortic valve [11]. Rarely, a fusion of the leaflets within the left AV valve (bridging and posterior leaflet) would lead to a double orifice valve. The combined area of the double orifice valve is always less than the single left AV valve area.

### 5.2 Left ventricular outflow tract (LVOT)

As described earlier, LVOT is wedged anteriorly and is narrow when compared to the aortic valve, irrespective of the type of AV septal defect. In partial form, where the superior bridging leaflet is attached to the crest of the septum, it is markedly narrow (**Figure 6**). This abnormality has been described as goose-neck deformity.

### 5.3 Chamber dominance

Depending on the overall flow from the atrioventricular orifices to respective ventricles, the chambers are usually the same size which is termed as 'balanced AVSD'. When a common AV valve opens more into the right ventricle or to the left ventricle, it would cause decreased growth of the contralateral ventricle and its great artery, leading to the term 'unbalanced AVSD'. In right ventricle dominant atrioventricular septal defect, left ventricle and aorta are hypoplastic depending on the amount of blood flow, but usually, the atrial and ventricular septal alignment is maintained. In left ventricular dominance, there will be hypoplasia of the right ventricle and pulmonary artery, typically with septal malalignment. This chamber dominance when it involves the atrium would give rise to double outlet atrium (**Figure 7**).

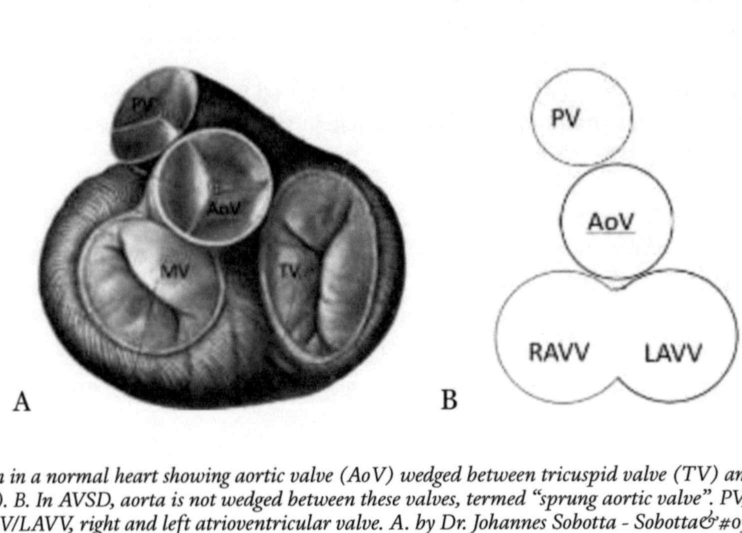


**Figure 6.**
*A. Diagram in a normal heart showing aortic valve (AoV) wedged between tricuspid valve (TV) and mitral valve (MV). B. In AVSD, aorta is not wedged between these valves, termed "sprung aortic valve". PV, pulmonary valve; RAVV/LAVV, right and left atrioventricular valve. A. by Dr. Johannes Sobotta - Sobotta's atlas and text-book of human anatomy 1906, public domain, https://commons.wikimedia.org/w/index.php?curid=29901804.*

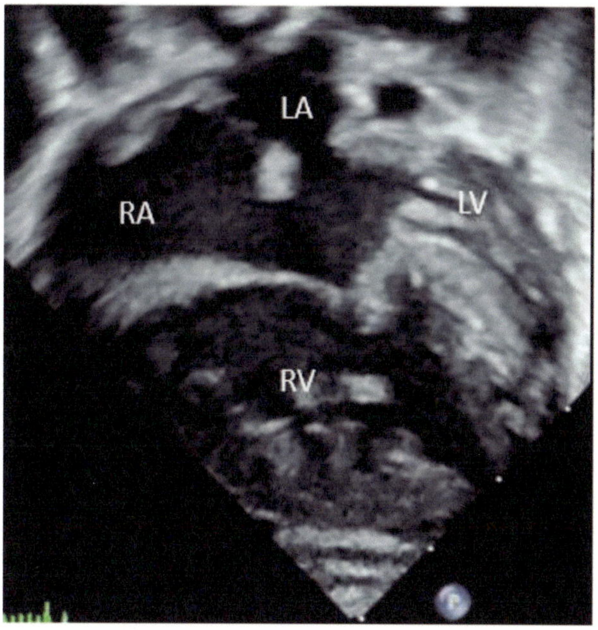


**Figure 7.**
*2D echocardiogram showing right ventricle (RV) dominant AVSD with severely hypoplastic left AV valve and ventricle (LV). Moderately dilated right atrium (RA) and RV with large primum ASD. LA, left atrium.*

### 5.4 Associated malformations

In partial atrioventricular septal defects, the most common associated malformation includes secundum ASD, patent ductus arteriosus and persistent left superior vena cava to coronary sinus [12].

Tetralogy of Fallot with pulmonary stenosis is found in one-tenth of the patients with common atrioventricular septal defect and in these patients, Rastelli type C is common. Among others, common atrium, double outlet right atrium, double inlet ventricle with discordant ventriculoarterial connections can be seen.

### 5.5 Atrioventricular conduction tissues

In normal hearts, AV node is located in the triangle of Koch which is formed by Tendon of Todaro, coronary sinus ostium and septal leaflet of the tricuspid valve [13–15]. In patients with AVSDs, because of deficient AV septum, the atria will meet the ventricle at the crux of the heart, shifting the AV node more posteriorly and inferiorly.

## 6. Embryology

In the past, failure of the fusion of endocardial cushions was thought to be the only reason for AV septal defects [16]. It could be the first step in the formation of these hearts, but not in entirety. Delamination of valve leaflets occurs late in development, with its formation occurring by undermining of the ventricular myocardium [17].

When the endocardial cushions fail to meet, subaortic outflow tract will not be normally wedged and there will be abnormal development of ventricular mass. Additionally, mesenchymal tissues surrounding the primum ostial foramen play a role in these defects [18, 19].

## 7. Pathophysiology

In patients with complete AVSD, there is one common AV valve with large atrial and inlet VSD (**Figure 8**). In intermediate form, there are two AV valve orifices, which are formed by a tongue of tissue between superior and inferior bridging leaflets. It has similar physiology as the complete form with large ASD and VSD. In partial AV septal defects, where there are two AV valve orifices with the bridging leaflet attached to ventricular septal crest, giving rise to only interatrial communication (**Figure 9A**). In some instances, there could be communication at the ventricular level from the chordal attachments which is described as a transitional type (**Figure 9B**). In all forms of AV septal defects, the left AV valve invariably has a cleft. Rarely there will be no septal communications seen with other common features of AVSD [8].

## 8. Clinical features

### 8.1 Partial AVSD

Usually, patients with partial AV septal defect (also called primum ASD) remain asymptomatic until early childhood. They rarely present early with failure to thrive depending on the size of the defect and severity of AV valve regurgitation. Patients with primum ASDs usually present earlier and with symptoms when compared with secundum ASDs. Auscultatory findings include widely split and fixed second heart

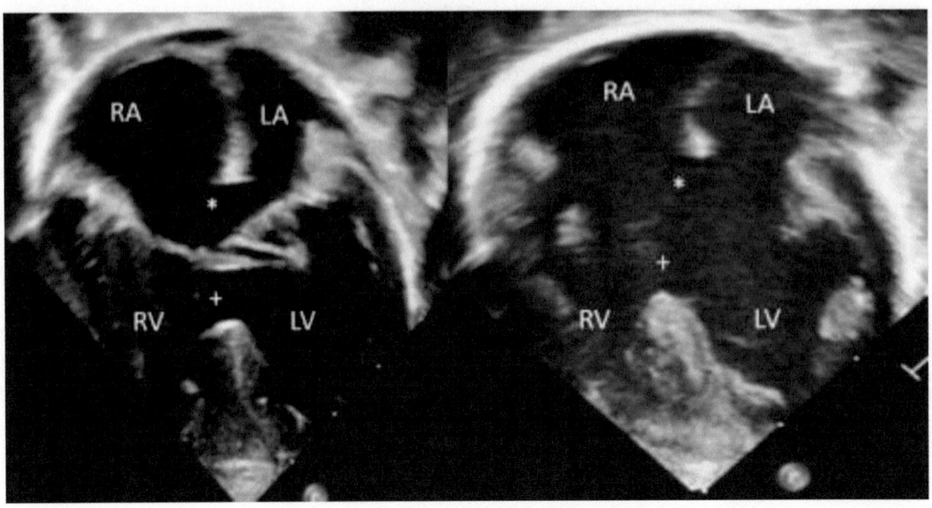


**Figure 8.**
*2D echocardiogram apical 4-chamber view: Complete balanced AVSD. A. When AV valve is closed, there is large primum atrial septal defect (ASD, *) and large inlet ventricular septal defect (VSD, +). Common AV valve and single orifice. B. with valve open. RA, right atrium; LA, left atrium; RV, right ventricle; LV, left ventricle.*

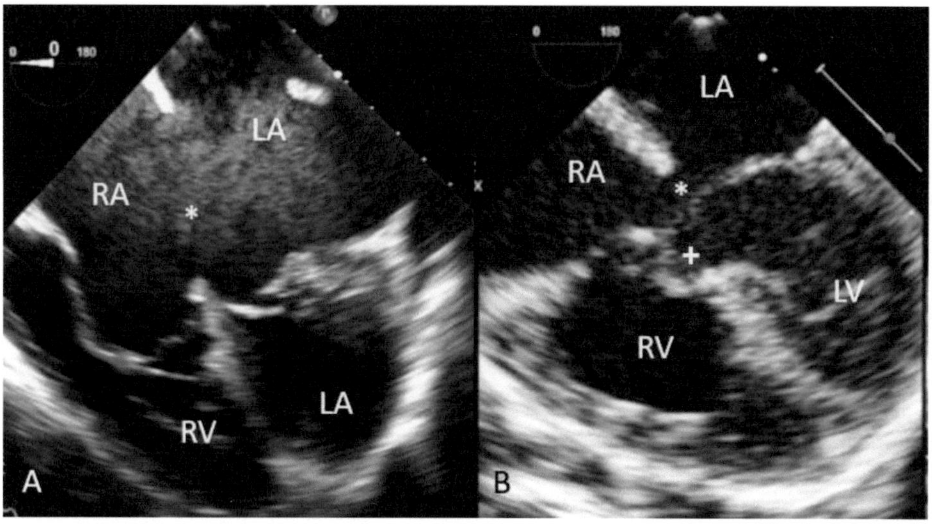


**Figure 9.**
*Transesophageal echocardiogram, four-chamber view. A. Partial AVSD with large primum atrial septal defect (ASD) (*). Note the valvar attachments to crest of the septum. B. Transitional AVSD with small primum ASD and inlet ventricular septal defect (+) covered by right AVV chordal attachments to the crest of ventricular septum. RA, right atrium; LA, left atrium; RV, right ventricle; LV, left ventricle.*

sound, crescendo- decrescendo systolic ejection murmur at the left upper sternal border from the increased flow across pulmonary valve, and holosystolic murmur at the apex from LAVV regurgitation. A mid-diastolic murmur may be heard at the apex if there is significant mitral regurgitation or at the left lower sternal border if there is a large atrial shunt.

### 8.2 Complete AVSD

Patients with complete AV septal defects present in the neonatal period after first few days/weeks of life when pulmonary vascular resistance falls. This is attributed to the large atrial and ventricular level shunts leading to pulmonary over circulation. There will be tachypnea, increased work of breathing, failure to gain weight. More often, they would require high-calorie nutrition, diuretics to decrease the preload. On exam, there will be accentuated first heart sound, with S1- coincident holosystolic murmur from LAVV regurgitation, widely split and fixed S2, crescendo- decrescendo systolic ejection murmur at the left upper sternal border from the increased flow across pulmonary valve and sometimes mid-diastolic murmur at apex.

## 9. Investigations

### 9.1 Electrocardiogram

As previously described, AV node is displaced posteriorly and inferiorly in these defects; this may result in prolongation of the PR interval. There will be a left superior deviation of the mean frontal plane vector. Biventricular hypertrophy is seen in complete and intermediate forms. Right ventricular hypertrophy is seen in the partial

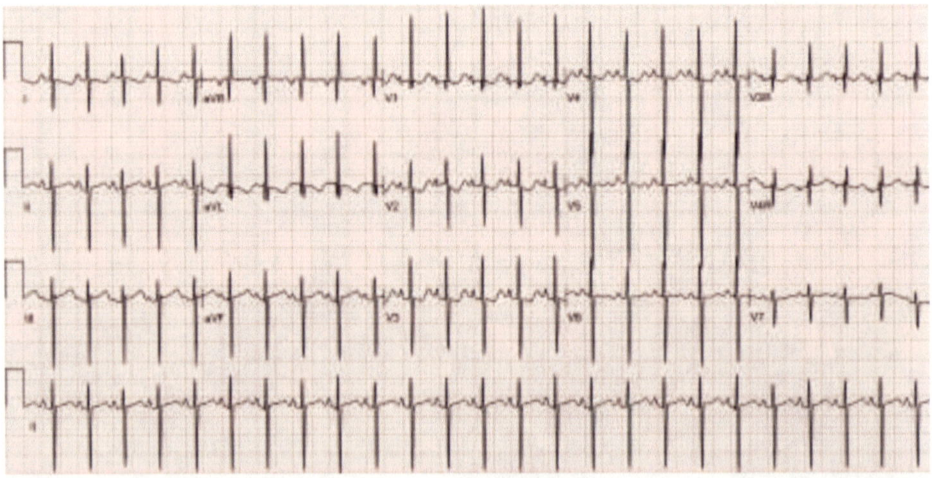

**Figure 10.**
*12-lead EKG in patient with CAVSD showing left superior axis deviation and right ventricular hypertrophy.*

form. If there is moderate to severe mitral insufficiency, left ventricular hypertrophy may be seen. Other abnormalities which might be seen are prolongation of PR interval (**Figure 10**) [20].

### 9.2 Chest roentgenogram

Chest roentgenogram shows cardiomegaly with increased pulmonary vascular markings. Features of pulmonary edema may be seen in subjects with congestive heart failure.

### 9.3 Echocardiography

Echocardiography is the primary diagnostic modality for the evaluation of atrioventricular septal AV defects [21]. Assessment of the ASD can be best done from a subcostal coronal and sagittal view. VSD could be best evaluated in the parasternal short axis. En-face view of the common AV valves is best achieved with a modified subcostal left anterior oblique view (**Figure 11**). This view also demonstrates the bridging leaflets, their attachments and helps with the Rastelli classification in patients with complete AVSDs. Subcostal short axis view would assess atrial or ventricular level unbalance. An Apical four-chamber view would augment the information on previously mentioned variables along with AV valve inflow and regurgitation. Overall, all the views complement each other to get comprehensive information, as in any other heart. Associated malformations like tetralogy of Fallot, coarctation, patent ductus arteriosus, arch sidedness should be evaluated using modified subcostal right anterior oblique/parasternal long axis and high parasternal/suprasternal views [22]. 3D echocardiography demonstrates a comprehensive and accurate assessment of the size and extent of the septal defects, size, number, and abnormalities of AV valve leaflets and their attachment sites, as well as the relation of the valvular structures to the great vessels [23]. Other findings such as double orifice left AV-valve, single papillary muscle should be evaluated.

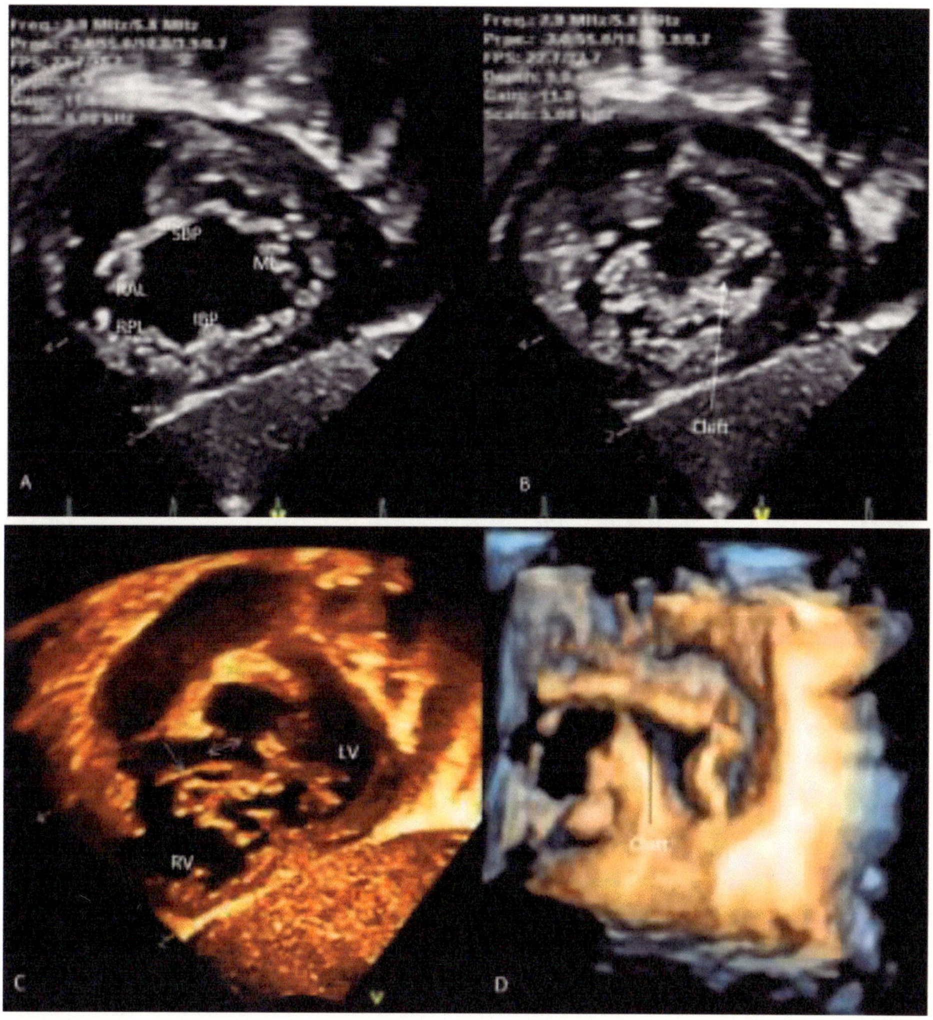


**Figure 11.**
*Echocardiogam left anterior oblique (LAO) view. 1. Rastelli type a with attachments of the anterior/superior bridging leaflet (SBL) to crest of venticular septum; B. when valve is closed, notice the cleft in LAVV valve; C. Rastelli type C with "free floating" anterior bridging leaflet (<–>) and chordal attachments to right ventricular (RV) free wall (–>); D. 3D image showing tri-foliate cleft LAVV. IBL, inferior bridging leaflet; ML, mural leaflet; RAL, right anterior leaflet; RPL, right posterior leaflet; ML, left mural leaflet; LV, left ventricle.*

In determining the balance of ventricles, a quantitative approach was proposed by Cohen et al. [24] using a subcostal sagittal view. In this view, they measured the area of AV valve over each ventricle and calculated a left/right ventricular ratio, also known as AV valve index (AVVI). Based on the index, patients were stratified either to single-ventricle or bi-ventricular repair pathways. Patients with an AVVI <0.67 and a large VSD would be considered for the single-ventricle pathway. This was modified to the left AV valve area/total area. An AVVI >0.6 is considered left ventricular dominant whereas AVVI <0.4 was considered right ventricular dominant. It is important after surgical repair to assess for residual defects, progressive LVOT obstruction, AVV stenosis and regurgitation, systolic function.

### 9.4 Cardiac catheterization

Cardiac catheterization is not frequently performed in AVSDs. However, it is helpful in assessing the hemodynamic information like the degree of shunting, pulmonary vascular resistance. One would see the characteristic "gooseneck appearance" from elongated LVOT on angiography. Patients with severely elevated PVR are poor candidates for full repair and may eventually be candidates for lung transplantation [25].

### 9.5 Advanced cardiac imaging

Cardiac computed tomography (CT) is particularly helpful to assess for any extracardiac defects or associated anomalies in these patients. Retrospective gated approach is useful for the evaluation of ventricular function and ventricular sizes, allows volumetric measurements, and also allows evaluation of ventricular function and wall motion. This may be of particular relevance in patients with hypoplastic ventricles and unbalanced AVSDs [26]. Cardiac magnetic resonance imaging (MRI) is an important tool to assess the degree of unbalance and guide for future surgical planning. These modalities have proven to decrease the amount of radiation exposure during cardiac catheterization [27].

## 10. Management

### 10.1 Medical management

Patients with complete defects present early with signs and symptoms of pulmonary over circulation such as tachypnea, increased work of breathing. In the neonatal period, when the pulmonary vascular resistance decreases, they require diuretics to help with pulmonary congestion and control heart failure along with optimizing nutrition. Occasionally they require afterload reducing agents if there is significant AV valve regurgitation and rarely inotropes. If heart failure or failure to thrive persists despite maximizing medical management, they would be referred for surgery. Based on the corrected gestational age, weight, type of atrioventricular septal defect and associated anomalies, surgical options vary which will be discussed below. As mentioned earlier, patients with partial atrioventricular septal defects usually show symptoms in childhood.

### 10.2 Surgical management

The goals of the surgery are to close the septal defect(s), repair the AV valve, construct two separate and competent AV valves, and avoid injury to conduction tissue.

1. Balanced atrioventricular septal defects

- Surgical Palliation

Palliation with main pulmonary artery band (PAB) is performed in babies less than 5 Kg who failed medical management. In the recent era, complete repair is done even in this weight range. Palliation is considered in patients who are premature, those deemed ineligible for definitive repair or with other co-morbidities. A recent study showed that PAB in complete AVSDs as a bridge to biventricular repair has similar survival as those for primary biventricular repair [28].

- Surgical Correction

Patients with complete AVSDs frequently require surgical repair in early infancy with a median age of 3.6 months at the time of repair [29]. Surgical repair is achieved by singe-patch, modified single-patch (Australian/Nunn) or two-patch techniques. A meta-analysis, which compared modified single-patch and two patch techniques showed no significant difference between two groups, but modified single-patch performed when there is small VSD had shorter cardiopulmonary bypass and aortic cross-clamp time [30]. Several other studies showed similar findings [31, 32–35]. The main advantages of the two-patch technique are maintaining planar alignment of AV valves, lower chances of narrowing of LVOT, not compromising ventricular volumes and preserving the integrity of bridging leaflets [36]. In the Pediatric Heart Network (PHN) study, earlier complete repair showed increased resource utilization with longer intensive care unit stay but no association with incidence of residual VSD or significant left AV valve regurgitation at six months of age (**Figure 12**). Moderate or greater left AV valve regurgitation was found in 22% at six months with the strongest predictor being moderate or greater left AV valve regurgitation at one month [32].

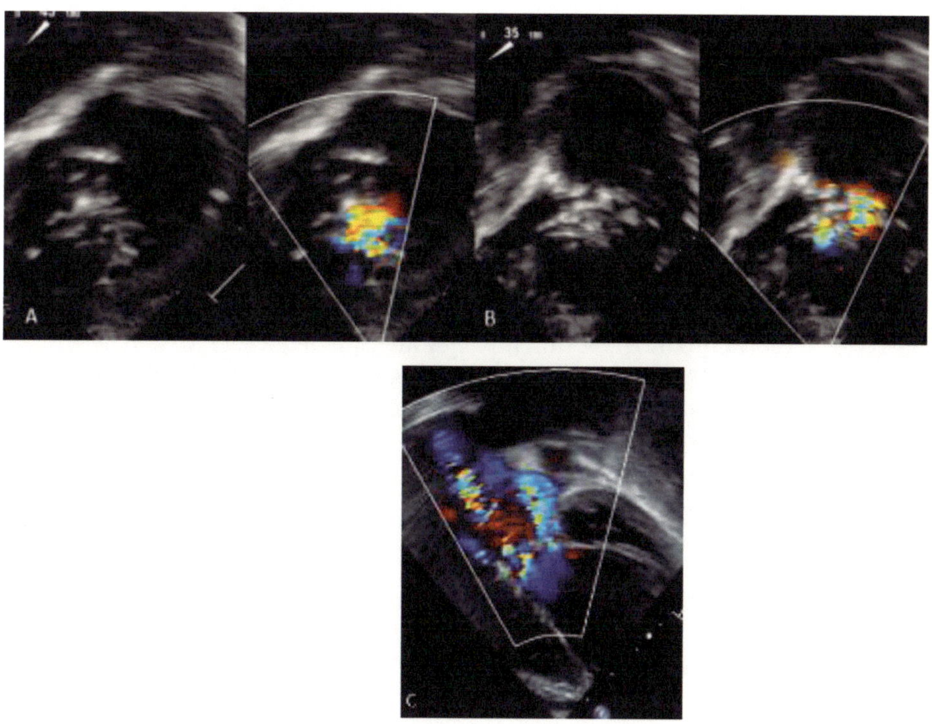


**Figure 12.**
*A, B: Intra-operative transesophageal echocardiogram, color compare deep transgastric view of left AV valve. A. Pre-operative image showing moderate regurgitation. B. Postoperative after left AVV repair. Note cleft is completely closed without any regurgitation. C. Transthoracic apical 4-chamber view of another patient with severe left AVV regurgitation in multiple jets.*

In the majority of the cases, cleft was closed, 93% in this study [37], it was partially closed, or left open in remaining cases.

Associated anomalies like patent ductus arteriosus, double orifice left AV valve parachute left AV valve should be addressed. Patients with complete AVSDs and tetralogy of Fallot associated with Down syndrome may need initial palliation with systemic to pulmonary artery shunt or right ventricular outflow tract (RVOT) stent placement and full repair at a later age. In a retrospective study [38], RVOT stenting showed a significant increase in median Z-score for both branch pulmonary arteries at a median follow-up of 255 days. Four patients out of 26 patients died during follow- up period, but none after the initial intervention. Another meta-analysis found no significant difference in the 6-year survival between staged palliation and primary repair, with higher rate of reintervention for RVOT who underwent staged repair [39].

In patients with partial and transitional AVSDs, there has been controversy regarding the age of surgical correction. A PHN study in 2010, showed good results at a median age of 1.8 years, with left AV valve regurgitation being most common and more frequently in children repaired after 4 years of age [12, 40, 41]. One patient out of 87 died in the hospital. Another review showed excellent results at median age of 1.5 years with LV outflow tract obstruction being most common reason for reoperation at their center [42]. Several other studies showed good long-term outcomes with 30-day and 5-, 10-, 20-, and 40-year survivals at 98%, 94%, 93%, 87%, and 76%, respectively. Approximately 3% of the patients in the Mayo group required permanent pacemaker [40, 41]. A minimally invasive right axillary approach has also been performed with good results in partial AVSD patients [43].

2. Unbalanced atrioventricular septal defects

Surgical techniques in patients with unbalanced AVSDs include single ventricle palliation, biventricular repair and 1.5 ventricular repair.

- Single Ventricle Palliation

Patients with severely hypoplastic right/left ventricle would be managed using staged single ventricle palliation. Initially, they are palliated with PAB and later undergo bidirectional Glenn around four to six months of age, if the pulmonary artery pressures are favorable. Around 2 to 3 years of age, extracardiac Fontan completion with or without fenestration is performed [44].

- One and half or bi-ventricular repair (BVR)

There are no clear selection criteria to stratify patients into either single or biventricular pathways. Several factors are taken into consideration such as hypoplastic ventricle end-diastolic volume (EDV) of >30 $mL/m^2$, normal ventricular function, adequate AV valve size and function, and low end-diastolic pressures on cardiac catheterization [45].

In select patients with right ventricular dominant AVSD, a staged left ventricular recruitment approach is considered, especially in patients with trisomy 21. It includes ASD closure or restriction, without VSD closure, septation of the common AV valve and banding of the main pulmonary artery [45, 46]. This strategy allows rehabilitation of the left ventricle. With this approach, patient would not be committed at an early age to either a single or bi-ventricular approach and it would give an opportunity to monitor for LV growth [45].

On the other hand, in patients with LV dominant AVSD with inadequate RV size, one and a half ventricular repair has been proposed with primary AVSD repair along with a bidirectional Glenn procedure [47]. This would allow growth of the hypoplastic right ventricle for future biventricular conversion. In some institutions, routine 3-D printing is done for all complex AVSD for pre-surgical planning which permitted biventricular repair in some patients who were previously deemed to be candidates for single ventricle palliation [48, 49].

## 11. Surgical outcomes

Even though the outcomes for partial AVSDs are excellent, approximately 10–15% of patients require additional operations. It is well known that pre-operative left AV valve regurgitation predicts the post-operative severity of regurgitation. Other factors are severely dysplastic valve, failure to close the cleft, age of initial surgery, left AV valve stenosis and LVOT obstruction [41]. A technical performance score (TPS) was proposed to grade residual lesions after partial and transitional AVSD repair. In that study, left AV valve regurgitation was the strongest predictor of in-hospital outcomes and unplanned reinterventions after discharge [50]. When compared to complete AVSD, LVOT obstruction occurs more frequently after repair of partial AVSD. Several technical strategies were proposed to decrease the likelihood of subaortic stenosis [51–53].

In complete AVSDs, late reoperation occurs in around 11–20% of patients with most common reason being left AV valve regurgitation [54, 55]. In these studies, freedom from further reoperation after the first reoperation was 63%, 48%, and 42% at 5, 10, and 15 years, respectively. On later follow-up (median 10.7 years, maximum 30 years), actuarial overall survival was 91%, 91%, and 86% at 5, 10, and 15 years, respectively [55]. A recent study showed improved outcomes with overall survival at 10, 15 and 20 years was 91.7%, 90.7% and 88.7%, respectively and freedom from reoperation was 82.7%, 81.1% and 77%, respectively [56].

## 12. Down syndrome

Around 36.5–66% of Down patients have pulmonary hypertension with congenital heart disease less than six months of age [5, 57]. There has been controversy about the extent of pulmonary vascular changes with Down and non-Down syndrome patients. There are studies which showed earlier development of pulmonary parenchymal hypoplasia and pulmonary vascular obstructive disease (PVOD) in this patient population [58–60]. In children with Down syndrome, Rastelli type A is most common. But when associated with tetralogy of Fallot, Rastelli type C is common. In unbalanced AVSDs, left ventricular dominance is more common [6]. It's known that this patient population tolerates single ventricle physiology poorly [61]. Nevertheless, surgical outcomes are not different for biventricular repair when compared with non-Down syndrome patients. Survival at 30 years was 85.6% for complete AVSD, in patients with trisomy 21 [62].

## 13. Conclusions

AVSDs are a group of disorders with deficient AV septum and abnormal AV valve morphology. It is the most common defect in Down syndrome. The definitive surgical repair has excellent outcomes in balanced AVSDs. For unbalanced AVSDs, it is a complex decision-making process and their repairs are usually categorized to single, one and half or bi- ventricular repair. For a select subset of patients, ventricular recruitment procedures improve the candidacy for future bi-ventricular circulation. Patients with Down syndrome should have similar surgical strategies as that of non-Down syndrome patients. The most common reason for reoperation is left AV valve regurgitation.

## Conflict of interest

The authors declare no conflict of interest.

## Author details

Rakesh Donthula[1*], Animisha Rudra[2*] and P. Syamasundar Rao[1*]

1 Division of Pediatric Cardiology, McGovern Medical School, Children's Memorial Hermann Hospital, Children's Heart Institute, The University of Texas Health Science Center at Houston, Houston, TX, USA

2 Kasturba Medical College, India

*Address all correspondence to: rakeshdonthulamd@gmail.com, rudraanimisha@gmail.com and p.syamasundar.rao@uth.tmc.edu

## References

[1] Mai CT et al. National population-based estimates for major birth defects, 2010-2014. Birth defects Research. 2019;**111**(18):1420-1435. DOI: 10.1002/BDR2.1589

[2] Egbe A, Uppu S, Stroustrup A, Lee S, Ho D, Srivastava S. Incidences and sociodemographics of specific congenital heart diseases in the United States of America: An evaluation of hospital discharge diagnoses. Pediatric Cardiology. 2014;**35**(6):975-982. DOI: 10.1007/s00246-014-0884-8

[3] Parker SE et al. Updated National Birth Prevalence estimates for selected birth defects in the United States, 2004-2006. Birth Defects Research. Part A, Clinical and Molecular Teratology. 2010;**88**(12):1008-1016. DOI: 10.1002/bdra.20735

[4] Stoll C, Dott B, Alembik Y, Roth M-P. Associated congenital anomalies among cases with down syndrome. European Journal of Medical Genetics. 2015;**58**(12):674-680. DOI: 10.1016/j.ejmg.2015.11.003

[5] Mourato FA, Villachan LRR, MattosS da S. "Prevalence and profile of congenital heart disease and pulmonary hypertension in down syndrome in a pediatric cardiology service." Revista Paulista de Pediatria. 2014;**32**(2):159-163. DOI: 10.1590/0103-0582201432218913

[6] Cetta HMF, Truong F, Minich D, Maleszewski LL, O'Leary JJ, Dearani PW, et al. Atrioventricular Septal Defects. In: Ninth FCHD, Allen RE, Shaddy DJ, Feltes PTF, editors. Moss and Adams&Apos; Heart Disease in Infants, Children, and Adolescents: Including the Fetus and Young Adult. Philadelphia: Lippincott Williams & Wilkins; 2016. pp. 757-782

[7] Tjark Ebels RHA, Tretter JT, Spicer DE. Atrioventricular septal defects. In: Fourth G, Wernovsky A, editors. Anderson's Pediatric Cardiology. Philadelphia: Elsevier Inc; 2019. pp. 521-554

[8] Silverman NH, Ho SY, Anderson RH, Smith A, Wilkinson JL. Atrioventricular septal defect with intact atrial and ventricular septal structures. International Journal of Cardiology. 1984;**5**(5):567-573. DOI: 10.1016/0167-5273(84)90167-0

[9] Ho SY, Russell G, Gerlis LM. Atrioventricular septal defect with intact septal structures in a 74-year-old. International Journal of Cardiology. 1990;**26**(3):371-373. DOI: 10.1016/0167-5273(90)90097-O

[10] Kaski JP, Wolfenden J, Josen M, Daubeney PEF, Shinebourne EA. Can atrioventricular septal defects exist with intact septal structures? Heart. 2006;**92**(6):832-835. DOI: 10.1136/HRT.2005.069278

[11] LaCorte MA, Cooper RS, Kauffman SL, Schiller MS, Golinko RJ, Griepp RB. Atrioventricular canal ventricular septal defect with cleft mitral valve. Angiographic and echocardiographic features. Pediatric Cardiology. 1982;**2**(4):289-295. DOI: 10.1007/{BF02426975}

[12] Minich LL et al. Partial and transitional atrioventricular septal defect outcomes. The Annals of Thoracic Surgery. 2010;**89**(2):530-536. DOI: 10.1016/j.athoracsur.2009.10.047

[13] Lev M. The architecture of the conduction system in congenital heart disease. I. Common atrioventricular orifice. AMA Archives of Pathology. 1958;**65**(2):174-191

[14] Feldt RH, DuShane JW, Titus JL. The atrioventricular conduction system in persistent common atrioventricular canal defect: Correlations with electrocardiogram. Circulation. 1970;**42**(3):437-444. DOI: 10.1161/01.cir.42.3.437

[15] Thiene G et al. Surgical anatomy and pathology of the conduction tissues in atrioventricular defects. The Journal of Thoracic and Cardiovascular Surgery. 1981;**82**(6):928-937

[16] LHS VM. Pathology and pathogenesis of endocardial cushion defects. Surgical implications. In: JC D, editor. Second Henry Ford Hospital International Symposium on Cardiac Surgery. New York: Appleton-Century-Crofts; 1977. pp. 201-207

[17] Ebels T, Tretter JT, Spicer DE, Anderson RH. 31 - Atrioventricular Septal Defects. Fourth ed. Philadelphia: Elsevier Ltd; 2022

[18] Goddeeris MM et al. Intracardiac septation requires hedgehog-dependent cellular contributions from outside the heart. Development. 2008;**135**(10):1887-1895. DOI: 10.1242/dev.016147

[19] Gutgesell HP, Huhta JC. Cardiac septation in atrioventricular canal defect. Journal of the American College of Cardiology. 1986;**8**(6):1421-1424. DOI: 10.1016/s0735-1097(86)80317-5

[20] Fournier A, Young M-L, Garcia OL, Tamer DF, Wolff GS. Electrophysiologic cardiac function before and after surgery in children with Atrioventricular Canal. The American Journal of Cardiology. 1986;**57**(13):1137-1141

[21] Snider RS, Serwer GA. Defects in cardiac septation. In: Snider RS, Serwer GA, editors. Echocardiography in Pediatric Heart Disease. St. Louis, MO: Mosby; 2009. pp. 277-289

[22] Cohen MS. Common Atrioventricular Canal defects. In: Lai WW, Mertens LL, Geva T, Cohen MS, editors. Echocardiography in Pediatric and Congenital Heart Disease. UK: John Wiley & Sons Ltd; 2016

[23] Singh A et al. Usefulness of live/real time three-dimensional transthoracic echocardiography in the assessment of atrioventricular septal defects. Echocardiography. 2006;**23**(7):598-608. DOI: 10.1111/j.1540-8175.2006.00268.x

[24] Cohen MS, Jacobs ML, Weinberg PM, Rychik J. Morphometric analysis of unbalanced common atrioventricular canal using two-dimensional echocardiography. Journal of the American College of Cardiology. 1996;**28**(4):1017-1023. DOI: 10.1016/S0735-1097(96)00262-8

[25] Rao PS, Harris AD. Recent advances in managing septal defects: Ventricular septal defects and atrioventricular septal defects [version 1; referees: 3 approved]. F1000Research. 2018;7:1-16. DOI: 10.12688/f1000research.14102.1

[26] Patel MD. Septal defects: Atrial septal defects, ventricular septal defects, atrioventricular septal defects, and unroofed coronary sinus. In: Adebo DA, editor. Pediatric Cardiac CT in Congenital Heart Disease. Switzerland: Springer; 2021

[27] Arar Y et al. {3D} advanced imaging overlay with rapid registration in {CHD} to reduce radiation and assist cardiac

catheterisation interventions. Cardiology in the Young. 2020;**30**(5):656-662. DOI: 10.1017/S1047951120000712

[28] Devlin PJ et al. Pulmonary artery banding in complete atrioventricular septal defect. The Journal of Thoracic and Cardiovascular Surgery. 2020;**159**(4):1493-1503.e3. DOI: 10.1016/j.jtcvs.2019.09.019

[29] Atz AM et al. Surgical management of complete atrioventricular septal defect: Associations with surgical technique, age, and trisomy 21. The Journal of Thoracic and Cardiovascular Surgery. 2011;**141**(6):1371-1379. DOI: 10.1016/j.jtcvs.2010.08.093

[30] Li D, Fan Q, Iwase T, Hirata Y, An Q. Modified single-patch technique versus two-patch technique for the repair of complete atrioventricular septal defect: A meta-analysis. Pediatric Cardiology. 2017;**38**(7):1456-1464. DOI: 10.1007/s00246-017-1684-8

[31] Loomba RS, Flores S, Villarreal EG, Bronicki RA, Anderson RH. Modified single-patch versus two-patch repair for atrioventricular septal defect: A systematic review and meta-analysis. World Journal for Pediatric and Congenital Heart Surgery. 2019;**10**(5):616-623. DOI: 10.1177/2150135119859882

[32] Fong LS, Winlaw DS, Orr Y. Is the modified single-patch repair superior to the double-patch repair of complete atrioventricular septal defects? Interactive Cardiovascular and Thoracic Surgery. 2019;**28**(3):427-431. DOI: 10.1093/icvts/ivy261

[33] Backer CL et al. Modified single patch: Are we still worried about subaortic stenosis? The Annals of Thoracic Surgery. 2015;**99**(5) discussion 1675:1671-1675. DOI: 10.1016/j.athoracsur.2015.01.032

[34] Ugaki S, Khoo NS, Ross DB, Rebeyka IM, Adatia I. Modified single-patch compared with two-patch repair of complete atrioventricular septal defect. The Annals of Thoracic Surgery. 2014;**97**(2):666-671. DOI: 10.1016/j.athoracsur.2013.09.084

[35] Bell D et al. Propensity-matched comparison of the long-term outcome of the Nunn and two-patch techniques for the repair of complete atrioventricular septal defects. European Journal of Cardio-Thoracic Surgery. 2020;**57**(1):85-91. DOI: 10.1093/ejcts/ezz124

[36] Das NPD, Dutta N, Das P. Repair of complete atrioventricular septal defect by two patch technique. CTS Net. 2020. DOI: 10.25373/ctsnet.12867356

[37] Xie O et al. Outcomes of repair of complete atrioventricular septal defect in the current era. European Journal of Cardio-Thoracic Surgery. 2014;**45**(4):610-617. DOI: 10.1093/ejcts/ezt444

[38] Abumehdi M et al. Short to medium term outcomes of right ventricular outflow tract stenting as initial palliation for symptomatic infants with complete atrioventricular septal defect with associated tetralogy of Fallot. Catheterization and Cardiovascular Interventions. 2020;**96**(7):1445-1453. DOI: 10.1002/ccd.29306

[39] Lenko E et al. Influence of staged repair and primary repair on outcomes in patients with complete atrioventricular septal defect and tetralogy of Fallot: A systematic review and meta-analysis. Interactive Cardiovascular and Thoracic Surgery. 2018;**26**(1):98-105. DOI: 10.1093/icvts/ivx267

[40] Mery CM et al. Contemporary results after repair of partial and transitional atrioventricular septal defects. The Journal of Thoracic and Cardiovascular

Surgery. 2019;**157**(3):1117-1127.e4. DOI: 10.1016/j.jtcvs.2018.10.154

[41] El-Najdawi EK et al. Operation for partial atrioventricular septal defect: A forty-year review. The Journal of Thoracic and Cardiovascular Surgery. 2000;**119**(5):880-889; discussion 889. DOI: 10.1016/S0022-5223(00)70082-1

[42] Devlin PJ, Backer CL, Eltayeb O, Mongé MC, Hauck AL, Costello JM. Repair of partial atrioventricular septal defect: Age and outcomes. The Annals of Thoracic Surgery. 2016;**102**(1):170-177. DOI: 10.1016/j.athoracsur.2016.01.085

[43] Dodge-Khatami J, Noor R, Riggs KW, Dodge-Khatami A. Mini right axillary thoracotomy for congenital heart defect repair can become a safe surgical routine. Cardiology in the Young. 2022:1-4. DOI: 10.1017/S1047951122000117

[44] Marcelletti C, Corno A, Giannico S, Marino B. Inferior vena cava-pulmonary artery extracardiac conduit. A new form of right heart bypass. The Journal of Thoracic and Cardiovascular Surgery. 1990;**100**(2):228-232

[45] Oladunjoye OO et al. Staged ventricular recruitment in patients with borderline ventricles and large ventricular septal defects. The Journal of Thoracic and Cardiovascular Surgery. 2018;**156**(1):254-264. DOI: 10.1016/j.jtcvs.2018.03.111

[46] Chiu P, Emani S. Left ventricular recruitment in patients with hypoplastic left heart syndrome. Seminars in Thoracic and Cardiovascular Surgery. Pediatric Cardiac Surgery Annual. 2021;**24**:30-36. DOI: 10.1053/j.pcsu.2021.03.001

[47] Cohen MS, Spray TL. Surgical management of unbalanced atrioventricular canal defect. Seminars in Thoracic and Cardiovascular Surgery. Pediatric Cardiac Surgery Annual. 2005;**8**(1):135-144. DOI: 10.1053/j.pcsu.2005.02.006

[48] Taqatqa AS, Vettukattil JJ. Atrioventricular septal defects: Pathology, imaging, and treatment options. Current Cardiology Reports. 2021;**23**(8):93. DOI: 10.1007/s11886-021-01523-1

[49] Vettukattil JJ, Mohammad Nijres B, Gosnell JM, Samuel BP, Haw MP. Three-dimensional printing for surgical planning in complex congenital heart disease. Journal of Cardiac Surgery. 2019;**34**(11):1363-1369. DOI: 10.1111/jocs.14180

[50] Tishler B, Gauvreau K, Colan SD, Del Nido P, Nathan M. Technical performance score predicts partial/transitional atrioventricular septal defect outcomes. The Annals of Thoracic Surgery. 2018;**105**(5):1461-1468. DOI: 10.1016/j.athoracsur.2017.11.043

[51] Van Arsdell GS et al. Subaortic stenosis in the spectrum of atrioventricular septal defects. Solutions may be complex and palliative. The Journal of Thoracic and Cardiovascular Surgery. 1995;**110**(5):1534-1541; discussion 1541. DOI: 10.1016/S0022-5223(95)70077-3

[52] Macé L, Dervanian P, Folliguet T, Verrier JF, Losay J, Neveax JY. Atrioventricular septal defect with subaortic stenosis: Extended valvular detachment and leaflet augmentation. The Journal of Thoracic and Cardiovascular Surgery. 1997;**113**(3):615-616. DOI: 10.1016/s0022-5223(97)70383-0

[53] van Son JA, Schneider P, Falk V. Repair of subaortic stenosis in

atrioventricular canal with absent or restrictive interventricular communication by patch augmentation of ventricular septum, resuspension of atrioventricular valves, and septal myectomy. Mayo Clinic Proceedings. 1997;**72**(3):220-224. DOI: 10.1016/S0025-6196(11)64752-6

[54] Pontailler M et al. Reoperations for left atrioventricular valve dysfunction after repair of atrioventricular septal defect. European Journal of Cardio-Thoracic Surgery. 2014;**45**(3):557-562; discussion 563. DOI: 10.1093/ejcts/ezt392

[55] Stulak JM et al. Reoperations after initial repair of complete atrioventricular septal defect. The Annals of Thoracic Surgery. 2009;**87**(6):1872-1877; discussion 1877. DOI: 10.1016/j.athoracsur.2009.02.048

[56] Fong LS et al. Predictors of reoperation and mortality after complete atrioventricular septal defect repair. European Journal of Cardio-Thoracic Surgery. 2021;**61**(1):45-53. DOI: 10.1093/ejcts/ezab221

[57] Alhuzaimi AN, Alotaibi NM, Alsuhaibani GI, Alanazi RK, Temsah M-H. Congenital heart defect and pulmonary hypertension in children with down syndrome: Clinical profile over two decades. Cureus. 2021;**13**(2):e13212. DOI: 10.7759/cureus.13212

[58] Cooney TP, Thurlbeck WM. Pulmonary hypoplasia in Down's syndrome. The New England Journal of Medicine. 1982;**307**(19):1170-1173. DOI: 10.1056/{NEJM198211043071902}

[59] Clapp S et al. Down's syndrome, complete atrioventricular canal, and pulmonary vascular obstructive disease. The Journal of Thoracic and Cardiovascular Surgery. 1990;**100**(1):115-121

[60] Bush DS, Ivy DD. Pulmonary hypertension in the population with down syndrome. Cardiol Therapeutics. 2022;**11**(1):33-47. DOI: 10.1007/S40119-021-00251-5

[61] Gupta-Malhotra M, Larson VEV, Rosengart RM, Guo H, Moller JH. Mortality after total cavopulmonary connection in children with the down syndrome. The American Journal of Cardiology. 2010;**105**(6):865-868. DOI: 10.1016/J.AMJCARD.2009.11.043

[62] Peterson JK et al. Long-term survival and causes of death in children with trisomy 21 after congenital heart surgery. The Journal of Pediatrics. 2021;**231**:246-253.e3. DOI: 10.1016/j.jpeds.2020.12.058

Chapter 7

# Hypoplastic Left Heart Syndrome

*Yolandee Bell-Cheddar, William Devine, Mario Castro-Medina, Raymond Morales, XinXiu Xu, Cecilia W. Lo and Jiuann-Huey Ivy Lin*

## Abstract

Hypoplastic left heart syndrome (HLHS) is a complex congenital heart disease (CHD) involving hypoplasia of the left ventricle (LV), aorta (Ao), and mitral valve. HLHS was uniformly fatal in the past, now survivable with 3-stage surgical palliation. However, there is high morbidity and mortality, with 25% of HLHS patients either dying or having a heart transplant within 1 year of age. The causes for such high morbidity and mortality are not well understood, but the majority of deaths are directly or indirectly related to cardiovascular/hemodynamics causes. Studies in a mouse model of HLHS uncover important contributing factors for single-ventricle patients such as the patient's intrinsic factors related to mitochondrial dysfunction, and derangements in the early stages of embryonic development. The HLHS mutant mice were noted to have metabolic dysfunction accompanied by cell cycle arrest and cardiomyocyte differentiation defects. Intrinsic cell defects may contribute to cardiac failure in the HLHS population. Moreover, strong evidence of the genetic etiology of HLHS has come from the observation that HLHS has a high recurrence risk and is associated with various chromosomal abnormalities. In this chapter, we will review the basic pathophysiology, pertinent pre-and post-operative managements of HLHS and recent advances derived from the HLHS mouse model.

**Keywords:** HLHS, cardiomyocyte, mitochondria, single ventricle, hemodynamics, complex genetics

## 1. Introduction

Hypoplastic left heart syndrome (HLHS) is a complex congenital heart disease (CHD) involving hypoplasia of the left ventricle (LV), aorta (Ao), and mitral valve (MV). While HLHS is relatively rare (prevalence 0.02%) [1], it accounts for 25% of CHD infant deaths [2]. The great surgical advancement in HLHS led to a transition from the only option of comfort care in the 1980s to a three-stage cardiac surgical palliation procedure offering a 50–70% five-year survival [2]. However, about 25% of HLHS patients either died or had a heart transplant within 1 year of their Norwood operation [3]. Most HLHS survivors suffer ongoing morbidity, with a substantial portion of these patients developing heart failure over time, as well as neurodevelopmental delay and neurocognitive impairment that can significantly degrade the health-related quality of life. The causes for such high morbidity and mortality are not well understood, but the majority of deaths are directly or indirectly related to cardiovascular causes [4]. While the causes for the poor cardiac outcomes are multifactorial, our study in a mouse model of HLHS uncovers important contributing factors related to mitochondrial dysfunction [5].

## 2. The morphologic Spectrum of hypoplastic left heart syndrome

Dr. Maurice Lev first described the hypoplastic left heart as hypoplasia of the aortic tract in 1952 [6]. However, the term HLHS was initially used by Noonan and Nadas in 1958 [7]. HLHS is a diagnosis that incorporates a spectrum of left ventricular inlet, ventricular and outlet obstructions that may include: aortic atresia or stenosis; mitral stenosis, atresia or agenesis (**Figure 1**); hypoplasia of the ascending aorta that may extend to the entire aortic arch; a non-apex forming left ventricle with variable degrees of left ventricular hypoplasia; commonly, a discrete coarctation of the aorta; and an intact ventricular septum in most patients [6–8].

A normal left ventricle has a mitral valve and gives rise to the aorta. Furthermore, the apical portion of a left ventricular septal surface shows finer trabeculations than a morphologic right ventricle, and the subarterial septal surface is smooth (**Figure 2a**). Hearts with HLHS show variability in the size of the left ventricle (**Figure 2b–d**), and the types of mitral valve malformations (**Figure 3b–e**) and aortic valve obstruction (**Figure 4b** and **c**) along with the varying degrees of hypoplasia of the ascending aorta and aortic arch (**Figure 5a** and **b**) with or without coarctation.

In classical HLHS, the left ventricle has an intact ventricular septum. Ventricular size may vary from a mild degree of hypoplasia to being morphologically absent with no discernible inlet or outlet. The hypoplastic ventricle is commonly muscle bound with a thick myocardial wall causing the hypoplastic left ventricle to bulge on the epicardial surface. The hypoplastic left ventricle almost universally shows endocardial fibroelastosis that, at times, can be quite prominent (**Figure 2b–d**). Additionally, the left atrium will demonstrate varying degrees of hypoplasia.

A normal mitral valve consists of an anterior and posterior leaflet with tension apparatus attached to papillary muscles (**Figure 3a**), and the anterior leaflet is in fibrous continuity with the aortic valve. In the setting of HLHS, mitral valve can vary from well-formed but miniature to dysplastic and stenotic to imperforate or congenitally absent (**Figure 3b–e**).

The normal aortic valve consists of three semilunar cusps (**Figure 4a**) and the aorta consists of the ascending aorta, aortic arch, isthmus, and descending aorta. Aortic valves in hearts with HLHS can vary from having three cusps to bicuspid and are dysplastic and stenotic or atretic. Hearts with HLHS can have ascending aortas that may uncommonly be mildly hypoplastic (**Figure 5a**), but most of the time they vary from moderately to extremely hypoplastic with an almost thread-like appearance (**Figure 5b**). The hypoplastic ascending aorta serves as a conduit to perfuse both coronary arteries in a retrograde manner. In addition, the aortic arch may be hypoplastic. Coarctation of the aorta - a shelf-like, circumferential, paraductal lesion - is common in the setting of HLHS and may be mild to severe. Furthermore, HLHS is ductal-dependent condition, and the arterial duct is usually widely patent and large (**Figure 5b**). The right heart is enlarged and shows right ventricular hypertrophy. A patent oval fossa or atrial septal defect (**Figure 5c**) is present. Sometimes, the flap valve of the oval fossa can show aneurysmal dilatation bulging into the right atrium.

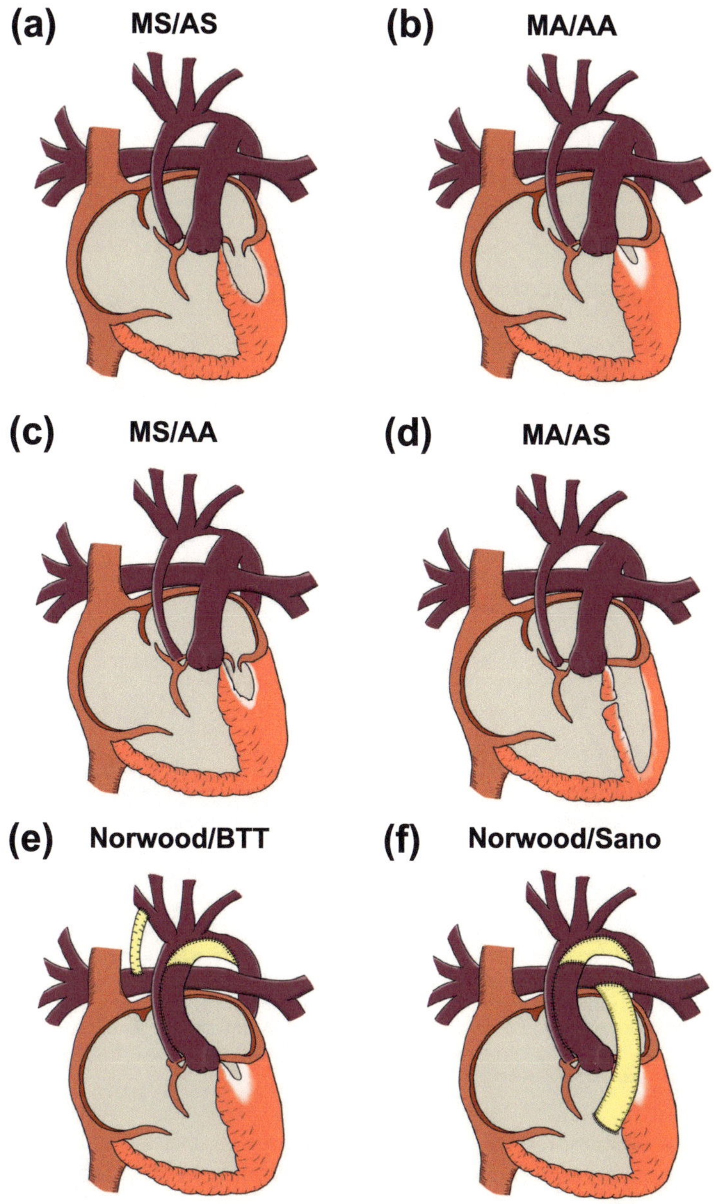


**Figure 1.**
*Illustration of 4 types of HLHS and Norwood procedure with modified BTT shunt (e) and Sano shunt (f). AA: aortic atresia, AS: aortic stenosis, BTT: Blalock-Taussig-Thomas shunt, MA: mitral atresia, MS: Mitral stenosis (graphic illustration by Dr. Raymond Morales).*

Hearts with premature closure of the oval fossa at an early gestational age result in malformations such as mitral atresia or stenosis and/or aortic atresia or stenosis, variable degrees of hypoplasia of the left ventricle, and endocardial fibroelastosis. The severity of the impact on the heart depends on the gestational timing of the closure or restriction of the oval fossa [9]. **Figure 6a–c** are images of a heart with premature closure of the oval fossa. Rarely, in patients born with premature closure of the oval

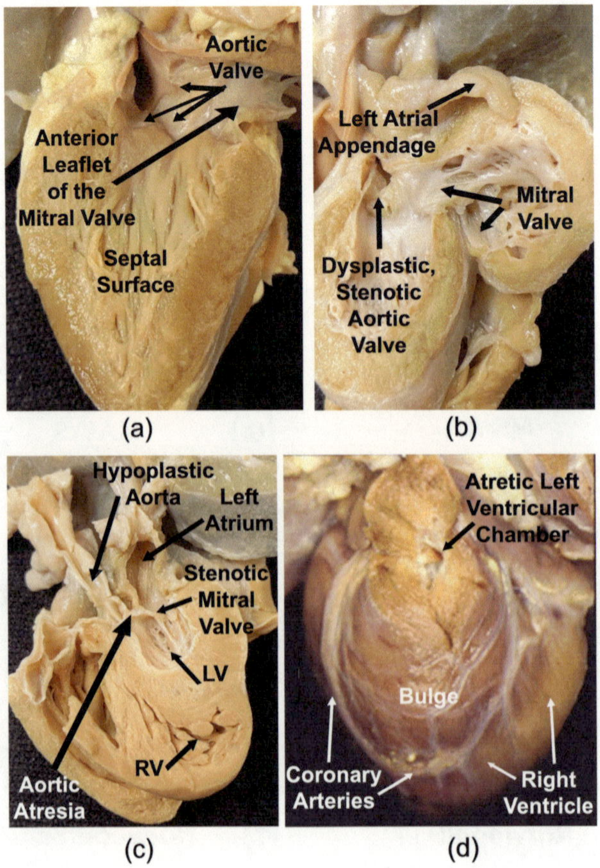


**Figure 2.**
*Variations in the degree of left ventricular hypoplasia in hearts with HLHS. (a) Septal view of a normal left ventricle, (b) hypoplastic left ventricle with a stenotic and dysplastic aortic valve and endocardial fibroelastosis, and (c) three-chamber view showing the muscle bound, non-apex forming hypoplastic left ventricle with endocardial fibroelastosis, mitral valve stenosis and aortic valvar atresia, (d) diminutive and atretic (no inlet or outlet) left ventricular chamber in a heart with aortic and mitral atresia, and the muscle bound left ventricular segment of the heart bulges on the epicardial surface, and the position of the left ventricle is outlined by the anterior and posterior descending coronary arteries.*

fossa and inflow obstruction such as mitral atresia and in cases of typical HLHS with inflow obstruction, an escape channel for the pulmonary venous return may be present [10]. This escape channel may be a levoatriocardinal vein that allows pulmonary blood to egress from the left atrium or a pulmonary vein and reaches the right atrium via the left innominate/superior caval veins (**Figure 6d**) [11]. Rarely the escape of pulmonary venous blood from the left atrium may be accomplished by partial or total anomalous pulmonary venous return [12].

A hypoplastic left ventricle with aortic stenosis and an intact ventricular septum (**Figure 7a**) is not classified as an HLHS. Furthermore, isolated cardiac malformations such as a right-dominant unbalanced atrioventricular septal defect (AVSD) (**Figure 7b**) or a heart with double outlet right ventricle (DORV) with its ventricular septal defect and mitral valve stenosis (**Figure 7c** and **d**), both of which have interventricular communications and a hypoplastic left ventricle are arguably not categorized as having HLHS because

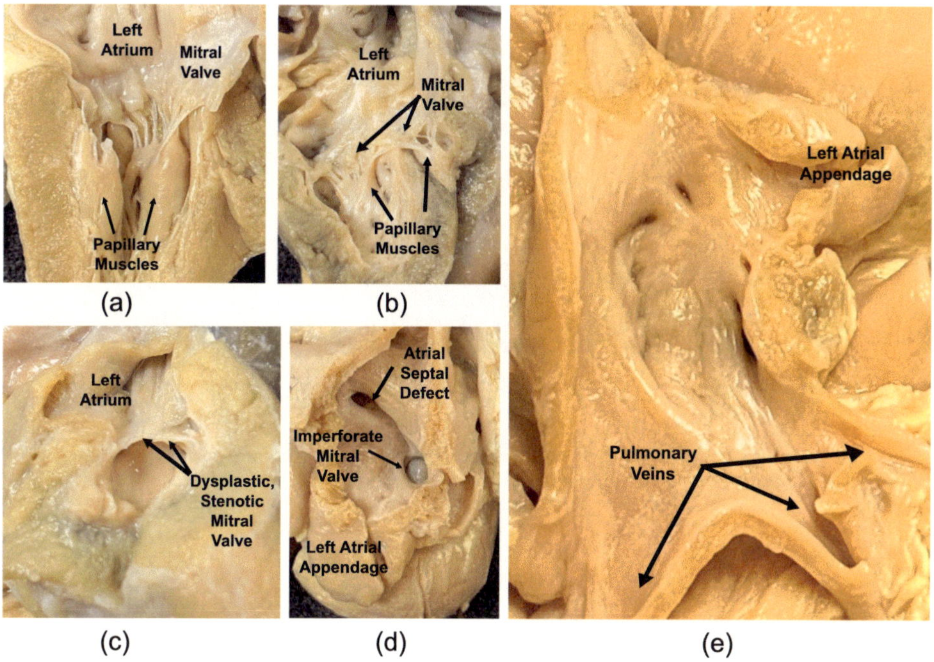


**Figure 3.**
*Variations in the condition of the mitral valve in hearts with HLHS. (a) Normal mitral valve, (b) normally configured but miniaturized mitral valve with slightly shortened and mildly thickened tension apparatus and mild diffuse endocardial fibroelastosis, (c) stenotic and dysplastic mitral valve in a heart with severe hypoplasia of the left ventricle and prominent endocardial fibroelastosis, (d) floor of the left atrium and an imperforate mitral valve, and (e) completely muscular floor of the left atrium without evidence of a mitral valve in a heart with mitral valve agenesis.*

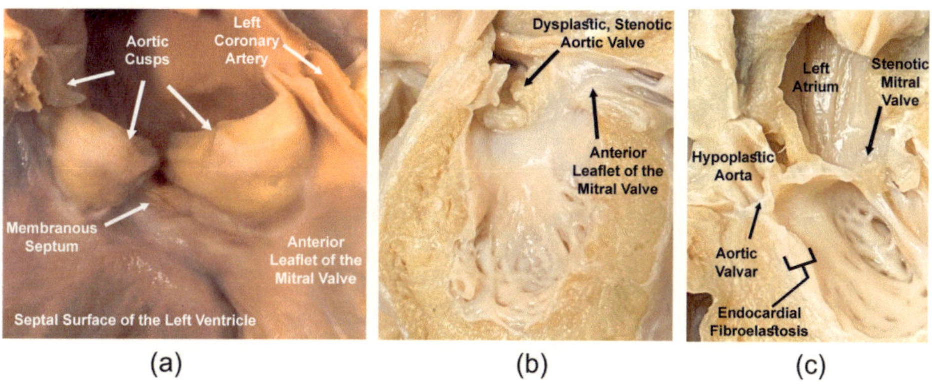


**Figure 4.**
*Aortic valve stenosis and atresia in the setting of HLHS. (a) Normal aortic valve, (b) tricuspid, stenotic and dysplastic aortic valve, and c) aortic valvar membranous atresia, mitral valve stenosis, and thick endocardial fibroelastosis.*

they do not meet the traditional definition. However, these types of hearts (right-dominant unbalanced AVSD and DORV) have been described as **HLHS variants** in addition to their hypoplastic left ventricles they had one or more of the expected left-sided obstructive

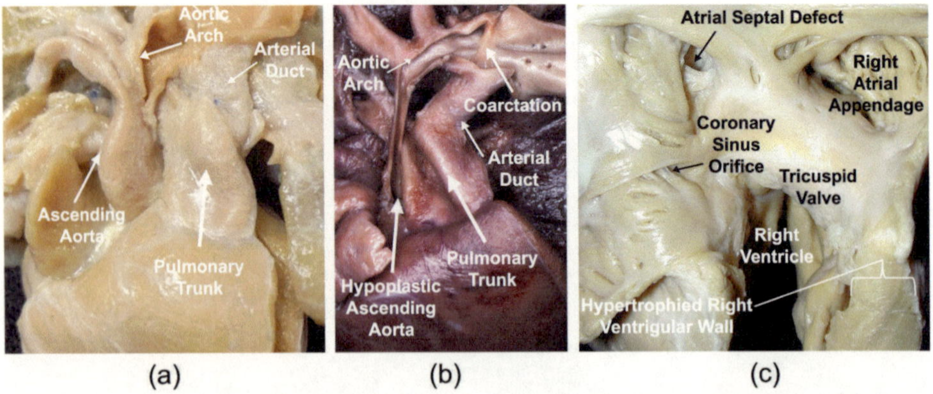


**Figure 5.**
*Supracardiac great arteries and the right side of specimens with HLHS. (a) Mildly hypoplastic ascending aorta and large arterial duct, (b) hypoplastic ascending aorta and proximal aortic arch, coarctation of the aorta at the level of a large arterial duct, (c) enlarged right heart with hypertrophy of the right ventricle and an atrial septal defect.*

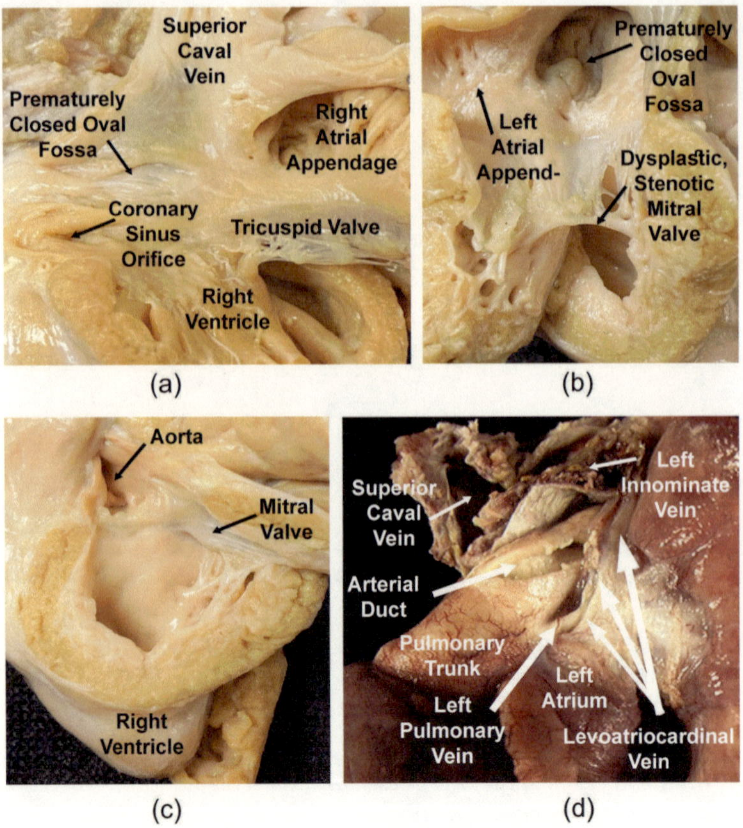


**Figure 6.**
*Right and left heart anatomy of a heart with premature closure of the oval fossa, and a specimen with a levoatriocardinal vein. (a) Septal surface of the right atrium illustrating the prematurely closed oval fossa, (b) dysplastic and stenotic mitral valve, (c) non-apex forming hypoplastic left ventricle with pronounced endocardial fibroelastosis, (d levoatriocardinal vein connecting the left atrium to the left innominate vein.*

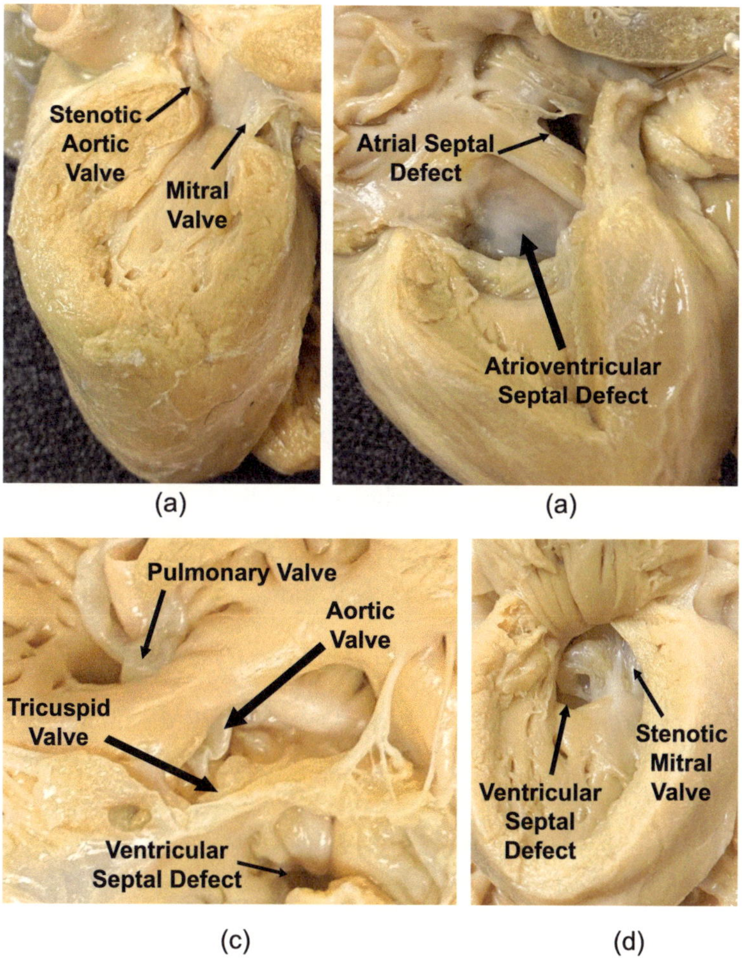


**Figure 7.**
*Specimens with hypoplastic left ventricles that do not meet the criteria of HLHS. (a) Aortic stenosis and intact ventricular septum, (b) right-dominant, unbalanced AVSD, and an atrial septal defect, (c) right ventricle view, DORV and a ventricular septal defect, (d) left ventricular view of C showing the hypoplastic left ventricle, ventricular septal defect, and the stenotic mitral valve.*

features seen in classical HLHS such as aortic stenosis/atresia or mitral valve atresia/stenosis, hypoplastic aorta or coarctation of the aorta. Hearts with a DORV or a right-dominant AVSD but had only aortic obstruction and a hypoplastic left ventricle that is physiology inadequate should not be classified as HLHS variants just because they require single ventricle surgical palliation such as the Norwood, bidirectional Glenn, and the Fontan procedures. The classifications of these types of hearts continue to be unsettled, and this is a reason the classification of HLHS variants needs to be based not only on morphology but also on genetic studies, and not on the need for single ventricle surgical palliation or describing them as HLHS variants just to make the cardiac malformations easier to understand for the clinician or others not trained in pediatric cardiology. Doing this may skew forthcoming studies concerning DORV, right-dominant unbalanced AVSD, and HLHS [13].

## 3. Surgical palliation of HLHS

The surgical palliation of HLHS consists of three, staged procedures: the Norwood, the Glenn, and the Fontan procedures.

The goal of the first two procedures is to prepare the heart for the final Fontan procedure. The ventricular function must be preserved by avoiding a pressure load (avoiding a pressure gradient in the aortic arch) or excessive load (correct-sized shunt), minimizing pulmonary vascular resistance (good-sized atrial communication), maintaining optimal pulmonary artery growth, and preserving the tricuspid valve function by avoiding ventricular dilatation associated with excessive volume work by the ventricle.

The first report of an attempted palliative operation for HLHS was in 1977 by Doty and Knott [14]. All the patients described died of poor right ventricular function or coronary ischemia. Norwood and associates reported the first successful palliative procedure that is still performed today [15].

The crucial components of this procedure can be divided into 3 steps:

1. Anastomosis of the main pulmonary artery with the ascending aorta to provide unobstructed right (systemic) ventricle outflow.

2. Atrial septectomy to allow unobstructed pulmonary venous drainage.

3. Systemic-to-pulmonary shunt as the source of controlled pulmonary blood flow using a Blalock-Taussing Shunt or Sano shunt (right ventricle to pulmonary artery conduit) [16–18].

The Norwood procedure is performed through median sternotomy; under moderate or deep hypothermia, using circulatory arrest or selective cerebral perfusion; the latter is currently the preferred option. Different materials are used for arch reconstruction; homograft is the most common material used, but there are other options including bovine pericardium, core-matrix, and femoral vein graft.

The systemic-to-pulmonary shunt can be performed by using the modified Blalock-Taussing-Thomas shunt (MBTT) (**Figure 1e**) or the right ventricle to pulmonary artery shunt (RVPA) which is named the Sano Shunt (**Figure 1f**).

MBTT shunt is made of polytetrafluoroethylene (PTFE, Gore-Tex): generally 3.5 mm for infants of 2.5–3.5 kg and 4 mm for larger infants.

The 5 mm RVPA shunt is used for neonates between approximately 2.3 and 3.5 kg. If PVR is high, a 6 mm RVPA shunt may be considered.

A randomized clinical trial comparing MBTT and RVPA at 15 North American Centers was performed which includes 275 patients with MBTT and 274 patients with RVPA shunt [16]. Compared with the MBTT group, the patients with RVPA shunt were associated with higher rates of transplantation-free survival at 12 months. By 14 months, the right ventricular end-diastolic volumes were similar in 2 groups [16], however, the RVPA shunt group had more unintended interventions and complications. Data collected over the follow-up period of 32 months showed a nonsignificant difference in transplantation-free survival between the two groups [16].

The second stage procedure is the bidirectional Glenn procedure that consists of a Cavo-pulmonary anastomosis which is usually is performed between 3 and 6 months of age. Viegas et al. reviewed 14 years of experience on 36 patients younger than

90-day-old and reported no mortality, but 90% of patients required Glenn patch augmentation. The indications to perform a Glenn procedure within the first 90 days of life are persistent hypoxemia, signs of ventricular dysfunction, and atrioventricular valve regurgitation [19].

Finally, the third stage procedure is total cavopulmonary connection or the modified Fontan procedure. There are two different surgical techniques for this procedure, namely, the lateral tunnel with intra-atrial PTFE graft and the extracardiac PTFE conduit; these procedures were popularized in an attempt to avoid late supraventricular arrhythmias [20]. The expandable Gore-Tex graft (Peca-labs) allows for dilatation of the Fontan conduit in the cardiac catheterization suite [21].

In 2002, Akintuerk et al. from Giessen, Germany were the first to describe the hybrid approach to HLHS, which is a combination of surgical intervention (application of bilateral branch pulmonary artery bands) and catheter intervention (placement of ductal stent) as primary palliation for neonates with HLHS [22]. In the United States, Galantowicz and Cheatham reported the results of this procedure in 2005 [23].

The results of the Norwood procedure have improved over the last few decades to where it is unethical not to offer this procedure to all newborns with HLHS; cardiac transplant is considered if there is any contraindication for the Norwood operation or Hybrid procedure.

## 4. Pre and post-operative care of HLHS

Adequate pre-operative management of HLHS requires knowledge of the fetal circulation in this disorder. In patients with aortic atresia and very severe aortic stenosis—in general, there is a lower $pO_2$ to the fetal brain with probably decreased blood flow to the brain as well. There is retrograde flow into coronaries in these instances and the ascending aorta is quite small. Normally the lungs will receive only 11% of the combined ventricular output [24], but the blood flow that the lungs see in HLHS fetus is usually higher [25]. In HLHS, it is conceivable that the relatively higher oxygen saturation could impact the normal microvascular development in the pulmonary artery and veins [26].

Postnatally, pulmonary venous return (normally fully saturated blood) must be routed to the right atrium. This mixes with desaturated blood in the right atrium and is ejected by the right ventricle. By default, the right ventricle supplies both systemic (through the PDA) and pulmonic circulations. Blood may need to flow retrograde to supply head and neck vessels and coronaries arteries. The delicate balance between systemic vascular resistance and pulmonic vascular resistance plays a major role. As suggested in the above section, ischemia of the brain and coronaries may occur.

In the postnatal period, we need an adequate interatrial communication, widely patent ductus arteriosus and a balanced pulmonary vascular resistance (PVR) to systemic vascular resistance (SVR). There is an inherent tendency for high pulmonary blood flow—in otherwise uncomplicated cases, with concurrent systemic steal. The right ventricle is volume overloaded at baseline. So, the immediate goals of pre-op care rest on preserving ductal patency and balancing PVR and SVR. One needs to be able to diagnose a high pulmonary to systemic flow ratio (Qp:Qs) state. Some of the clinical manifestations include hypotension, decreased urine output, delayed capillary refill, and lactic acidosis. Patients may also present with tachypnea, increased work of breathing, and respiratory distress.

### 4.1 Keeping the duct patent

The ductus arteriosus can be kept patent via the use of prostaglandin $E_1$ ($PGE_1$). The previously described starting dose range of 0.05–0.10 mcg/kg/min [27] has fallen out of favor to a lower starting dose of 0.01 mcg/kg/min [28]. It is most probable that these previously higher doses were the starting doses for patients who had not been prenatally diagnosed; and who came to medical attention later in the neonatal period. The risk of precipitating apnea is higher at higher starting doses. The recommended maintenance dose of PGE is 0.01–0.04 mcg/kg/min. At our institution, we will use doses as low as 0.003 mcg/kg/min–0.005 mcg/kg/min while patients await surgical repair. There are still institutions that will maintain their patients on $PGE_1$ for prolonged periods of time.

The other means by which the ductus arteriosus can be maintained patent is through stenting of the ductus arteriosus. For patients with HLHS, this is generally done as part of the Hybrid procedure.

### 4.2 Limiting pulmonary blood flow

Pulmonary blood flow may be limited by manipulating pulmonary vascular resistance. This may be done by the use of sub-ambient oxygen otherwise called hypoxemic mixture [29]. The literature on this is sparse; particularly there are no randomized controlled trials. There has been hesitation to use this widely due to concerns about the cellular effect of hypoxemic mixture on tissue oxygenation. The other concern is that a non-intubated patient receiving a hypoxic mixture may hypoventilate or become apneic due to prostaglandin administration; therefore, the $PaO_2$ levels may fall drastically [30]. The use of a hypoxemic mixture requires vigilance in terms of frequent checking of blood gases—to look at $PaO_2$ and base deficit. Attempts to maintain Qp:Qs of approximately 1:1, with an ideal goal for $PaO_2$ of 35–45 mmHg should be made. A useful thing to be aware of is that a central line placed in the right atrium of a patient with HLHS and aortic atresia is generally representative of an arterial gas in such patients. Hypoxemic mixture can be administered via high flow nasal cannula or via oxy-hood or a combination of both or through the endotracheal tube of an intubated patient.

Adjusting the ventilator settings of an intubated patient to allow for higher $PaCO_2$ will also restrict pulmonary blood flow, as well as blending $CO_2$ into the circuit [31, 32]. The latter is also not commonly practiced.

### 4.3 Optimization of systemic circulation

One can increase systemic circulation by use of afterload reduction agents such as milrinone—which can be titrated to effect as we monitor saturations; clinical cardiac output, base deficit, lactate levels, and $PaO_2$ [2]. Optimization of oxygen-carrying capacity by keeping hematocrit >40% is also ideal. Ultimately, if all these maneuvers fail and one still needs to wait for intervention, then muscle relaxation of the patient may need to be considered in order to decrease metabolic demand, fully take over respiratory support and manipulated $PaCO_2$.

Some of the maneuvers to limit pulmonary blood flow and increase systemic circulation are listed in the table below.

| Limiting pulmonary blood flow | Augmenting systemic blood flow |
|---|---|
| Hypoxemic mixture | Good intravascular volume |
| $PaCO_2$ | Increasing oxygen-carrying capacity |
| Intubation and mechanical ventilation | Milrinone (afterload reduction) |
| Muscle relaxation | Muscle relaxation |

### 4.4 Special considerations

Neonates with a restrictive atrial septum are usually quite ill-appearing with hypoxia and heart failure. The keys to management prior to cardiac catheterization intervention are intubation; ventilation; maintaining good blood volume; inotropic support in the form of a dopamine infusion or epinephrine infusion and continuing prostaglandin. It should be noted that increasing the PGE may worsen the clinical picture as there may be a transient increase in the blood return to the left atrium with no egress. Administration of sodium bicarbonate to mitigate the acidotic milieu and alerting the cardiac catheterization team as well as the surgical team are crucial. The atrial level communication in a patient with HLHS is superior in position and often times the tissue is very thick. As such, the cardiac catheterization intervention to establish atrial level patency can be challenging. If a balloon atrial septostomy cannot be effectively performed, then static ballooning may be done (alternatively stent implantation across the restrictive PFO) and if that fails, the surgical opening of the atrial septum is indicated. Blalock-Hanlon procedure (described in 1948 by Alfred Blalock and C. Rollins Hanlon) [33] is not usually performed for HLHS patients.

Infants with moderate-to-severe tricuspid valve insufficiency and/or poor right ventricular function from the very beginning pose an especially high degree of challenge for the cardiac intensive care physician. Some considerations in their management include ventilation; institution of diuretics; inotropic support; heart failure/cardiac transplant evaluation and supportive care/palliation team care involvement.

The patient with HLHS and severe pulmonary venous obstruction will develop marked hypoxemia over time. This hypoxemia may progress after a period of apparent well-being. The goal for these patients until surgical intervention—is to intubate, provide hyper-ventilation, increase $FiO_2$, and increase SVR using inotropic support. A severe degree of pulmonary venous obstruction is a surgical emergency and may require rescue via extracorporeal membrane oxygenation (ECMO).

### 4.5 Non-cardiac pre-op management

Genetic evaluation should include chromosome microarray and whole-exome sequencing, if indicated. A screening renal and head ultrasound is also recommended. Feeding the patient with HLHS pre-operatively is also important. Those with relatively balanced circulations—should feed by mouth. For those in whom we may be concerned about their systemic circulation—total parenteral nutrition may be the judicious approach to avoid complications such as necrotizing enterocolitis [2].

### 4.6 Post-operative management of the HLHS

The post-operative management of the HLHS patient is dependent on which initial procedure is undertaken. In general, there are three first-stage palliation procedures—Norwood procedure with MBTT shunt; Norwood procedure with Sano shunt; and the Hybrid procedure as mentioned in the above section.

The initial management of patients with Norwood MBTT shunt revolves again around achieving that fine balance between pulmonary and systemic flows. If the shunt is relatively large, the patient may have too much pulmonary blood flow and all the maneuvers to limit those as described in the prior section may be instituted. If the shunt placed is long or narrow and relatively resistive and or patient has high pulmonary artery pressure or PVR, then one may find oneself in the situation where there is a need to increase the SVR (use of epinephrine, norepinephrine, vasopressin, calcium) to drive flow through the shunt; to administer volume; and, in extreme cases, to Administrator pulmonary vasodilators in the form of inhaled nitric oxide. These maneuvers are intended to be temporary as the infant's circulation adapts. The management of these patients post-operatively requires great skill and expertise. One also needs to ensure patency of the shunt by administering anticoagulation—usually in the form of heparin drip—which could later be transitioned to Enoxaparin or Aspirin or both. The regimen of anticoagulation is institution-dependent.

The patients who undergo the Norwood procedure and Sano modification are, in general, less cerebrally challenging to care for. Their cardiac output is highly dependent on pre-load and single ventricular function and less so on a potentially tenuous balance between Qp and Qs. Volume administration and inotropic support generally are sufficient.

Both procedures require judicious monitoring and aggressive treatment of dysrhythmias.

### 4.7 Hybrid procedure

The Hybrid procedure involves placement of a PDA stent and bilateral PA bands and, if needed, atrial septostomy [22, 23]. The management of patients post-operatively after a Hybrid procedure can be very similar to the way we manage patients post a Norwood procedure and MBTT shunt. Balancing Qp:Qs is important. Keen attention should be paid to the maintenance of duct patency with anticoagulation and/or anti-platelet therapies.

Patients should be observed closely for signs of stent migration either into the pulmonary artery or the aorta as well as for the possibility of PA band migration. Retrograde arch obstruction from the migration of the stent can be screened through daily 4-limb blood pressure measurements. Intermittent echocardiographic assessment can assist in early diagnosis.

### 4.8 Second stage palliation

The Glenn procedure is the second stage in the HLHS palliation. By far, it is much less challenging to manage these patients post-operatively. The expectation is that these patients will exit the operating room extubated. If the patient had a reassuring pre-Glenn catheterization study, then the hope is that this would have translated into a successful procedure.

In terms of the respiratory system, post-operative care lies in the avoidance of high positive end-expiratory pressure (PEEP) and high PVR states. Through avoidance of hyperventilation, one may manipulate PaCO2 to optimize flow in the Glenn circulation should the patient be intubated. Augment cardiac inotropy, if necessary. Oftentimes, a combination of milrinone and epinephrine drips post-operatively works well. Pain control and, later, effective diuresis are also important. Cerebral congestion from the new passive circulation to the pulmonary arteries can be a source of significant patient discomfort. Simple maneuvers such as elevating the head of the bed can contribute to great patient comfort by using gravity to promote anterograde blood flow from the cerebral to the pulmonary circulation.

Monitoring these patients for desaturation relative to their physiology is also important; and assessing for the common causes of a desaturated Glenn patient is crucial. The desaturated Glenn patient may pose a serious dilemma for the ICU team. The use of 100% $FiO_2$ and inhaled nitric oxide can be employed. Ultimately, the patient may need to be intubated. In such instances, cardiac catheterization procedure should be pursued to investigate the possible causes. Ensuring adequate hemoglobin levels for Glenn's physiology is important. If the patient requires additional pulmonary blood flow, then an aortopulmonary shunt may be added to the system [34].

These patients require monitoring for high chest tube output and pleural effusions/chylothorax.

### 4.9 Third stage

The third stage of palliation is called the Fontan procedure or total cavo-pulmonary anastomosis. Similar to the Glenn procedure, acute post-operative management includes avoidance of high PEEP, and high PVR triggers. The majority of Fontan patients will return from the operating room extubated. Typically, the saturations in a patient post Fontan procedure will be around 92–95%—barring the presence of collaterals or pulmonary vein desaturations. They are preload dependent—at some institutions, the initial post-operative fluid management involves giving patient one and half times maintenance fluid volume. After the first 24–36 h, effective diuresis is then initiated.

Inotropic support may involve the use of epinephrine, milrinone, and/or dopamine. Most recently, the potential beneficial use of vasopressin post-operatively has been explored [35].

Arrhythmias are not infrequent. Postoperatively Fontan patients should be observed for supraventricular tachyarrhythmias of all forms (atrial tachyarrhythmias, re-entry tachyarrhythmias, and junctional arrhythmias).

Like in the Glenn patients, the post-operative Fontan patients require monitoring for high chest tube output and pleural effusions/chylothorax.

Any evidence of an acutely failing Fontan physiology [36, 37] should be anticipated and acted upon expeditiously. If there is evidence of an acutely failed Fontan physiology—serious consideration should be given to taking down the Fontan circuit [38].

## 5. Possible etiologies for HLHS

### 5.1 Reduced blood flow—"no flow, no growth" is a possible etiology of hypoplastic left heart syndrome

Reduced blood flow through the left side of the developing heart is the most prevalent hypothesis in the causation of HLHS. Abnormal blood flow has a negative effect on the shear forces applied to the developing heart which in turn impacts the growth of the left ventricle. Any experimental manipulation to decrease left ventricular preload during embryonic development by either obstructing the left atrioventricular canal flow [39], inserting a balloon in the left atrium [25], or by placing an occluder in the foramen ovale [40] resulted in cardiac phenotypes of HLHS in chick embryos and fetal lambs. This hypothesis is further supported by the observation of the HLHS phenotypes in human fetuses with foramen ovale restriction [41] and premature closure of foramen ovale (**Figure 6**).

### 5.2 Fetal aortic valve stenosis and HLHS

A group of fetuses with aortic valve stenosis with dilated or normal-sized left ventricles in mid-gestation were found to develop into HLHS [42, 43]. In this group of patients, the aortic stenosis in the developing heart resulted in left ventricular dysfunction, myocardial damage, and decreased left ventricular flow which led to HLHS after birth [43, 44]. However, after successful aortic valvuloplasty for aortic stenosis in human fetus, some patients did not have an improvement in their left ventricle growth and ended up with single ventricle palliation [42]. Therefore, intrinsic defects of left ventricular cardiomyocytes cannot be excluded.

## 6. Complex genetics in HLHS

Strong evidence of the genetic etiology of HLHS came from the observation that HLHS has a high recurrence risk [45] and is associated with various chromosomal abnormalities [46, 47]. Identifying the genetic causes of HLHS may yield deeper insights into the molecular mechanism driving the pathogenesis of HLHS. In families with HLHS, often bicuspid aortic valve (BAV) is also observed, indicating a genetic link between these two congenital heart lesions [48]. Paradoxically, BAV is the most common CHD (prevalence 1–2%) and is clinically important because of the morbidity and mortality of associated phenotypes, specifically aortic valve disease and aortic aneurysm/dissection (aortopathy). Indeed, BAV underlies aortic valve disease in >50% of patients of all ages undergoing valve surgery [49]. The recurrence of left-sided congenital heart defects in first-degree relatives of a proband of HLHS is about 10–15%, suggestive of a strong but heterogeneous genetic component [45, 47, 50–52]. In addition, there are approximately 30% of fetuses with HLHS that have extracardiac abnormalities [53]. Analysis from the Society of Thoracic Surgeons database from 2002 to 2006 demonstrated mortality after Norwood procedure was significantly worse in HLHS neonates with non-cardiac abnormalities and/or syndromes with higher unfavorable results in patients with chromosomal defects [54].

### 6.1 Possible genetic etiologies associated with HLHS

1. Syndromes with HLHS as a cardiac phenotype: Holt-Oram syndrome caused by TBX 5 mutations [55], Rubinstein Taybi syndrome caused by CREB binding protein mutation [56, 57], Smith-Lemli-Opitz syndrome [58], and Noonan syndrome [59, 60].

2. Chromosomal abnormalities: chromosomal abnormalities were noted in 10% of HLHS including trisomy 13 [61, 62], trisomy 18 [62, 63], trisomy 21 [62, 64],

Turner syndrome [62, 65], and DiGeorge syndrome [62, 64]. Turner syndrome with HLHS is associated with significant mortality [54, 66].

3. Copy number variants: Jacobsen syndrome (11q24-qter deletion) [67], Alagille syndrome (20p12.2-p12.3 deletion) [68], dup 1q21.1, dup 16p13.11, dup 15q11.2-13, dup 22q11.2, and del 2q23.1 [69], del14q23.3 [70]. Copy number variants were reported to be associated with more than 10% of single ventricle lesions including HLHS [71–73]. However, copy number variants of undetermined significance in neonates with HLHS are not associated with worse clinical outcomes [73].

4. Gene mutations: Notch1 [72, 74, 75], Nkx2.5 [72, 75, 76], HAND1 [72, 75, 77], GJA1 [78], Lrp2 [79], SMAD3 [80], ERBB4 [81], PROX1 [82]. Pathological mutations in cardiomyopathy-associated genes-MYBPC3, RYR2 and MYH6 were noted in HLHS patients with cardiomyopathy which suggests a shared clinical and genetic pathway between HLHS and cardiomyopathy [83].

### 6.2 Cell intrinsic defects in the pathogenesis of HLHS

The complex genetics of HLHS is further supported by analysis of HLHS mutant mice through the usage of a large-forward genetic screen [5]. Lo et al. recovered 8 HLHS mutant lines with exome sequencing demonstrating no shared mutations among the 8 HLHS lines [5, 84] (**Figure 8**). The results indicate that HLHS is genetically heterogeneous with a multi-genetic etiology. Through extensive analysis of one HLHS mutant line, *Ohia* identified defects in mitochondrial bioenergetics, nitric oxide (NO) metabolism, and cell cycle regulation [5]. The *Ohia* HLHS mouse model exhibits mid-to-late gestation lethality with heart failure characterized by severe pericardial effusion with poor cardiac contractility. This is associated with decreased cardiomyocyte proliferation and increased apoptosis [5]. Ultrastructural analysis showed the myocardium with poorly organized thin myofilaments and altered mitochondrial morphology [5]. Dynamic changes in mitochondria morphology play an important role in the developmentally regulated metabolic switch from glycolysis to oxidative phosphorylation, a process that also plays a critical role in regulating cardiomyocyte differentiation [85]. This entails closure of the mitochondrial permeability transition pore (mPTP) and formation of a mitochondrial transmembrane potential ($\Delta\Psi_m$) mediating oxidative phosphorylation. Using primary cardiomyocyte explants from the E14.5 *Ohia* HLHS mouse heart, Lo et al. measured the $\Delta\Psi_m$, in cardiomyocytes from the right (RV) and left ventricle (LV). A reduction was observed in both the RV and LV cardiomyocytes. To determine whether the abnormal open state of the mPTP is a cell-autonomous defect, mouse induced pluripotent stem cell-derived cardiomyocytes (iPSC-CM) were used to verify the cardiomyocyte and mitochondrial defects. Those studies indicate that the mitochondrial dysfunction, and proliferation and differentiation defects observed in the *Ohia* HLHS heart tissue are cell autonomous. Hence, the feasibility to model HLHS-HF in iPSC-CM is suggested by studies of the mouse model of HLHS [5]. Furthermore, modeling using human iPSC-CM showed early heart failure (HF) patient iPSC-CM have increased apoptosis, redox stress, and failed antioxidant response. This was associated with mitochondrial permeability transition pore (mPTP) opening, mitochondrial hyper-fusion, and respiration defects. In contrast, iPSC-CM from patients without early-HF had a hyper-elevated antioxidant response with increased mitochondrial fission and mitophagy. Single-cell transcriptomics also showed dichotomization by HF outcome with mitochondrial

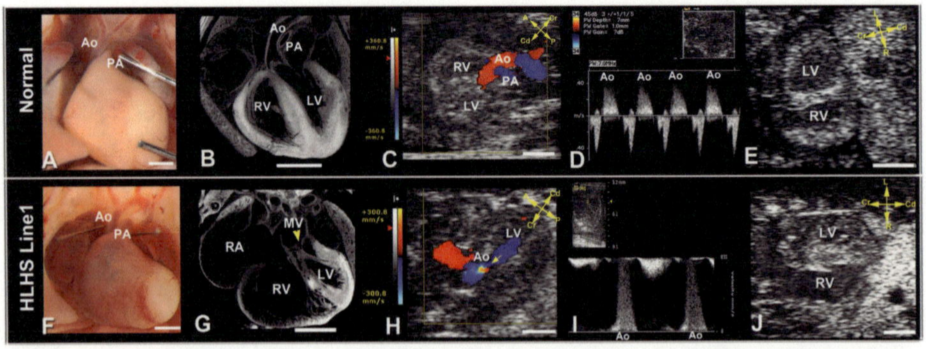


**Figure 8.**
Ohia *HLHS phenotypes. (A, F) newborn (P0) or E16.5 hearts from wild-type (A) and HLHS mutants (F). Hypoplastic aorta and LV are visible in the HLHS mutant. (B, G)) Histopathology showing the cardiac anatomy of HLHS mutant (G) and littermate control (B) at birth (P0) and E14.5. Compared with controls, the HLHS mutant exhibited hypoplastic aorta and aortic valve atresia, hypertrophied LV with no lumen, and MV stenosis, arrowhead. (C–E, H–J) Ultrasound color-flow imaging of normal fetus (C–E), showing robust flow from the aorta (Ao) and pulmonary artery (PA). In the HLHS mutant (H–J), the aorta showed only a narrow flow stream, whereas the pulmonary artery showed robust flow. 2D imaging revealed hypoplastic LV (H), as compared with the normal-sized LV in the control (C) (modified with permission from reference 5).*

dysfunction and endoplasmic reticulum (ER) stress associated with early-HF. Importantly, oxidative stress and apoptosis associated with early-HF were rescued by sildenafil inhibition of mPTP opening or TUDCA suppression of ER stress. Together, these findings support a new paradigm for modeling clinical outcomes in iPSC-CM, demonstrating that uncompensated mitochondrial oxidative stress underlies early-HF in HLHS [86].

## 6.3 Increased mitochondrial oxygen consumption is associated with poor cardiac outcomes in HLHS patients

Oxygen consumption rate (OCR) from peripheral blood mononuclear cells in 16 biventricular-CHD (BV-CHD) patients, 20 single ventricle-CHD (SV-CHD) patients, and 22 healthy controls without CHD demonstrated higher respiratory maximum and reserve in single ventricle patients with poor cardiac outcome (death or cardiac death) [87]. Apart from that, we observed a lower OCR in HLHS patients with cardiac dysfunction compared with normal controls [87]. Of the 8 SV-CHD patients with Fontan completion, we observed significantly higher OCR in 4 patients with poor cardiac outcomes (death or cardiac death) (**Figure 9a** and **b**). These changes were observed in two related respiratory parameters—respiratory maximum and respiratory reserve. In contrast, SV-CHD patients with normal cardiac function showed significantly lower OCR when compared to either SV-CHD patients with HF, BV-CHD patients, or healthy controls (**Figure 9a** and **b**). Given SV-CHD with systemic RV are known to have worse clinical outcomes than SV-CHD patients with systemic LV [88–90], we reanalyzed the data focusing on only SV patients with HLHS (systemic RV), either with or without HF. This analysis yielded similar findings with significantly higher respiratory maximum and reserve observed in the post-Fontan HLHS patients with HF. However, we observed a lower OCR in HLHS patients without HF (**Figure 9c** and **d**). In addition, there is no difference between post-Fontan SV or HLHS patients either with or without HF when compared to BV-CHD patients or control subjects in basal glycolysis by measurement ECAR. Heart tissue from *Ohia* mutant mice with HLHS showed elevated

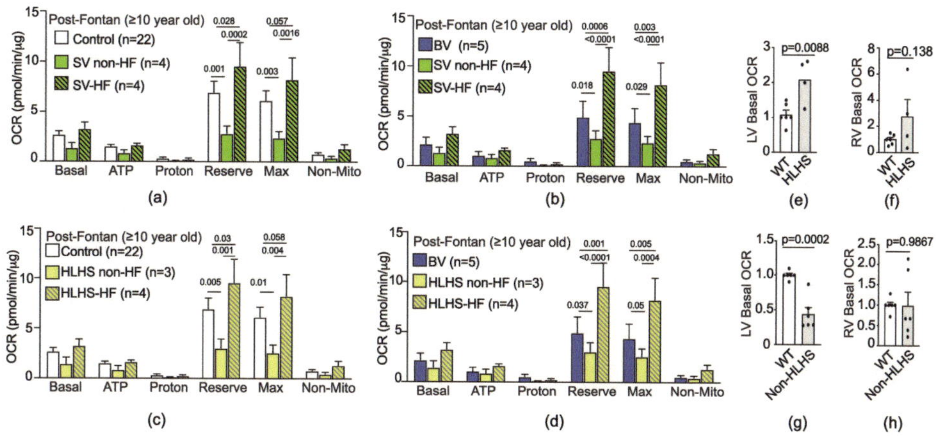

**Figure 9.**
*Mitochondrial respiration in SV-CHD patients and* Ohia *HLHS mutant mouse heart. (a, b) Mitochondrial respiration in the PBMCs of SV-CHD patients ≥10 years old with and without HF vs. age-matched controls (a) and BV-CHD patients (b). (c, d) Mitochondrial respiration in the PBMCs of HLHS-CHD patients ≥10 years old with and without HF vs. age-matched controls (c) and BV-CHD patients (d). (e–h) Basal OCR in LV and RV heart tissue from E14.5-16.5* Ohia *line with* Sap130/Pcdha9 *mutations known to cause HLHS. This analysis was obtained using the Seahorse Analyzer. (e, f) Data was obtained from litters comprising wild-type (WT) (n = 7) and HLHS (n = 4). (g, h) Quantitively analysis of 5 Sap130/Pcdha9 mutants with normal cardiac anatomy without HLHS (e, f) and six WT controls. (a–d) Mean ± SEM with one-way ANOVA test. Subjects' numbers are indicated in the legend for the graphs. (e–h) Bar graphs show mean ± SEM with Student's t-test. Each dot represents one mouse embryo's heart tissue (modified with permission from reference [81]).*

basal respiration (**Figure 9e** and **f**). This is also associated with HF, shown by in utero echocardiography observation of poor cardiac contractility, low cardiac output, and severe pericardial effusion in the *Ohia* HLHS fetal mice [5]. In contrast, genetically identical *Ohia* mutants without CHD showed reduced basal respiration but entirely normal cardiac function (**Figure 9g** and **h**). Together these findings suggest intrinsic metabolic defects in patients with HLHS with a shared genetic etiology with their structural heart defects. These results are supported by studies demonstrating that mitochondrial metabolism [91] plays an important role in heart development and the regulation of cardiomyocyte differentiation [85]. These findings suggest systemic defects impact mitochondrial respiration in SV-CHD patients.

### 6.4 The complex genetics driving the cardiac and neurodevelopmental outcomes in HLHS patients

Many studies have shown patients with complex CHD, especially those with HLHS, have impaired neurodevelopment associated with developmental delay, learning disabilities, behavioral deficits, and cognitive impairment [92–97]. The etiology of the cognitive impairment in HLHS had been generally assumed to arise from hypoxic injury (prior to palliation) and/or complications from medical/surgical management. Clinical studies analyzing various risk elements (cardiopulmonary bypass time, hypothermia, etc) in the Single Ventricle Reconstruction Trial showed such factors can explain some of variance in HLHS outcomes which suggests patient intrinsic factors may contribute to the cause of the poor neurodevelopmental outcomes in SV-CHD patients [92]. A shared genetic etiology for CHD and brain abnormalities has been indicated by a large-scale human genomic study [98] as well as studies of HLHS mutant mouse models. Mouse models of HLHS were also observed to exhibit brain abnormalities, suggesting that mutations causing the cardiac lesion in HLHS can also cause brain defects that could contribute to the poor neurodevelopmental outcome in HLHS patients [99–101]. The brain phenotypes observed in the HLHS mice included microcephaly, which has also been reported in HLHS patients [99, 101]. Also seen were other brain abnormalities largely confined to forebrain structures, including the cerebral cortex, hippocampus, corpus callosum, cerebellum, and olfactory bulbs. In contrast, the midbrain and hindbrain structures were mostly spared. These findings suggest abnormal brain development with regional brain dysplasia may drive the neurodevelopmental delay and neurocognitive impairment associated with HLHS.

## 7. Summary and conclusion

A diagnosis of HLHS was once uniformly lethal, but now survivable with multi-stage surgical palliation. However, it is still associated with significant morbidity and mortality. Through clinical research and animal models, our understanding of the pathophysiology and underlying mechanisms is actively evolving to improve outcomes for this vulnerable population of patients.

## Acknowledgements

We thank Miss Olivia Phillips for her computer assistance in preparing the figures.

## Disclosure

The contributing authors declare no competing interests in this article.

## Author details

Yolandee Bell-Cheddar[1], William Devine[2], Mario Castro-Medina[3], Raymond Morales[1], XinXiu Xu[2], Cecilia W. Lo[2] and Jiuann-Huey Ivy Lin[1,2]*

1 Department of Critical Care Medicine, University of Pittsburgh, Pittsburgh, PA, USA

2 Department of Developmental Biology, University of Pittsburgh, Pittsburgh, PA, USA

3 Department of Surgery, University of Pittsburgh, Pittsburgh, PA, USA

*Address all correspondence to: jiuannhuey.lin5@upmc.edu

## References


[1] Reller MD et al. Prevalence of congenital heart defects in metropolitan Atlanta, 1998-2005. The Journal of Pediatrics. 2008;**153**(6):807-813

[2] Feinstein JA et al. Hypoplastic left heart syndrome: Current considerations and expectations. Journal of the American College of Cardiology. 2012;**59**( Suppl. 1):S1-S42

[3] Alsoufi B et al. Impact of patient characteristics and anatomy on results of Norwood operation for hypoplastic left heart syndrome. The Annals of Thoracic Surgery. 2015;**100**(2):591-598

[4] Ohye RG et al. Cause, timing, and location of death in the single ventricle reconstruction trial. The Journal of Thoracic and Cardiovascular Surgery. 2012;**144**(4):907-914

[5] Liu X et al. The complex genetics of hypoplastic left heart syndrome. Nature Genetics. 2017;**49**(7):1152-1159

[6] Lev M. Pathologic anatomy and interrelationship of hypoplasia of the aortic tract complexes. Laboratory Investigation. 1952;**1**(1):61-70

[7] Noonan JA, Nadas AS. The hypoplastic left heart syndrome; an analysis of 101 cases. Pediatric Clinics of North America. 1958;**5**(4):1029-1056

[8] Anderson RH, Spicer DE, Crucean A. Clarification of the definition of hypoplastic left heart syndrome. Nature Reviews Cardiology. 2021;**18**(3):147-148

[9] Chrysostomou C, Romaguera RL, Rodriguez MM. Giant aneurysm of the atrial septum associated with premature closure of foramen ovale. Cardiovascular Ultrasound. 2005;**3**(1):20

[10] Bernstein HS et al. The levoatriocardinal vein: Morphology and echocardiographic identification of the pulmonary-systemic connection. Journal of the American College of Cardiology. 1995;**26**(4):995-1001

[11] Vlahos AP et al. Hypoplastic left heart syndrome with intact or highly restrictive atrial septum: Outcome after neonatal transcatheter atrial septostomy. Circulation. 2004;**109**(19):2326-2330

[12] Seliem MA, Chin AJ, Norwood WI. Patterns of anomalous pulmonary venous connection/drainage in hypoplastic left heart syndrome: Diagnostic role of doppler color flow mapping and surgical implications. Journal of the American College of Cardiology. 1992;**19**(1):135-141

[13] Hayes DA et al. Beyond hypoplastic left heart syndrome: The Spectrum of congenital heart disease associated with left ventricular hypoplasia. Current Pediatrics Reports. 2013;**1**(2):102-108

[14] Doty DB, Knott HW. Hypoplastic left heart syndrome. Experience with an operation to establish functionally normal circulation. The Journal of Thoracic and Cardiovascular Surgery. 1977;**74**(4):624-630

[15] Norwood WI, Lang P, Hansen DD. Physiologic repair of aortic atresia-hypoplastic left heart syndrome. The New England Journal of Medicine. 1983;**308**(1):23-26

[16] Ohye RG et al. Comparison of shunt types in the Norwood procedure for single-ventricle lesions. New England Journal of Medicine. 2010;**362**(21):1980-1992

[17] Sano S et al. Right ventricle-pulmonary artery shunt in first-stage

palliation of hypoplastic left heart syndrome. The Journal of Thoracic and Cardiovascular Surgery. 2003;**126**(2):504-509 discussion 509-10

[18] Sano S et al. Outcome of right ventricle-to-pulmonary artery shunt in first-stage palliation of hypoplastic left heart syndrome: A multi-institutional study. The Annals of Thoracic Surgery. 2004;**78**(6):1951-1957 discussion 1957-8

[19] Viegas M et al. Bidirectional Glenn procedure in patients less than 3 months of age: A 14-year experience. The Annals of Thoracic Surgery. 2020;**110**(2):622-629

[20] Ben Ali W et al. Extracardiac versus lateral tunnel Fontan: A meta-analysis of long-term results. The Annals of Thoracic Surgery. 2019;**107**(3):837-843

[21] Loneker AE et al. Mechanical and microstructural analysis of a radially expandable vascular conduit for neonatal and pediatric cardiovascular surgery. Journal of Biomedical Materials Research. Part B, Applied Biomaterials. 2018;**106**(2):659-671

[22] Galantowicz M et al. Hybrid approach for hypoplastic left heart syndrome: Intermediate results after the learning curve. The Annals of Thoracic Surgery. 2008;**85**(6):2063-2070 discussion 2070-1

[23] Galantowicz M, Cheatham JP. Lessons learned from the development of a new hybrid strategy for the management of hypoplastic left heart syndrome. Pediatric Cardiology. 2005;**26**(2):190-199

[24] Mielke G, Benda N. Cardiac output and central distribution of blood flow in the human fetus. Circulation. 2001;**103**(12):1662-1668

[25] Fishman NH et al. Models of congenital heart disease in fetal lambs. Circulation. 1978;**58**(2):354-364

[26] Rudolph AM. Aortic atresia, mitral atrsia, and hypoplastic left ventrcile. In: Congenital Diseases of the Heart—Clinical-Physiological Consideration. Hoboken, New Jersey, United States: Wiley-Blackwell; 2009. pp. 257-288

[27] Freed MD et al. Prostaglandin E1 infants with ductus arteriosus-dependent congenital heart disease. Circulation. 1981;**64**(5):899-905

[28] Vari D et al. Low-dose prostaglandin E1 is safe and effective for critical congenital heart disease: Is it time to revisit the dosing guidelines? Cardiology in the Young. 2021;**31**(1):63-70

[29] Tabbutt S et al. Impact of inspired gas mixtures on preoperative infants with hypoplastic left heart syndrome during controlled ventilation. Circulation. 2001;**104**(12 Suppl. 1):I159-I164

[30] Sharma S, Hashmi MF, Burns B. Alveolar Gas Equation. Treasure Island (FL): StatPearls; 2022

[31] Jobes DR et al. Carbon dioxide prevents pulmonary overcirculation in hypoplastic left heart syndrome. The Annals of Thoracic Surgery. 1992;**54**(1):150-151

[32] Mora GA et al. Experimental model of single ventricle. Influence of carbon dioxide on pulmonary vascular dynamics. Circulation. 1994;**90** (5 Pt 2):II43-II46

[33] Herrmann V et al. The Blalock-Hanlon procedure. Simple transposition of the great arteries. Archives of Surgery. 1975;**110**(11):1387-1390

[34] Casella SL et al. Targeted increase in pulmonary blood flow in a bidirectional Glenn circulation. Seminars in Thoracic and Cardiovascular Surgery. 2018;**30**(2):182-188

[35] Kumar TK et al. Vasopressin after the Fontan operation. World Journal for Pediatric and Congenital Heart Surgery. 2016;**7**(1):43-48

[36] Rychik J et al. Evaluation and management of the child and adult with fontan circulation: A scientific statement from the american heart association. Circulation. 2019:**140**:6 CIR0000000000000696

[37] Deal BJ, Jacobs ML. Management of the failing Fontan circulation. Heart. 2012;**98**(14):1098-1104

[38] Almond CS et al. Outcome after Fontan failure and takedown to an intermediate palliative circulation. The Annals of Thoracic Surgery. 2007;**84**(3):880-887

[39] Harh JY et al. Experimental production of hypoplastic left heart syndrome in the chick embryo. The American Journal of Cardiology. 1973;**31**(1):51-56

[40] Wong FY et al. Induction of left ventricular hypoplasia by occluding the foramen ovale in the fetal lamb. Scientific Reports. 2020;**10**(1):880

[41] Hahn E, Keller R. Foramen Ovale restriction in a late gestation fetus resembling hypoplastic left heart syndrome. JACC: Case Reports. 2021;**3**(5):721-723

[42] McElhinney DB et al. Predictors of technical success and postnatal biventricular outcome after in utero aortic valvuloplasty for aortic stenosis with evolving hypoplastic left heart syndrome. Circulation. 2009;**120**(15):1482-1490

[43] Makikallio K et al. Fetal aortic valve stenosis and the evolution of hypoplastic left heart syndrome: Patient selection for fetal intervention. Circulation. 2006;**113**(11):1401-1405

[44] Hawkins JA, Clark EB, Doty DB. Morphologic characteristics of aortic atresia: Implications for fetal hemodynamics. International Journal of Cardiology. 1986;**10**(2):127-132

[45] Hinton RB Jr et al. Hypoplastic left heart syndrome is heritable. Journal of the American College of Cardiology. 2007;**50**(16):1590-1595

[46] Grossfeld PD. The genetics of hypoplastic left heart syndrome. Cardiology in the Young. 1999;**9**(6):627-632

[47] Benson DW, Martin LJ, Lo CW. Genetics of hypoplastic left heart syndrome. The Journal of Pediatrics. 2016;**173**:25-31

[48] Hinton RB et al. Hypoplastic left heart syndrome links to chromosomes 10q and 6q and is genetically related to bicuspid aortic valve. Journal of the American College of Cardiology. 2009;**53**(12):1065-1071

[49] Borger MA et al. The American Association for Thoracic Surgery consensus guidelines on bicuspid aortic valve-related aortopathy: Full online-only version. The Journal of Thoracic and Cardiovascular Surgery. 2018;**156**(2):e41-e74

[50] Loffredo CA et al. Prevalence of congenital cardiovascular malformations among relatives of infants with hypoplastic left heart, coarctation of the aorta, and d-transposition of the great arteries. American Journal of Medical Genetics. Part A. 2004;**124A**(3):225-230

[51] Brenner JI et al. Cardiac malformations in relatives of infants with hypoplastic left-heart syndrome. American Journal of Diseases of Children. 1989;**143**(12):1492-1494

[52] Gill HK et al. Patterns of recurrence of congenital heart disease: An analysis of

6,640 consecutive pregnancies evaluated by detailed fetal echocardiography. Journal of the American College of Cardiology. 2003;**42**(5):923-929

[53] Natowicz M et al. Genetic disorders and major extracardiac anomalies associated with the hypoplastic left heart syndrome. Pediatrics. 1988;**82**(5):698-706

[54] Patel A et al. Impact of noncardiac congenital and genetic abnormalities on outcomes in hypoplastic left heart syndrome. The Annals of Thoracic Surgery. 2010;**89**(6):1805-1813 discussion 1813-4

[55] Bruneau BG et al. Chamber-specific cardiac expression of Tbx5 and heart defects in Holt-Oram syndrome. Developmental Biology. 1999;**211**(1):100-108

[56] Hanauer D, Argilla M, Wallerstein R. Rubinstein-Taybi syndrome and hypoplastic left heart. American Journal of Medical Genetics. 2002;**112**(1):109-111

[57] Bartsch O et al. FISH studies in 45 patients with Rubinstein-Taybi syndrome: Deletions associated with polysplenia, hypoplastic left heart and death in infancy. European Journal of Human Genetics. 1999;7(7):748-756

[58] Kohler HG. Brief clinical report: Familial neonatally lethal syndrome of hypoplastic left heart, absent pulmonary lobation, polydactyly, and talipes, probably smith-Lemli-Opitz (RSH) syndrome. American Journal of Medical Genetics. 1983;**14**(3):423-428

[59] Antonelli D, Antonelli J, Rosenfeld T. Noonan's syndrome associated with hypoplastic left heart. Cardiology. 1990;**77**(1):62-65

[60] Schulz S et al. Prenatal diagnosis of hypoplastic left heart syndrome associated with Noonan syndrome and de novo RAF1 mutation. Prenatal Diagnosis. 2012;**32**(10):1016-1018

[61] Chen M, Shih JC, Wang BT. Trisomy 13 manifested as hypoplastic left heart and other structural abnormalities. Prenatal Diagnosis. 2003;**23**(13):1102-1103

[62] Allen RH, Benson CB, Haug LW. Pregnancy outcome of fetuses with a diagnosis of hypoplastic left ventricle on prenatal sonography. Journal of Ultrasound in Medicine. 2005;**24**(9):1199-1203

[63] Kukora S et al. Infant with trisomy 18 and hypoplastic left heart syndrome. Pediatrics. 2019;**143**(5):e20183779

[64] Zakaria D et al. Chromosomal abnormalities affect the surgical outcome in infants with hypoplastic left heart syndrome: A large cohort analysis. Pediatric Cardiology. 2018;**39**(1):11-18

[65] Madriago E et al. Frequency and outcomes of cardiac operations and catheter interventions in turner syndrome. The American Journal of Cardiology. 2012;**110**(4):580-585

[66] Lara DA et al. A population-based analysis of mortality in patients with turner syndrome and hypoplastic left heart syndrome using the Texas birth defects registry. Congenital Heart Disease. 2017;**12**(1):105-112

[67] Mattina T, Perrotta CS, Grossfeld P. Jacobsen syndrome. Orphanet Journal of Rare Diseases. 2009;**4**(1):9

[68] Robert ML et al. Alagille syndrome with deletion 20p12.2-p12.3 and hypoplastic left heart. Clinical Dysmorphology. 2007;**16**(4):241-246

[69] Warburton D et al. The contribution of de novo and rare inherited copy

number changes to congenital heart disease in an unselected sample of children with conotruncal defects or hypoplastic left heart disease. Human Genetics. 2014;**133**(1):11-27

[70] Payne AR et al. Submicroscopic chromosomal copy number variations identified in children with hypoplastic left heart syndrome. Pediatric Cardiology. 2012;**33**(5):757-763

[71] Carey AS et al. Effect of copy number variants on outcomes for infants with single ventricle heart defects. Circulation. Cardiovascular Genetics. 2013;**6**(5):444-451

[72] Iascone M et al. Identification of de novo mutations and rare variants in hypoplastic left heart syndrome. Clinical Genetics. 2012;**81**(6):542-554

[73] Dailey-Schwartz AL et al. Copy number variants of undetermined significance are not associated with worse clinical outcomes in hypoplastic left heart syndrome. The Journal of Pediatrics. 2018;**202**:206-211.e2

[74] Theis JL et al. Compound heterozygous NOTCH1 mutations underlie impaired cardiogenesis in a patient with hypoplastic left heart syndrome. Human Genetics. 2015;**134**(9):1003-1011

[75] Kobayashi J et al. Directed differentiation of patient-specific induced pluripotent stem cells identifies the transcriptional repression and epigenetic modification of NKX2-5, HAND1, and NOTCH1 in hypoplastic left heart syndrome. PLoS One. 2014;**9**(7):e102796

[76] Elliott DA et al. Cardiac homeobox gene NKX2-5 mutations and congenital heart disease: Associations with atrial septal defect and hypoplastic left heart syndrome. Journal of the American College of Cardiology. 2003;**41**(11):2072-2076

[77] Reamon-Buettner SM et al. A loss-of-function mutation in the binding domain of HAND1 predicts hypoplasia of the human hearts. Human Molecular Genetics. 2008;**17**(10):1397-1405

[78] Dasgupta C et al. Identification of connexin43 (alpha1) gap junction gene mutations in patients with hypoplastic left heart syndrome by denaturing gradient gel electrophoresis (DGGE). Mutation Research. 2001;**479**(1-2):173-186

[79] Theis JL et al. Patient-specific genomics and cross-species functional analysis implicate LRP2 in hypoplastic left heart syndrome. eLife. 2020;**9**:e59554

[80] Fitzgerald KK et al. Novel SMAD3 mutation in a patient with hypoplastic left heart syndrome with significant aortic aneurysm. Case Reports in Genetics. 2014;**2014**:591516

[81] McBride KL et al. Association of common variants in ERBB4 with congenital left ventricular outflow tract obstruction defects. Birth Defects Research. Part A, Clinical and Molecular Teratology. 2011;**91**(3):162-168

[82] Gill HK et al. Separation of the PROX1 gene from upstream conserved elements in a complex inversion/translocation patient with hypoplastic left heart. European Journal of Human Genetics. 2009;**17**(11):1423-1431

[83] Theis JL et al. Genetic association between hypoplastic left heart syndrome and cardiomyopathies. Circulation: Genomic and Precision Medicine. 2021;**14**(1):e003126

[84] Li Y et al. Global genetic analysis in mice unveils central role for cilia in congenital heart disease. Nature. 2015;**521**(7553):520-524

[85] Hom JR et al. The permeability transition pore controls cardiac

mitochondrial maturation and myocyte differentiation. Developmental Cell. 2011;**21**(3):469-478

[86] Xu X, Jin K, Bais AS, Zhu W, Yagi H, Feinstein TN, Nguyen PK, Criscione JD, Liu X, Beutner G, Karunakaran KB, Rao KS, He H, Adams P, Kuo CK, Kostka D, Pryhuber GS, Shiva S, Ganapathiraju MK, Porter GA Jr, Lin JI, Aronow B, Lo CW. Uncompensated mitochondrial oxidative stress underlies heart failure in an iPSC-derived model of congenital heart disease. Cell Stem Cell. 2022 Apr 7:S1934-5909(22)00101-1. DOI: 10.1016/j.stem.2022.03.003. Epub ahead of print. PMID: 35395180

[87] Xu X et al. Mitochondrial respiration defects in single-ventricle congenital heart disease. Frontiers in Cardiovascular Medicine. 2021;**8**:734388

[88] Hinton RB, Ware SM. Heart failure in pediatric patients with congenital heart disease. Circulation Research. 2017;**120**(6):978-994

[89] Lamour JM et al. The effect of age, diagnosis, and previous surgery in children and adults undergoing heart transplantation for congenital heart disease. Journal of the American College of Cardiology. 2009;**54**(2):160-165

[90] Adams PS et al. Low nasal NO in congenital heart disease with systemic right ventricle and postcardiac transplantation. Journal of the American Heart Association. 2017;**6**(12):e007447

[91] Nakano H et al. Glucose inhibits cardiac muscle maturation through nucleotide biosynthesis. eLife. 2017;**6**:e29330

[92] Newburger JW et al. Early developmental outcome in children with hypoplastic left heart syndrome and related anomalies: The single ventricle reconstruction trial. Circulation. 2012;**125**(17):2081-2091

[93] Wernovsky G. Current insights regarding neurological and developmental abnormalities in children and young adults with complex congenital cardiac disease. Cardiology in the Young. 2006;**16**(Suppl. 1):92-104

[94] Mahle WT et al. Neurodevelopmental outcome and lifestyle assessment in school-aged and adolescent children with hypoplastic left heart syndrome. Pediatrics. 2000;**105**(5):1082-1089

[95] Donofrio MT, Duplessis AJ, Limperopoulos C. Impact of congenital heart disease on fetal brain development and injury. Current Opinion in Pediatrics. 2011;**23**(5):502-511

[96] Campbell MJ et al. Neuromotor performance in infants before and after early open-heart surgery and risk factors for delayed development at 6 months of age. Cardiology in the Young. 2019;**29**(2):100-109

[97] Limperopoulos C et al. Neurodevelopmental status of newborns and infants with congenital heart defects before and after open heart surgery. The Journal of Pediatrics. 2000;**137**(5):638-645

[98] Homsy J et al. De novo mutations in congenital heart disease with neurodevelopmental and other congenital anomalies. Science. 2015;**350**(6265):1262-1266

[99] Hinton RB et al. Prenatal head growth and white matter injury in hypoplastic left heart syndrome. Pediatric Research. 2008;**64**(4):364-369

[100] Clouchoux C et al. Delayed cortical development in fetuses with complex congenital heart disease. Cerebral Cortex. 2013;**23**(12):2932-2943

[101] Glauser TA et al. Congenital brain anomalies associated with the hypoplastic left heart syndrome. Pediatrics. 1990;**85**(6):984-990

Chapter 8

# Ebstein's Anomaly

*Luciana Da Fonseca Da Silva, William A. Devine, Tarek Alsaied, Justin Yeh, Jiuann-Huey Ivy Lin and Jose Da Silva*

## Abstract

Ebstein's anomaly of the tricuspid valve is a cardiac malformation characterized by downward displacement of the septal and inferior tricuspid valve (TV) leaflets, redundant anterior leaflets with a sail-like morphology, dilation of the true right atrioventricular annulus, TV regurgitation, and dilation of the right atrium and ventricle. The wide variety of anatomic and pathophysiologic presentations of Ebstein's anomaly has made it difficult to achieve uniform results with surgical repair, resulting in the development of many different surgical techniques for its repair. In 1993, Da Silva et al. developed a surgical technique involving cone reconstruction of the TV. This operation aims to undo most of the anatomic TV defects that occurred during embryologic development and to create a cone-like structure from all available leaflet tissue. The result mimics normal TV anatomy, which is an improvement compared to previously described procedures that result in a monocusp valve coaptation with the ventricular septum. In this chapter, we review the surgical maneuvers that we have used to obtain the best functional TV in cases with several anatomic variations of Ebstein's anomaly. The cone procedure for reconstruction for Ebstein's anomaly can be performed with low mortality and morbidity. This tricuspid valve repair is effective and durable for the majority of patients.

**Keywords:** Ebstein's anomaly, tricuspid valve, delamination, circular shunt, Starne's procedure, cone procedure

## 1. Introduction

Ebstein's anomaly of the tricuspid valve is a rare congenital heart malformation that accounts for about 0.5% of all congenital heart defects and 0.005% of all live births [1, 2]. In a report from the Society of Thoracic Surgery (STS) Congenital Heart Surgery Database from 2010 to 2016, there were 494 patients with Ebstein's anomaly who received index operations in 95 centers [3]. Given the low incidence of this defect, some centers will have limited experience managing patients with Ebstein's anomaly, suggesting the potential importance of regionalizing care in patients with more complex physiology. Ebstein's anomaly was first described by Wilhelm Ebstein with the autopsy findings of abnormal tricuspid valves in 1866 [4]. The patient, Joseph Prescher, was a 19-year-old worker who presented with cyanosis, dyspnea, palpitations, cardiomegaly, and distended jugular veins [4]. Ebstein's anomaly is more than an issue with inferior displacement and rotation of the tricuspid valve, as this anomaly may also involve abnormalities of the right ventricular myocardium and in some cases the left ventricle [5]. This malformation is thought to be due to the defects in the process of "delamination from the underlying myocardium" [6] during the development of the tricuspid valve. Presentation of this malformation varies widely from neonates in extremes to an incidental finding during physical examination in an otherwise asymptomatic adult secondary to the anatomic severity of the tricuspid valve and the associated heart malformations [7].

## 2. Morphology of Ebstein's anomaly of the tricuspid valve

### 2.1 Ebstein's anomaly is an anomaly with both myocardial and valvular defects

The chief distinguishing feature of an Ebstein's malformation is the positioning of the hinge point of the tricuspid valve into the right ventricular cavity with an apical and anterior rotated appearance toward the right ventricular outflow tract rather than at its normal location at the atrioventricular junction or annulus, and this is due to failure of the septal and inferior leaflets to delaminate from the underlying myocardium. In addition, Ebstein's malformation is often accompanied by valvar dysplasia, anomalies of the tension apparatus, and myocardial anomalies, and in severe cases, the dilated thin-walled, atrialized inlet component is divided from the apical tubercular and outlet components by a muscular shelf. Furthermore, an Ebstein's anomaly may be associated with an atrial septal defect, pulmonary atresia, or congenitally corrected transposition of the great arteries (ccTGA) and less commonly with pulmonary stenosis, a ventricular septal defect, or an atrioventricular septal defect [1, 8].

A normal morphologic right ventricle (**Figure 1a** and **b**) is divided into inlet, apical trabecular, and outlet components and has a tricuspid valve with its orifice pointing toward the ventricular apex. The tricuspid valve consists of three leaflets designated anterior-superior, inferior, and septal, and its hinge point is located at the annulus. In addition, the tension apparatus of the septal leaflet is attached to the coarsely

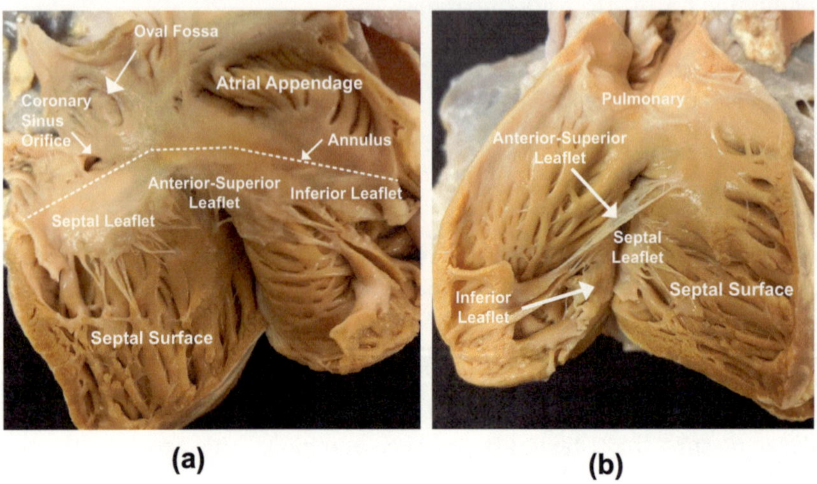


**Figure 1.**
*Morphology of the right side of a normal heart. (a) Septal surfaces of the right atrium, inlet, and apical components of the ventricle and tricuspid valve. (b) Right ventricular outlet and pulmonary valve and pulmonary trunk.*

trabeculated septal surface, and the pulmonary valve is supported by a complete muscular sleeve separating it from the tricuspid valve.

With an Ebstein's anomaly, the extent of the area of failed delamination, and the appearance of atrioventricular valve rotation may vary from mild to severe, and the functional orifice of the tricuspid valve opens toward the ventricular outflow tract. In addition, there is variability in the condition of the tricuspid valve leaflets. The delaminated anterior-superior leaflet may be small or severely deformed with fenestrations, and its tendinous cords can be short and thickened, and in other cases, the leaflet tissue may be redundant and located within the right ventricular outflow tract possibly resulting in an element of obstruction. Moreover, the inferior and septal leaflet tissue can be hypoplastic and dysplastic. However, in some cases, the inferior leaflet may be large and curtain-like with fenestrations, some of which may have a fan-like appearance. **Figure 2** shows the un-delaminated areas of the septal and inferior leaflets. The functional orifice of the tricuspid valve shows the appearance of slight rotation away from the apical component and toward the outlet component. Both the septal and inferior leaflets are dysplastic at the level of their hinge points. The anterior-superior leaflet is dysplastic with thickened tendonous cords. The right ventricular inlet component shows slight atrialization.

**Figure 3a** shows the severe form of Ebstein's anomaly with the hinge point located well within the right ventricular chamber and located on a muscular shelf that separates the inlet and apical trabecular components. Proximal to this muscular shelf, the heart shows marked atrialization and dilatation and the septal surface is smooth with loss of trabeculations. The atrialization in hearts with Ebstein's anomaly can vary from almost non-existent to severe. In severe cases, the atrialized right ventricle can be greatly dilated and affect the shape and function of the left ventricle (**Figure 3b**) [8–10].

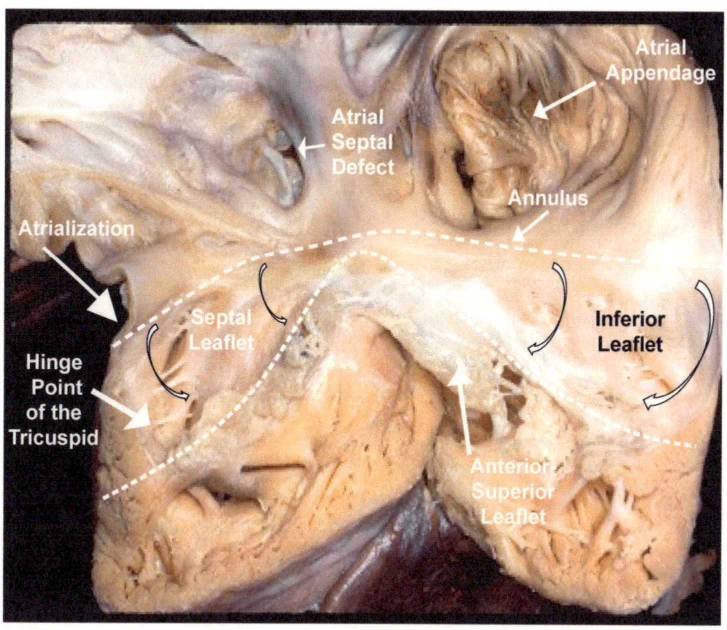


**Figure 2.**
*Right side of a heart with a moderate Ebstein's anomaly showing the septal and inferior leaflets of the tricuspid valve failure to delaminate from the ventricular wall and a rotational appearing displacement of their hinge points, slight atrialization of the inlet to the right ventricle and a small atrial septal defect at the site of the oval fossa.*

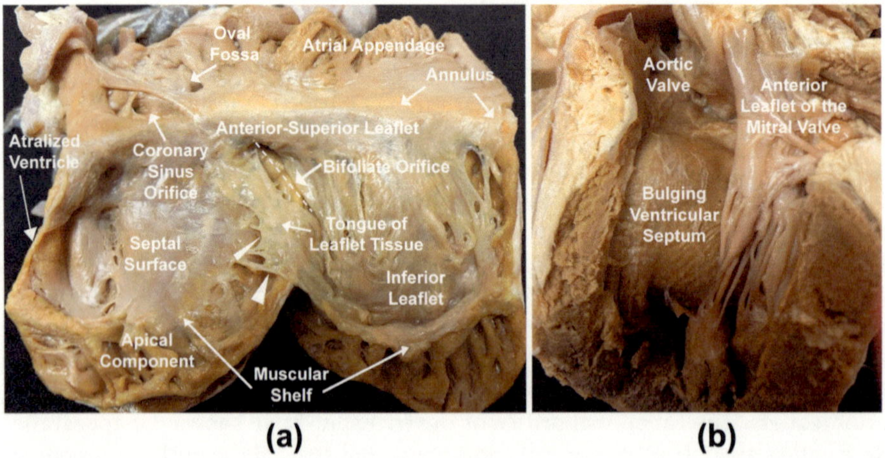


**Figure 3.**
*Heart specimens with severe Ebstein's anomaly. (a) Right side showing severe dilatation and marked atrialization of the inlet of the right ventricle with failed delamination of the septal leaflet showing a smooth septal surface and the muscular shelf. The inferior leaflet is curtain-like with short chords attaching it to the muscular shelf. The functional orifice is bifoliate and faces the pulmonary outlet. The dash line shows the solitary zone of apposition, and the arrow heads show the second outlet from the right ventricle. (b) Shows the left ventricle with the septum bulging into the left ventricular cavity because of a severe Ebstein's anomaly of the right side of the heart.*

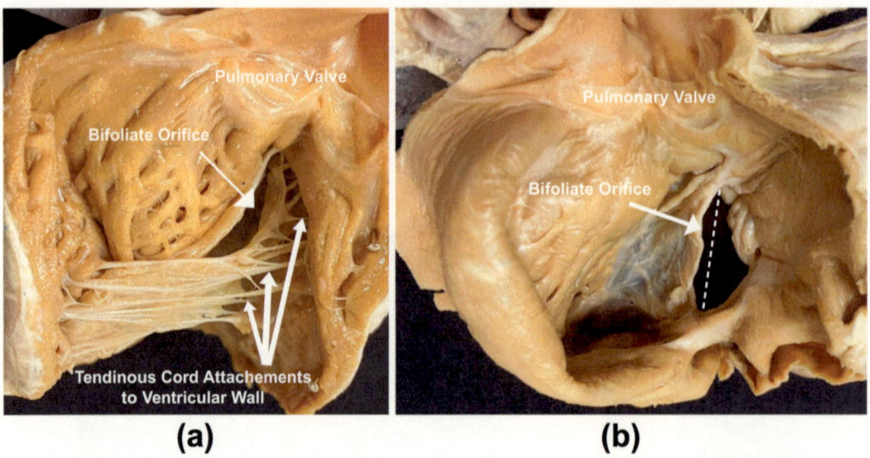


**Figure 4.**
*The outlet components of two hearts with severe Ebstein's anomaly. (a) Shows the bifoliate functional orifice of the tricuspid valve along with multiple tendinous cords attached to the ventricular wall at the junction between the atralized inlet and the functional parts of the right ventricle, the apical trabecular and outlet components. (b) A view of the outlet component from the arterial side showing the functional bifoliate orifice, the only outlet from the inlet and apical components of the right ventricle, directed toward the pulmonary valve. The dash line shows the solitary zone of apposition.*

This heart illustrated in **Figure 3a** shows two exits from the right ventricle. One outlet from the inlet component is through a functional orifice that faces the pulmonary outlet, and this orifice is a bifoliate opening that functionally closes along a solitary zone of apposition. This bifoliate orifice is created by a tongue of valvar tissue joining the anterior-superior to the inferior leaflets. A second exit from the right ventricle is through the proximal outlet component and between tendinous cords.

In some cases of Ebstein's anomaly, the functional bifoliate outlet orifice leaflet can show multiple tendinous cord attachments to the ventricular wall at the junction between the atralized inlet and the apical trabecular and outlet components (**Figure 4a**), or the bifoliate functional orifice may be the only outlet from the right ventricle (**Figure 4b**).

Besides atrial septal defects, Ebstein's malformations have an association with pulmonary atresia. **Figure 5a** shows the right side of a heart with Ebstein's anomaly, which is markedly dilated, shows severe atrialization of the inlet and a very dysplastic atrioventricular valvar leaflet tissue. **Figure 5b** shows the outlet from this right ventricle illustrating the pulmonary atresia and redundant dysplastic atrioventricular valve leaflet tissue.

### 2.2 Ebsteinoid malformation and congenitally corrected transposition of great arteries

Some patients with congenitally corrected transposition of the great arteries exhibit Ebstein-like malformation of the left-sided morphologic tricuspid valve. Ebstein's malformation in the setting of the discordant atrioventricular and discordant ventriculo-arterial connections (ccTGA) is less severe than in cases with normal concordant connections. Because Ebstein's anomaly in the setting of ccTGA is not completely the same as in hearts with concordant connections, it has been suggested that it should be called an Ebsteinoid anomaly. **Figure 5c** is an example of a heart with ccTGA and an Ebsteinoid malformation in a left-sided morphologic right ventricle.

### 2.3 Classification

In 1988, Carpentier et al. reported the most described morphological classification [11] (**Figure 6**) [7].

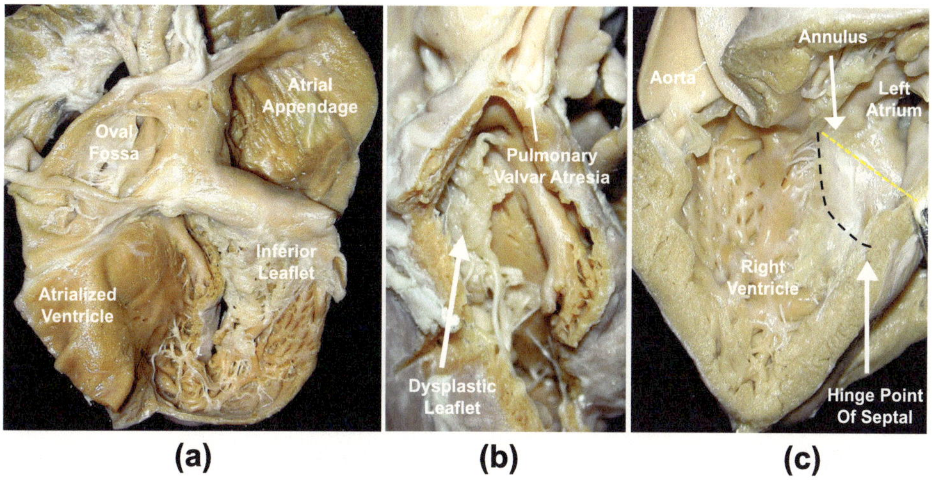


**Figure 5.**
*Cardiac specimen with Ebstein's anomaly and pulmonary atresia and a specimen with congenitally corrected transposition of the great arteries and an Ebsteinoid anomaly. (a) Shows the right side of a markedly dilated heart with Ebstein's anomaly with failure of delamination of the septal leaflet and pulmonary valvar atresia. (b) Shows the outlet component of this heart showing the dysplastic leaflets of the atrioventricular valve and pulmonary valvar atresia. (c) Shows the septal surface of a left-sided morphologic right ventricle with congenitally corrected transposition of the great arteries (atrioventricular discordant and ventriculo-arterial discordant connections) with an Ebsteinoid anomaly. (Images 5a and 5b used with Robert H. Anderson's permission).*

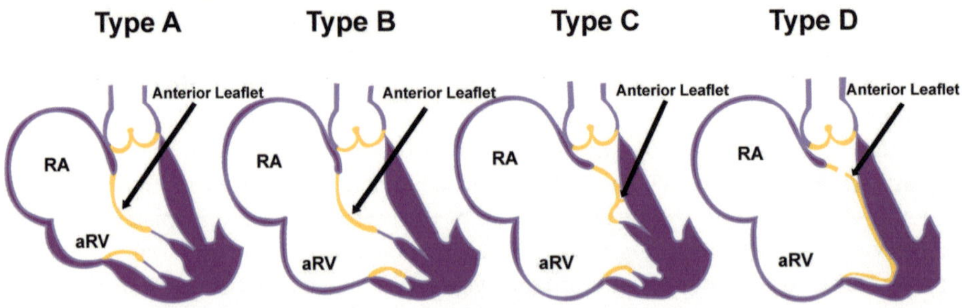


| | A | B | C | D |
|---|---|---|---|---|
| Septal/Posterior Leaflet Displacement | Mild | Moderate | Severe | Extremely Severe (Tricuspid Valve Sac) |
| Anterior Leaflet | Normal Morphology and Mobility | Abnormal Attachments with Normal Mobility | Partial Adhesions to the Ventricular Free Wall and Restricted Motion | Severe Adhesions to the Ventricular Wall |
| "Atrialized" Ventricle | Small/Preserved Function | Moderate/Reduced Function | Large/Reduced Function | Very Large/Minimal Function |
| Functional Ventricle | Normal/Preserved Function | Reduced/Preserved Function | Small/Reduced Function | Infundibulum/Depressed Function |

**Figure 6.**
*Carpentier classification of Ebstein's anomaly. RA: right atrium, ARV: atrialized right ventricle; FRV: functional right ventricle (modified with permission from reference [7]).*

Type A: Mild apical displacement of the tricuspid valve leaflets with the adequate functional right ventricle.

Type B: Moderate apical displacement of the tricuspid leaflets with a moderate reduced size but adequate functional right ventricular volume with freely mobile anterior leaflet.

Type C: Severe apical displacement of the tricuspid valve leaflets with a small functional right ventricle. Anterior leaflet movement is restricted due to abnormal chordal attachments that cause right ventricular outflow tract obstruction.

Type D: Complete non-delamination of the tricuspid valve leaflets with almost complete atrialization of the right ventricle, only infundibular portion of the right ventricle remaining: "Tricuspid sac".

## 3. Genetics

The molecular mechanisms underpinning the failed delamination of the tricuspid valve in Ebstein's anomaly are unknown [12]. Genetic factors resulting in Ebstein's anomaly may be related to the mutations *in myosin heavy chain 7 (MYH7)* and *NKX2.5*. One study reports heterozygous mutations in MYH7 were noted in eight of 141 (6%) patients with Ebstein's anomaly. Ebstein's anomaly with left ventricular noncompaction (LVNC) had a higher frequency of MYH7 mutations (6 out of 8) than Ebstein's anomaly without LVNC [13]. A heterozygous missense mutation in MYH7 was identified in two siblings with familial Ebstein's anomaly and LVNC [14]. Ebstein's anomaly is noted to be the cardiac phenotypes for mutations involving NKX2.5 [15]. Genetic anomalies or syndromes were detected in 19 of 243 fetuses (11%) in a multi-center study. Eleven patients were confirmed with Trisomy 21, two patients were noted to have CHARGE syndrome, and two patients were noted to have a 1p36 deletion [16]. There was no association between Ebstein's anomaly with genetic abnormalities and mortality [16].

## 4. Environment

Maternal use of lithium during the first trimester was associated with an increased risk of congenital heart defects (2.41%), including Ebstein's anomaly [17].

## 5. Pathophysiology

The presentation and pathophysiology of Ebstein's anomaly depend on the severity of the morphology and associated congenital heart defects. Symptomatic neonates generally present with cyanosis, cardiomegaly, arrhythmias, and congestive heart failure [18]. At the extreme end in Carpentier type C and D of Ebstein's anomaly, there is severe displacement of the tricuspid valve that results in severe tricuspid regurgitation and an ineffective functional right ventricle. With the physiological elevation in pulmonary vascular resistance typically seen in neonates, the small and ineffective functional right ventricle is unable to generate antegrade pulmonary blood flow, especially when the ductus arteriosus is still patent, which leads to "functional pulmonary atresia." True anatomic pulmonary valve atresia is also associated with Ebstein's anomaly and requires a patent ductus (PDA) to provide pulmonary blood flow.

Another serious condition observed in neonatal Ebstein's patients is a "circular shunt," where there is ineffective systemic output due to recirculation of blood with a poorly functioning right ventricle and severe tricuspid regurgitation in association with an atrial septal defect and a patent ductus arteriosus. Retrograde flow from the ductus arteriosus (**Figure** 7 arrow 1) through a regurgitant pulmonary valve

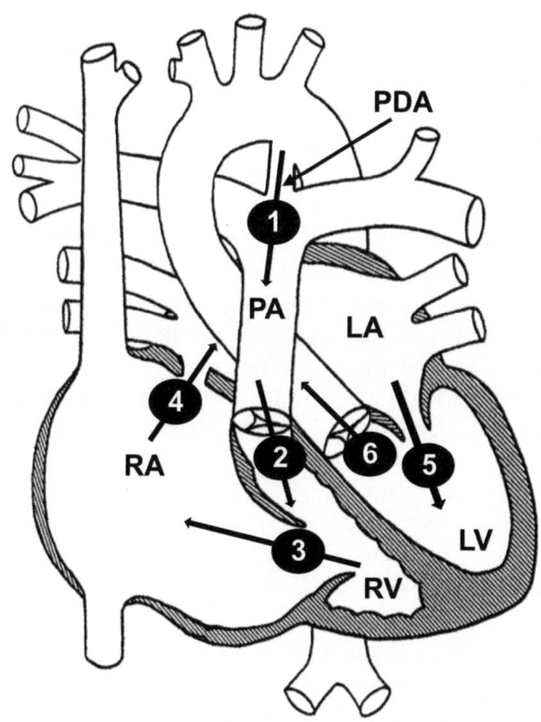


**Figure 7.**
*Diagram illustrating the "circular shunt" physiology.*

(**Figure** 7 arrow 2) circulates into the right atrium due to severe tricuspid regurgitation (**Figure** 7 arrow 3) and then passes into the left heart (**Figure** 7 arrow 5, 6) through an atrial septal defect (**Figure** 7 arrow 4) for another cycle through this circular shunt via the ductus arteriosus (**Figure** 7). High perinatal mortality is associated with the presence of a "circular shunt"; in utero NSAIDs constrict the ductus arteriosus improving fetal survival and resulting in greater gestational age at delivery [19]. In neonates, a "circular shunt" creates unstable hemodynamics with severe hypoxia and low-cardiac-output syndrome. Patients may be temporized with mechanical ventilation and inotropic support, but more definitive correction of the physiology with surgical intervention, typically the Starnes procedure may be required [7].

The goal of medical treatment during the neonatal period is to assist with the generation of antegrade pulmonary blood flow by supporting the functional right ventricle. Antegrade pulmonary flow improves as the pulmonary vascular resistance falls and can be augmented by the initiation of pulmonary vasodilators, such as inhaled nitric oxide (iNO). Prostaglandin infusion is crucial to maintain patent ductus in neonates with anatomic pulmonary atresia. A trial of withdrawing prostaglandin may be required to assess for the presence of functional pulmonary atresia. Early prostaglandin withdrawal may also be necessary for neonates with a "circular shunt." With less severe forms of Ebstein's anomaly (Carpentier type A and B), the functional right ventricular can generate antegrade pulmonary blood flow. These neonates may recover out of the neonatal period without any intervention. Such neonates need to be followed into infancy as the tricuspid regurgitation may worsen over time leading to worsening cardiomegaly from worsening right atrial dilatation and thinning out of the atrialized right ventricle [7].

In the neonatal period, cyanosis due to inadequate pulmonary flow and/or right to left shunting, as well as congestive heart failure are the main issues. Neonates with adequate antegrade pulmonary blood flow and a reasonable size functional right ventricle are candidates for a biventricular repair beyond the neonatal period.

Neonates with pulmonary atresia fall into two groups: true anatomic pulmonary valve atresia and "functional pulmonary atresia." In neonates with Ebstein's anomaly and anatomic pulmonary atresia, initial prostaglandin administration followed by either stenting of the ductus arteriosus or placement of a surgical Blalock-Tausig shunt may be the option to get out of the neonatal period in patients with an adequate functional right ventricle. When the functional right ventricle is small, patients may undergo a Starne's repair followed subsequently by a Cone procedure and/or a Fontan procedure.

Neonates with functional pulmonary atresia are often very unstable, as some patients may develop a "circular shunt" with retrograde flow back through the pulmonary valve. Such neonates usually present in extremis and need a Starne's repair. The strategy for stable patients depends again on the size of the functional right ventricle.

## 6. Diagnostic studies

### 6.1 Echocardiogram

Echocardiography remains the mainstay in the diagnosis of patients with Ebstein's anomaly and guides management decisions regarding surgical strategy. Each patient with the Ebstein anomaly should undergo a comprehensive transthoracic echocardiogram that allows evaluation of the right atrial size, right ventricular size, and function, the accurate anatomy of the tricuspid valve, the right ventricular outflow tract, the pulmonary valve, the atrial and ventricular septum, and left ventricle. This evaluation

| | |
|---|---|
| Tricuspid valve anatomy and function | • Inferior displacement of septal and posterior/inferior leaflets<br>• Attachments/tethering of leaflets<br>• Rotation of the tricuspid valve orifice toward the right ventricular outflow tract.<br>• Coaptation point of TV leaflets<br>• TV function – stenosis and insufficiency<br>• Muscularization of leaflets |
| Right ventricle | • Size of atrialized RV<br>• Functional RV size<br>• Abnormal appearing RV myocardium<br>• RV function (2D wall motion, tissue Doppler measurements, TR gradient, 3D measures)<br>• Abnormalities of right ventricular outflow tract |
| Pulmonary valve | • Pulmonary valve morphology<br>• Pulmonary atresia (functional or anatomy)<br>• Insufficiency<br>• Pulmonary stenosis<br>• Supra-valvar pulmonic stenosis |
| Right atrium | • Atrial septal defect<br>• Right atrial size |
| Left ventricle | • Compression/abnormal geometry<br>• LV diastolic dysfunction<br>• Abnormal septal wall motion<br>• Left ventricular non-compaction |
| Associated lesions | • Ventricular septal defect<br>• Congenitally corrected TGA |

*LV, left ventricle; RV, right ventricle; TGA, transposition of the great arteries; TV, tricuspid valve.*

**Table 1.**
*Checklist for echocardiography in Ebstein anomaly.*

is crucial for decision-making before surgical repair [20]. **Table 1** summarizes the important details elucidated by echocardiogram that need to be evaluated in patients with Ebstein's anomaly.

The most sensitive and specific echocardiographic finding to diagnose Ebstein's anomaly is the apical displacement of the septal leaflet of the tricuspid valve. This can be best seen in apical four-chamber views by echocardiography. When indexed to the body surface area, the distance between the hinge point of the septal leaflet of the tricuspid valve and the anterior leaflet of the mitral valve is called the displacement index. A displacement index above 8 mm/m$^2$ is considered diagnostic of Ebstein's anomaly (**Figure 8**) [21]. However, it is important to note that there are rare cases of "atypical Ebstein" anomaly with normal displacement index [22]. Additionally, there are some cases with a displacement of the anterior leaflet of the tricuspid valve [23]. The evaluation of the tricuspid valve leaflets and attachments can be best performed from an apical view with sweeps posteriorly toward the coronary sinus and anteriorly toward the ventricular outflow tracts. In addition to the displacement, this will clarify septal attachments. It is common to have tethering attachments of the septal and posterior/inferior leaflets of the tricuspid valve to the right ventricular wall. In some cases, the posterior/inferior leaflet is muscularized with muscular attachments to the right ventricular free wall (**Figure 9**). These attachments are called the linear attachments of the tricuspid valve and they have implications for surgical repair [24]. As the anterior leaflet is usually the larger leaflet and is often sail-like, describing this leaflet's

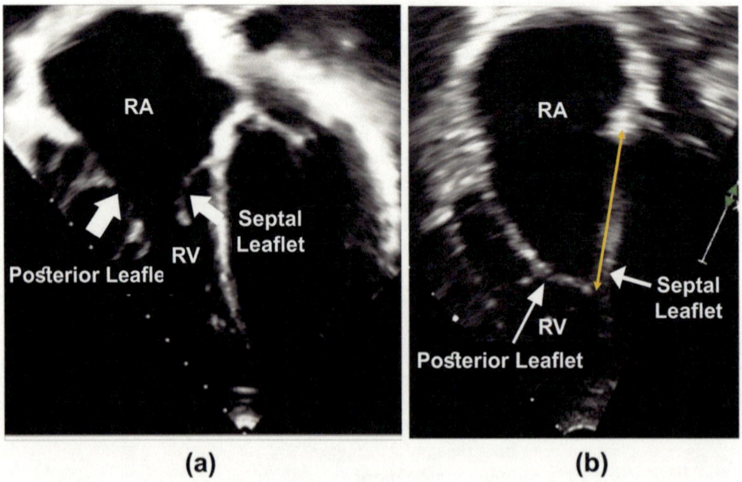


**Figure 8.**
*Apical four-chamber view measuring the displacement of the tricuspid valve which is mild in the left panel and severe in the right panel.*

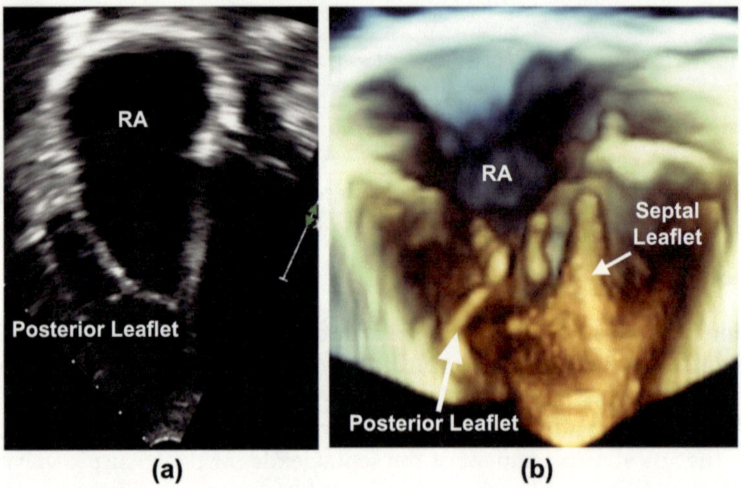


**Figure 9.**
*Muscularization and abnormal attachments of the posterior/inferior leaflet of the tricuspid valve by 2D echocardiography and 3D echocardiography showing the muscular "linear" attachments.*

size and attachments is important to help surgical planning. The parasternal long-axis views allow for an accurate description of the anterior and posterior/inferior leaflets (**Figure 10**). It is important to note that often, there is a fusion of the anterior and posterior/inferior leaflets creating a bileaflet tricuspid valve, as discussed above. Three-dimensional echocardiography can give important insights into the valve anatomy in many patients and should be used when possible. The tricuspid valve is also often severely rotated toward the right ventricular outflow tract, and this can be seen by parasternal long and short axis views (**Figure 11**). Additional important features include the annular size, which is often dilated. Also, muscularization and dysplasia of the tricuspid valve leaflets should be evaluated.

After evaluating the anatomical features of the tricuspid valve, it is important to evaluate the tricuspid valve function using multiple views. Grading of the tricuspid

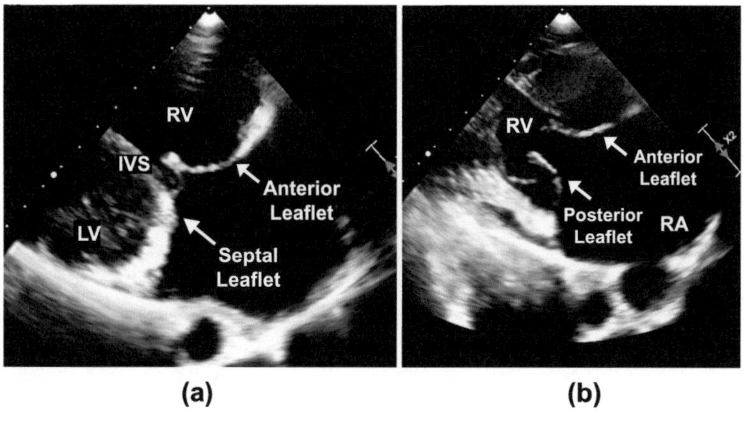


**Figure 10.**
*Parasternal long-axis view with a focus on the tricuspid valve showing the anterior and septal leaflet on the left panel and the posterior/inferior and anterior leaflet on the right panel.*

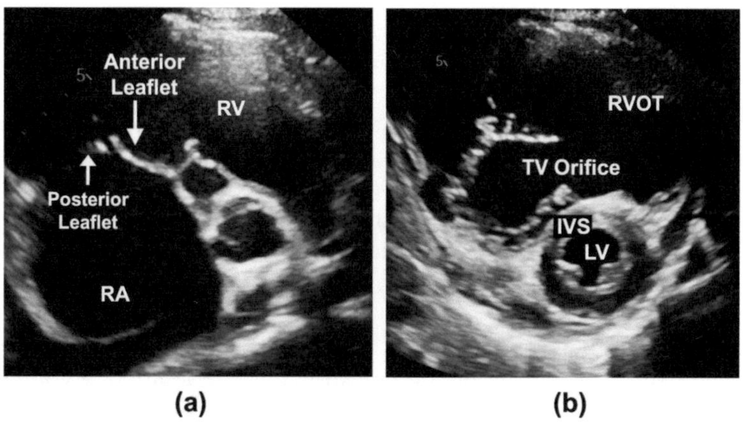


**Figure 11.**
*Parasternal short axis view showing the anatomy of the tricuspid valve leaflets and the rotation of the tricuspid valve orifice toward the right ventricular outflow tract. LV: left ventricle, RVOT: right ventricular outflow tract, TV: tricuspid valve.*

regurgitation depends on the width of the vena contracta and can be challenging in the malformed valve. Using multiple views helps to clarify the severity of tricuspid regurgitation. The classification can be graded as trivial, mild, moderate, or severe. A width below 3 mm in multiple views is considered mild, while a width of more than 7 mm is considered severe (**Figure 12**). It is important to note that these criteria are derived from older patients and may not apply to the infant. Furthermore, the evaluation can be challenging when multiple jets exist. In infants, the percentage of the vena contract width to the tricuspid valve annulus is used with a width below 10% considered as mild while above 30% considered as severe [25]. It is also important to note that the orientation of the regurgitant jet can be unusual due to the rotation of the valve and thus using multiple views and sweeps will be essential to clarify the inflow and regurgitation jets. By continuous wave doppler, the tricuspid regurgitation jet velocity is reported as a measure of the ability of the right ventricle to generate pressure. Also, evaluation by Doppler to assess the degree of tricuspid stenosis is

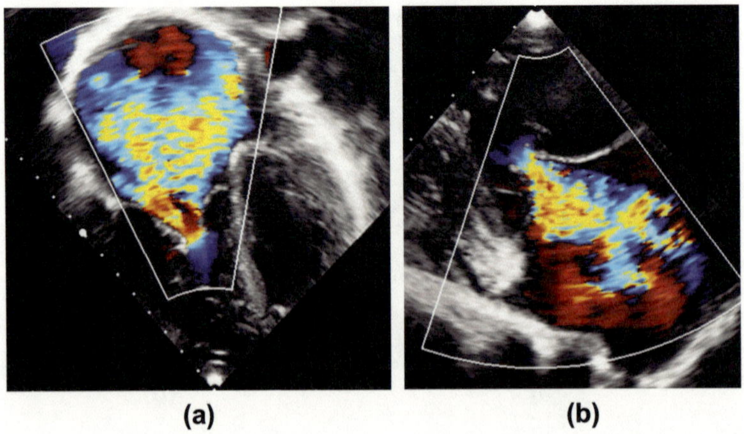

**Figure 12.**
*Apical four chamber and parasternal short-axis views showing a patient with Ebstein anomaly and severe tricuspid regurgitation.*

important, as some patients may have a significant degree of narrowing of the tricuspid valve orifice. Post tricuspid valve repair or replacement, a mild gradient <6 mmHg is common and should be followed.

An echocardiographic grading system for determining the severity of neonatal Ebstein, The Great Ormond Street score (Celermajer index), is calculated by dividing the combined area of the right atrium and atrialized right ventricle by the combined area of the functioning right ventricle and left heart. At the end of diastole, the measures are taken in the apical four-chamber view. Patients with a ratio of <1 had a 92% survival rate and those with a ratio of >1.5 had a 100% mortality rate [26].

For a variety of reasons, quantifying RV function in the Ebstein anomaly is difficult by two-dimensional echocardiography. Although evaluation of RV volume and function is always challenging by 2D echocardiogram, it is even more difficult to assess in Ebstein's anomaly. The RV is frequently enlarged (both the atrialized and functional portions) to the point where imaging it totally in one plane is challenging. Although experienced observers may classify right ventricular activity based on qualitative evidence, intraobserver and interobserver variability is very common. To assess ventricular function, the fractional area change (FAC) of the RV can be calculated. This can be determined by tracing the systolic and diastolic areas in the apical four-chamber view or from the systolic and diastolic areas in the apical four-chamber image. This is limited by the inability to visualize the dilated RV in one image in Ebstein patients [25, 27]. Tricuspid Annular Plane Systolic Excursion (TAPSE) has also been used to evaluate the right ventricular function and poses a challenge in Ebstein's anomaly given the abnormal tricuspid valve annulus and morphology. Tissue Doppler systolic wave S′ of the tricuspid valve has similar challenges [28].

The atrial septum should also be evaluated. Atrial septal defect or patent foramen ovale is very common. Evaluating the size and direction of shunting should be performed. This can be best seen from subcostal coronal and sagittal views. Right to left flow across the atrial septum may result in desaturation at rest or with exercise [29].

The right ventricular outflow tract should also be carefully evaluated. In severe Ebstein cases, the RV outflow tract can become a large part of the functional right ventricle. The function of the pulmonary valve should be evaluated for pulmonary stenosis and regurgitation. This can be achieved from parasternal and subcostal views. There may be true or functional pulmonary valve atresia; the latter is common especially in the immediate neonatal period when there is transient pulmonary hypertension. The presence of a pulmonary insufficiency jet on color Doppler imaging would indicate the functional type of the pulmonary valve atresia.

### 6.2 Cardiac magnetic resonance imaging

Multimodality imaging can provide crucial preoperative information, such as a functional and structural assessment of the right ventricle and the tricuspid valve anomaly. This data helps with surgical planning and preoperative counseling. Multimodality imaging can provide personalized details of distinct components of the tricuspid valve. While echocardiography provides correct valvar anatomical details and assessment of right ventricular pressure, cardiac magnetic resonance (CMR) enables a more accurate evaluation of the regurgitant fraction and right ventricular function, which complements the information provided by echocardiography.

Before the cone operation, CMR enables functional and anatomical examination of the RV and tricuspid valve abnormality, which is crucial for surgical planning [30]. Preoperative CMR offered extra information in more than three-quarters of patients, according to a study by Johnson et al., with 69% of the findings changing surgical therapy [31] . Leaflet attachments of the posterior/inferior and anterior leaflets to the RV wall can also be assessed using CMR. There are two types of attachments—focal attachments and linear attachments. Normal attachments, such as focal attachments, allow unobstructed communication between the atrialized and functional RV. Linear attachments occur when the leaflet is completely or partially attached to a muscle shelf at the joint (**Figure 13**).

Additionally, CMR can measure the degree of displacement and rotation of the tricuspid valve and can also measure the Great Ormond Street Hospital score

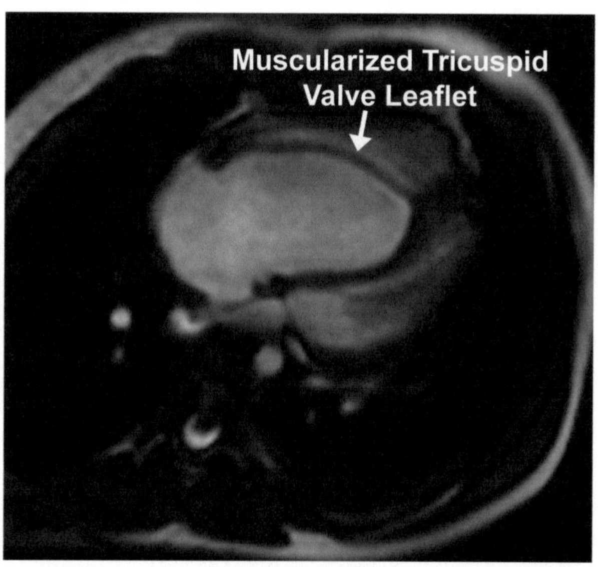


**Figure 13.**
*Cardiac MRI image showing the muscularization of the tricuspid valve leaflet on a four-chamber view.*

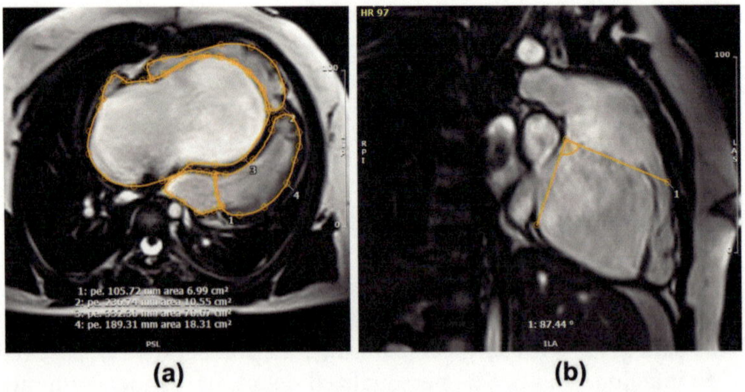


**Figure 14.**
*Cardiac MRI image in four-chamber view showing the calculation of the great Ormond street hospital index using the right atrium and atrialized right ventricle area divided by the sum of the functional right ventricle, left atrium, and left ventricle.*

(**Figure 14**). Most importantly, CMR gives an accurate assessment of chamber size including atrialized and functional right ventricle and RV function. CMR is the gold standard for RV size and function and overcomes the limitations of 2D echocardiography to measure RV size and function.

### 6.3 Computed tomography (CT)

CT provides excellent spatial resolution and fast image acquisition. This makes it ideal to image the coronary arteries and vascular anatomy. CT scans are used frequently in procedural planning for a ductus arteriosus stent [32]. The downside of CT scans is exposured to radiation. With improved CT technology using lower radiation and better temporal resolution.

## 7. Surgical treatment

### 7.1 Historical evolution

In the beginning, the surgical procedures for Ebstein's anomaly treatment included systemic-pulmonary anastomosis (Blalock-Taussig and Potts-Smith) closure of atrial septal defect, and anastomosis of the superior vena cava to the right pulmonary artery (Glenn operation, bidirectional cavopulmonary shunt (BCPS)) [33–36].

In 1960, Weinberg et al. reported the first successful Glenn operation for Ebstein's anomaly [36]. However, despite the reported improvement of cyanosis and reductions in the patients' symptoms, Weinberg et al. were cautious in their conclusions, leaving open questions regarding the procedure's effectiveness.

In 1962, Barnard and Schrire reported valve replacement in a patient with Ebstein's anomaly who was the first survivor of tricuspid valve regurgitation correction [37]. In this procedure, part of the valve prosthesis ring was sutured in the right atrium proximally to the coronary sinus—a maneuver intended to avoid atrioventricular block.

In 1964, Hardy et al. [38] reported the first successful performance of tricuspid valve repair with transverse plication of the RV atrialized portion. The technique utilized by Hardy et al. had been previously described by Hunter and Lillehei in 1956 [39]. Bahnson et al., at the University of Pittsburgh, published the successful application of the same repair technique and described important anatomical findings in Ebstein's anomaly specimens in 1965 [40].

The tricuspid valve replacement presented less-than-ideal results with 54% mortality reported by the international cooperative study published in 1974 [41]. Similarly, poor results were also reported by Lillehei et al. [42] and in the published experience of the Mayo Clinic [43].

Danielson et al. developed a modification of Hardy's technique, to which was added the posterior tricuspid annuloplasty and the right atrium reduction plasty [44]. Similar to Hunter and Lilelehei's technique, this procedure comprises transverse plication of the atrialized portion of the RV, leading to an approximation of the displaced leaflets and the true tricuspid annulus, obliterating the atrialized right ventricle. Next, the posterior part of the tricuspid annulus is plicated to further reduce the tricuspid annulus circumference. This technique became one of the most used surgical repair techniques for the treatment of Ebstein's anomaly. The Mayo Clinic group accumulated a great deal of experience with Danielson's procedure, however, 36–65% of cases still required tricuspid valve replacement [45–47].

In 2006, the Mayo Clinic reported their 30-year experience with the treatment of 186 children under 12 years old with Ebstein's anomaly [48]. Valve repair using Danielson's technique had a mortality rate of only 5.8% but this repair was possible in only 52 patients (28%), highlighting the limitations of this procedure. In 117 patients (62%), the TV was replaced by prosthesis, while other approaches were used in the remaining 17 children [48].

In 1988, Carpentier et al. [11] described a new technique for valve repair. In contrast to the transverse plication of the atrialized right ventricular chamber described by Danielson et al. (19), Carpentier's procedure involved vertical plication of the atrialized right ventricle. Furthermore, they brought the tricuspid valve leaflets to the anatomically correct level, thus achieving good right ventricular morphology. The tricuspid valve annulus was remodeled and reinforced with a prosthetic ring.

Carpentier's group applied this procedure to the vast majority of anatomical presentations of the disease, but their initial series showed a high hospital mortality rate of 14%, as well as frequent long-term complications [11]. The experience of the Carpentier group, representing the second-largest published series, included an overall mortality rate of 9% [49].

Quaegebeur et al. [50] performed a slight modification in this operation without the use of prosthetic ring. They reported that there was no hospital death, but still observed a high incidence of moderate and severe tricuspid regurgitation.

Many additional surgical techniques were developed, but the wide variety of anatomical and pathophysiological presentations of Ebstein's anomaly makes it difficult to achieve uniform results with surgical repair. Among them, we highlighted the Hetzer and the Sebening procedures [51, 52]. Some of these techniques were used to treat many patients and are still used in a few centers and in specific anatomical situations.

Sarris et al. [53] reported the collective results of 179 operations from 13 institutions associated with the European Congenital Heart Surgeons Association, which showed a 13.3% in-hospital mortality rate. However, it should be noted that this rate included operations in newborns, which constitute a higher-risk group. Despite using a variety of available TV repair techniques, they accomplished tricuspid valve repair in only 27.3% of patients, with a hospital mortality rate of 7.1% for this procedure.

### 7.2 The Da Silva Cone procedure

Starting in 1989, we developed and routinely used a new surgical technique that was initially called conical reconstruction of the TV [54]. The surgical goals of this method included undoing most of the tricuspid valve anatomical defects that occurred during embryological development and creating a cone-like structure from all available leaflet tissue. This procedure is illustrated in **Figure 15** and aimed to cover 360° of the right AV junction with leaflet tissue, allowing leaflet-to-leaflet coaptation [55]. The result is intended to mimic the normal TV anatomy, with leaflet-to-leaflet coaptation, in contrast to previously applied procedures in which a monocusp valve coapts with the ventricular septum muscle [11, 44, 50, 51].

The first 40 patients who underwent this new procedure had a 2.5% mortality rate and none required tricuspid valve replacement. Early postoperative echocardiograms showed a significant reduction of TV regurgitation, while the medium-term follow-up examinations showed substantial clinical improvement and a low incidence of reoperation [56]. We next performed a study with a larger number of patients and longer follow-up [57], with a focus on investigating the need for valve replacement and the recurrence of TV valve failure, which are the problems observed with the techniques of Danielson and Carpentier, respectively [11, 44, 45]. There were four deaths in 52 enrolled patients (7.69%) during the 57 months of mean follow-up with improved tricuspid regurgitation. In addition, the functional area of the right ventricle increased from 8.53 $cm^2/m^2$ to 21.01 $cm^2/m^2$ after surgery [57].

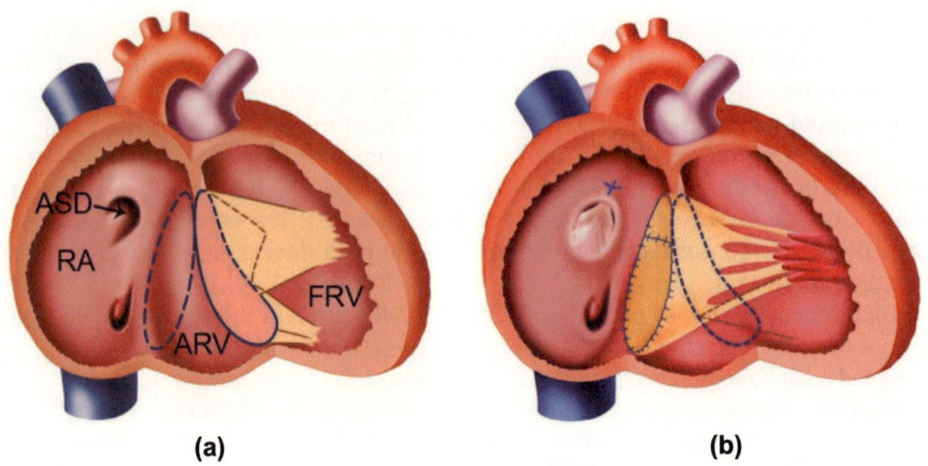


**Figure 15.**
*Ebstein's anomaly heart illustration (a) shows the displacement of the septal and posterior leaflets of the tricuspid valve, dividing the right ventricle into two chambers—atrialized right ventricle (proximal to the tricuspid valve) and the functional right ventricle (distal to the tricuspid valve). The cone procedure illustration (b) depicts the tricuspid valve leaflet mobilized and reconstructed in a cone-like shape and reattached to the normal atrioventricular junction, and the atrial septal defect closed in a valved fashion with a single stitch. ASD = atrial septal defect, RA = right atrium, ARV = atrialized right ventricle, functional right ventricle (Modified with permission from reference [55]).*

Below, we review the surgical maneuvers that we have used to obtain the best functional tricuspid valve repair in several anatomical variations of Ebstein's anomaly.

### 7.3 Surgical technique

The operation is performed via median sternotomy, with the institution of a cardiopulmonary bypass through aortic and bicaval cannulation. For myocardial protection, moderate systemic hypothermia (25–28°C) and cold antegrade blood cardioplegia are used, and a subsequent cardioplegia dose is applied at a suitable interval during the cross-clamp period. The main pulmonary artery can be closed by snare placement to maintain a dry RV during valve repair. This also facilitates examination of the TV after repair, when the RV is filled with a saline solution via a bulb syringe or catheter placed inside the RV [58].

The main steps of the cone operation are described below:

*Step 1: Exposure and assessment of the tricuspid valve.*

This is accomplished by transverse right atriotomy with the placement of stay sutures just above the true valve annulus at the 10, 12, and 3 o'clock positions. The sutures at the 10 and 12 o'clock positions go through the pericardium to avoid annular plane distortion. The left heart is vented by the insertion of a catheter across the patent foramen ovale (PFO) or atrial septal defect (ASD).

*Step 2: Mobilization of the tricuspid valve.*

The surgical methods used to achieve TV mobilization in cases of Ebstein's anomaly are chosen according to the degree of anterior leaflet tethering, septal leaflet size, degree of delamination failure of the inferior and septal leaflets, and the axis of the tricuspid opening in relation to the right ventricle outflow tract (RVOT) and to the RV apex. TV mobilization is accomplished by complete sectioning of the abnormal tethering tissues between the tricuspid leaflets and ventricular wall, leaving the leaflet tissues attached to the ventricle only at its distal margin (by normal papillary muscle, cords, or directly to muscle). In most cases, the majority of leaflet tissue is detached circumferentially, except at the 10–12 o'clock positions. This portion usually is attached to the true annulus without tethering to the ventricular wall, thus allowing free movement. In special situations, the leaflets are detached in the full circumference, allowing complete mobilization of the valve. Aggressive detachment of the leaflet down to its distal point is a critical component of this procedure, to free an adequate amount of tissue for cone construction. This also allows sufficient mobility of the leaflet body in the constructed cone, enabling adequate movement during systole and closure with a good coaptation surface.

The anterior and inferior leaflets of the tricuspid valve are mobilized as a single piece (**Figure 16**), starting with an incision at its proximal attachment to the atrioventricular junction (12 o'clock position) and moving clockwise, toward the displaced inferior leaflet. The incision terminates when the inferior leaflet is completely released from its abnormal proximal attachment to the RV wall. This step provides access to the space between these leaflets and the RV wall, allowing the sectioning of all abnormal papillary muscle, myocardial bridges, and chordal tissues that tether these leaflets to the RV wall. The anterior papillary muscle, which is usually positioned at the anteroposterior commissure, must be freed from its more proximal attachment to the RV wall, retaining only the supports near the RV apex. In some cases, the posterior leaflet must be completely released from its abnormal attachments to the RV to allow its medial rotation to join the septal leaflet, composing the septal aspect of the cone.

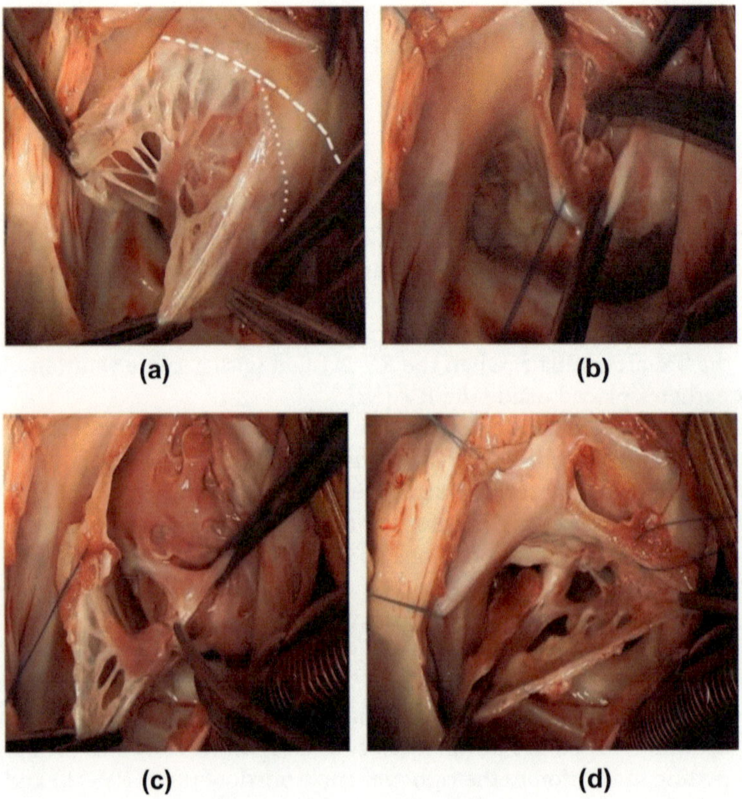

**Figure 16.**
*Anterior and posterior leaflets of the tricuspid valve mobilized as a single piece. (a) Anterior and posterior leaflets anatomy—dotted line shows the displaced and the dashed line shows the true tricuspid annulus, (b) anterior leaflet mobilization, (c) section of posterior leaflet proximal connection to RV wall, and (d) the completely mobilized anterior and posterior leaflets (with permission from reference [58]).*

The TV anteroseptal commissure is approached with the goal of creating a space between the ventricular septum and the septal aspect of the cone, and of moving the opening axis of the tricuspid valve toward the RV apex. An incision is made at the proximal attachment line of the anterior leaflet, approximately 1 cm anterior to the anteroseptal commissure. This incision is continued counterclockwise down to the septal leaflet, which is mobilized to its lateral limit (**Figure 17**). Stay sutures are placed at the leaflet's proximal edge, exposing the subvalvular apparatus of the septal aspect of the anterior leaflet, septal leaflet, and the anteroseptal commissure. The tissues holding the proximal portion of these leaflets to the septum are divided. If the tricuspid valve opens toward the RV outflow tract, it is necessary to mobilize or cut the papillary muscle abnormally attached to the RVOT. The medial papillary muscle is usually related to the anterior and septal leaflet at its commissure, but in some cases, it is fused to the septum and can be deeply freed improving the mobility of that area of the future cone.

*Step 3: Cone construction.*

The cone is constructed using all available mobilized tissue, via the vertical suturing of leaflets—both inferior to septal and septal to anterior. A 5-0 polypropylene running suture technique is used for adults, while a 6-0 polypropylene interrupted suture

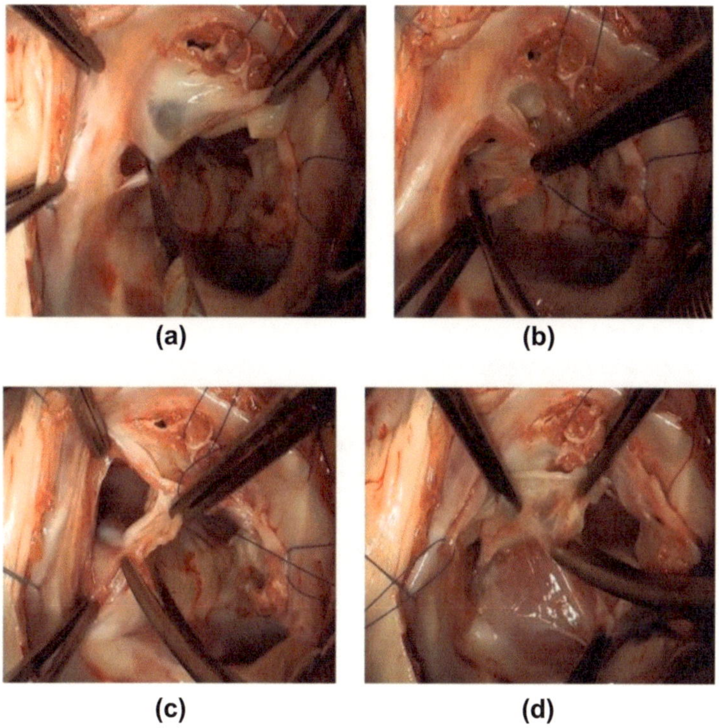

**Figure 17.**
*Anteroseptal commissure mobilization. (a) An incision is made at the proximal attachment line of the anterior leaflet continues anticlockwise (b), mobilizes the medial papillary muscle (c), and reaches the septal leaflet (d), which is mobilized as deep as possible (with permission from reference [58]).*

technique is applied in children. The cone tends to be narrower posteriorly where there is typically less available leaflet tissue, and thus this area must be widened by vertical incision and horizontal suturing of the leaflet tissue in the constructed cone. The septal leaflet is incorporated into the cone such that the septal part of the cone is longer than the septal vertical distance between the final TV hinge line to its distal attachment to the ventricular septum. Importantly, this allows the septal component of the cone to move anteriorly in the process of coaptation with the anterior component of the cone during systole. Furthermore, this prevents tension at the suture line in the septal aspect of the annular attachment of the cone. If there is not enough leaflet tissue, a piece of the autologous pericardium can be added to this region.

The principal methods of septal leaflet incorporation into the cone are as follows:

1. Placing a vertical suture to join the septal leaflet superior edge to the septal edge of the anterior leaflet, followed by the placement of a second suture line uniting the septal leaflet inferior edge with the lateral edge of the posterior leaflet (**Figure 18a–c**). This approach is used for septal leaflets that are large after having been mobilized.

2. Combining the septal leaflet with the completely detached posterior leaflet. These leaflet plication and combining maneuvers increase the cone's depth and reduce its proximal circumference (**Figure 18d** and **e**).

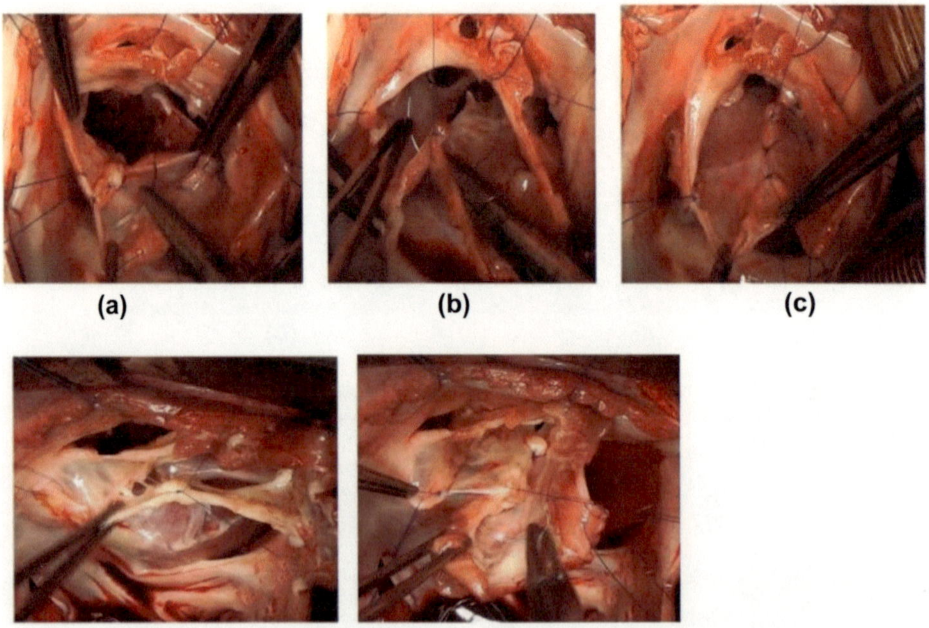


**Figure 18.**
*Septal leaflet incorporation: (a) a vertical suture joins the septal leaflet superior edge to the medial edge of the anterior leaflet, (b) and (c) a second suture line unites the septal leaflet inferior edge to the lateral edge of the posterior leaflet. In cases with a small septal leaflet, it is combined with the completely detached posterior leaflet by a vertical suture (d), followed by a horizontal suture (e). V = vertical suture, H = horizontal suture (with permission from reference [58]).*

*Step 4: Plication of the right ventricle and the true tricuspid annulus.*

This step begins with vertical plication of the thin and attenuated RV-free wall. This portion of the atrialized RV is usually aneurysmal and its limits are defined by the triangle formed by the line of attachment of the displaced inferior tricuspid leaflet, the posterior ventricular septal edge, and the posterolateral area of the true tricuspid annulus. RV plication begins with the placement of a 4-0 polypropylene stitch at the distal apex of this triangular-shaped area, and the suture is continued toward the atrioventricular junction, excluding all of the aneurysmal atrialized RV. Initially, for vertical RV plication, we used a 4-0 polypropylene running suture in two layers with gentle superficial bites to avoid coronary injury or distortion. Recently, we modified this technique, placing interrupted 4.0 polypropylene sutures in multiple places to achieve the vertical plication of the RV atrialized portion. This interrupted suture technique is more often used in children. The vertical plication reduces the true tricuspid annulus at the atrioventricular junction. If further reduction is required, sutures are placed first at the anteroseptal and then at the anteroposterior position of the true tricuspid annulus. The true tricuspid annulus must be reduced such that it matches the proximal circumference of the cone. These multiple plications are important to prevent the right coronary artery distortion or kinking that can occur with a large TV annular reduction at a single site. Additional plication with interrupted sutures is applied to the area where the leaflets were tethered to the RV wall, to prevent anterior wall bulging and dilation of the RV. This maneuver mimics the usual trabeculation of the RV.

*Step 5: Fenestration of the Cone apex.*

The linear attachment of the leaflets can cause obstruction of blood inflow to the RV. To prevent obstruction, fenestrations of the 1/3 distal attachments of the leaflets and division of papillary muscles are usually applied.

*Step 6: Cone attachment to the true tricuspid annulus.*

The cone is attached proximally to the true annulus over 360 degrees and with no tension in the horizontal or vertical plane (**Figures 19** and **20**). The proximal cone circumference must be correctly matched to the true annular dimension. If necessary, the true annulus can be further reduced by separate plication at 2–3 o'clock and 9 o'clock, and the cone proximal circumference can be reduced by leaflet plication. The initial attachment and assessment are performed with the placement of 5-0 polypropylene single sutures to achieve an even distribution of the valve in the tricuspid annulus. The suture line is then completed with a running suture. To reduce the risk of heart block, special care should be taken when suturing the area of the annulus just medial to the coronary sinus. In this area, the valve can be sutured in a proximal position, in the Todaro's tendon. In patients with a fragile adult-size annulus, the use of a prosthetic ring may be considered for reinforcement.

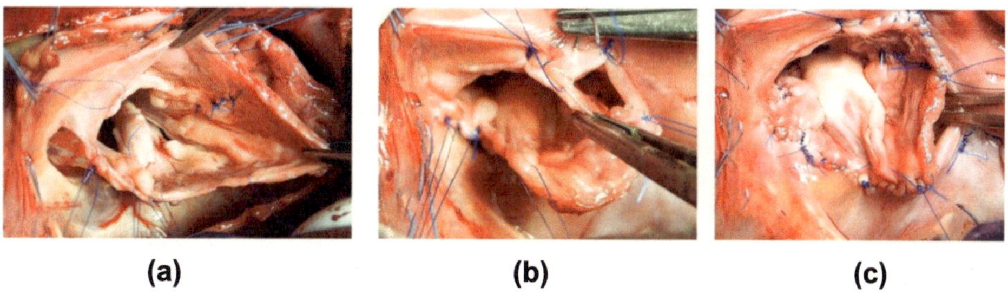


**Figure 19.**
*Cone attachment to the true tricuspid annulus. The constructed cone (a) is reattached to the true tricuspid annulus starting at the anterior position (b) and completing the attachment (c), taking superficial bites when suturing near the atrioventricular node area (arrow) (with permission from reference [58]).*

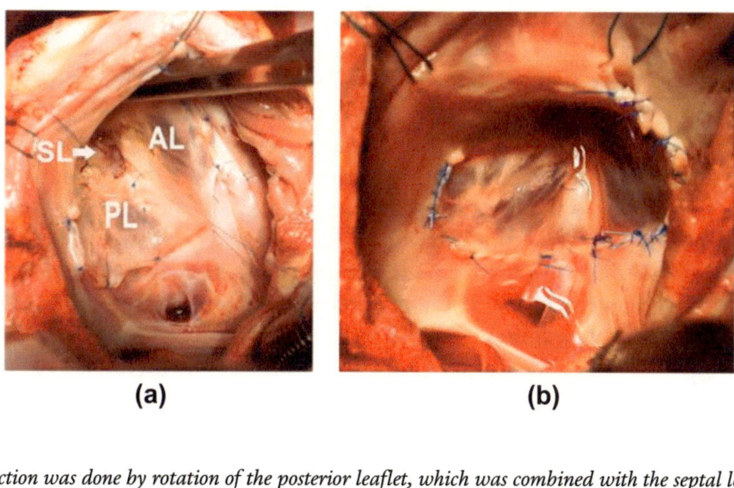


**Figure 20.**
*Cone construction was done by rotation of the posterior leaflet, which was combined with the septal leaflet (a), before attachment to the true tricuspid annulus (b). AL = anterior leaflet, PL = posterior leaflet and SL = septal leaflet (with permission from reference [58]).*

*Step 7: Atrial septal defect treatment.*

The ASD/PFO are closed in a valved fashion, such that blood can be shunted from right to left in the event of postoperative RV failure. The opening size of the resulting orifice should be proportional to the degree of RV dysfunction or enlargement. This can be accomplished with the single-stitch technique in cases of PFO or by using a polytetrafluoroethylene (PTFE) patch with an extension flap positioned inside the left atrium to allow unidirectional blood flow toward the left atrium. In cases of severe RV dysfunction, the single-stitch technique (**Figure 20**) can be performed with placement near the PFO anterior corner, which will result in a less restrictive PFO. In cases of RV dysfunction, some authors recommend the bidirectional Glenn procedure as an adjunct to Ebstein's anomaly repair [53, 59–62]. We have considered using the Glenn procedure in some patients, as we will describe in the neonatal section.

### 7.4 Special anatomic types of Ebstein's anomaly

In some anatomical situations, the three leaflets are connected at the commissures and there is a well-formed distal attachment of the TV to the RV. In such cases, the TV leaflets are mobilized from their displaced hinge line and the TV is released from its abnormal connections to the RV wall. Next, some plications are made at the distal and proximal edges of the TV, reducing its proximal and distal circumferences, and widening the septal and posterior leaflets to give it a cone shape.

The cone technique can also be used to treat patients presenting with Ebstein's anomaly with Carpentier's type D anatomy. **Figure 21** depicts one of our patients who was successfully repaired by taking down the leaflets as a single piece, retaining only the distal direct attachment of the leaflet to the RV. Vertical fenestrations were provided at the distal third of this large leaflet. Then the lateral and medial edges of this leaflet were sutured together, creating a cone-like structure. As in all other cases, the cone was revised and any holes/fenestrations in the proximal 2/3 of the cone's membranous tissues were closed to achieve a similar circumferential depth and to prevent regurgitation leaks. Furthermore, natural, or surgically created fenestrations should be present at the distal 1/3 of the cone to permit unrestricted forward blood flow in diastole.

### 7.5 Important notes on Da Silva cone technique

The mechanism of tricuspid insufficiency in Ebstein's anomaly is usually related to restrictive leaflet movements. This occurs due to failure of leaflet delamination that results in more distal hinge line attachment to the RV, as well as to the presence of muscular bridges and abnormal papillary muscles that tether the TV leaflets to the RV wall, restricting their movements. Creating a competent tricuspid valve using the cone technique requires extensive mobilization of the displaced or tethered leaflets. Otherwise, the repair will result in leaflet coaptation failure or excessive tension in the leaflet suture line due to pulling of the leaflet that remained improperly attached to the free RV wall, which will be subject to strong tension when the RV is filled. An understanding of these concepts is essential to minimize the incidence of tricuspid insufficiency after the cone procedure and to prevent postoperative dehiscence of the suture line due to diastolic tension. The septal leaflet is frequently incorporated into the septal aspect of the cone, in combination with the posterior tricuspid leaflet. This is a very important component of the cone technique, as it helps prevent both stenosis and insufficiency of the tricuspid valve.

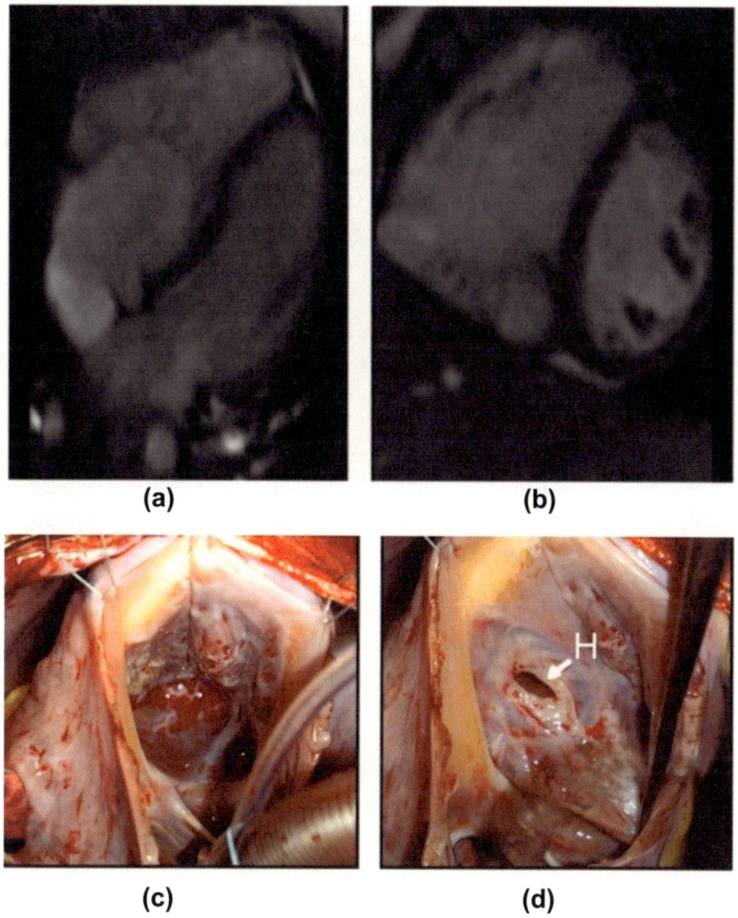


**Figure 21.**
*Preoperative magnetic resonance images and intraoperative photos depicts the heart's anatomy of a 4-year-old girl with type D Ebstein's anomaly (Carpentier's classification). Images (a) (b), and (c) show that the tricuspid valve leaflets are tethered to the right ventricle wall and image d shows that there is only a small hole-H communicating the atrialized to the functional right ventricle (with permission from reference [58]).*

## 7.6 Bidirectional Glenn procedure to improve postoperative cardiac output

It is expected that some RV dysfunction will be evident early after the cone procedure due to RV wall damage related to surgical maneuvers superimposed on varying degrees of RV impairment from the Ebstein's malformation itself. Additionally, myocardial injury may be caused by the extended ischemic time required to perform this somewhat complex operation. With this in mind, we have routinely used a valved ASD that allows blood flow from the right to the left atrium, aiming to reduce RV preload and increase LV preload, thereby helping to prevent low cardiac output due to severe RV dysfunction in the early postoperative period. In most patients, the ASD stays functionally closed from the beginning of the postoperative course. However, approximately 10% of cases evolve with right-to-left blood shunting that can cause a substantial drop in oxygen saturation. In such cases, oxygen saturation usually increases in a few days as RV function improves. Additionally, the resulting RV decompression may prevent excessive tension at the tricuspid valve, decreasing the risk of suture dehiscence and TV regurgitation.

In some studies, the problems related to postoperative RV dysfunction have been addressed by diverting the superior caval blood flow to the right pulmonary artery. Chauvaud et al. [59] used this bidirectional cavopulmonary shunt (BCPS)—also called the Glenn procedure—as an adjunctive procedure to Carpentier's operation in patients with Ebstein's anomaly and severe right ventricular dysfunction (36% of procedures). They reported that this combination of procedures led to improved results. Other studies have also reported the use of this technique to reduce RV preload in cases of severe RV dysfunction, thus significantly reducing mortality caused by RV failure [60, 61]. Quinonez et al. [62] also reported the creation of a BCPS as an adjunctive procedure with surgical treatment of Ebstein's anomaly in 14 patients from the Mayo Clinic (TV replacement in 13 and TV repair in 1). In most cases, this approach was planned in anticipation of RV failure, but it was also sometimes performed as a salvage procedure when faced with postoperative hemodynamic instability. Considering the serious clinical situation of the included patients, the study results were excellent with only one death, outlining the importance of this procedure for a subset of patients. Liu et al. [63] also reported the use of the BCPS procedure in addition to the cone operation in a series of young patients. This group applied BCPS procedure to 67% of patients with Ebstein's anomaly (20 of 30), which drew our attention. However, their series of young patients had good clinical outcomes at mid-term follow-up. We think this method can be used in children to improve pulmonary circulation in case of residual tricuspid regurgitation after the cone repair. We also believe that it is important to employ one of these two methods after the cone operation to prevent low postoperative cardiac output and to protect the dysfunctional RV from distension. We preferentially use the valved closure of ASD. Despite initial cyanosis in some patients and the possibility of paradoxical thromboembolism, RV dysfunction is completely or partially reversible with time and, consequently, oxygen saturation progressively improves [57]. While the BCPS has the advantage of providing better oxygenation, we do not routinely use it because it may be associated with pulsations of the head and neck veins and other complications [61]. In case of low oxygen saturation (<75%) we add a BCPS for older patients or a small (3.0-mm) modified Blalock-Taussig (BT) shunt. We tend to anticoagulated patients who present a dilated RV and/or right-to-left atrial shunting.

The cone procedure for reconstruction of the TV in Ebstein's malformation usually provides a full coaptation of the leaflets, resulting in effective and durable tricuspid regurgitation repair in the majority of patients. Therefore, its use has been expanded to patients who previously underwent other types of Ebstein's anomaly treatment.

### 7.7 Surgical treatment in neonatal Ebstein's anomaly

Despite recent medical advances, it remains difficult to manage critically ill neonates with Ebstein's anomaly. A multicenter study conducted at excellent hospitals reported that surgical or catheter interventions carried high mortality (30%) in newborns with critical Ebstein's anomaly [16]. Additionally, multivariable analysis showed that the lack of antegrade pulmonary valve flow or the presence of pulmonary regurgitation at the time of diagnosis were powerful hemodynamic risk indicators [16]. That study emphasized the necessity for careful surgical management of this group of patients.

Newborns with Ebstein's anomaly presenting a dependency on prostaglandins or mechanical ventilation, worsening cyanosis or heart failure, anatomic pulmonary atresia, a circular shunt, will require surgical intervention during the neonatal period [7].

The primary cone repair of neonatal Ebstein's anomaly is a complex procedure due to the delicate valve tissues and the associated lung immaturity. It can be applied only to a small subgroup of older (over 2-week-old), and stable patients with a favorable TV morphology, such as a large and mobile anterior leaflet, a reasonably sized functional RV with good systolic function, and good pulmonary artery and valve anatomy [64]. In that situation, the procedure by an experienced surgeon would be indicated to correct a severe regurgitation that would limit the pulmonary flow and cause cyanosis. In a few situations, where the tricuspid valve presents more complex anatomy in patients with inadequate forward pulmonary flow, with cyanosis, but without expressive cardiomegaly, or septal impingement to the left ventricle, a PDA stent or a BT shunt can be the initial surgical approach. This stenting procedure has the goal to allow the child to develop the pulmonary circulation and the RV for the next step, which is the Cone procedure applied at 4 or 5 months, resulting in a biventricular repair.

However, the great majority of newborns with Ebstein's anomaly presenting with heart failure should be addressed with the Starnes procedure that, by decompressing the left ventricle and giving more space to the lungs, offers a better outcome for these very sick babies [65].

The surgical palliation with the Starnes procedure consists of excluding the malformed right ventricle with a fenestrated patch sewn at the anatomic level of the tricuspid valve annulus and creation of a systemic to pulmonary artery shunt to provide the pulmonary blood flow. This procedure allows the decompression of the malformed right ventricle, but also ameliorates the septal impingement to the left, with a significant effect on the systemic left ventricle, which reassumes the globular shape after the Starnes. Any pulmonary insufficiency should be contained, and the coronary sinus must stay on the atrial side of the patch to assure effective decompression of the right ventricle. The atrial communication is enlarged and a reduction atrioplasty opens space inside the chest for the lung development [66]. The modified Starnes procedure is adequate for neonates who are hemodynamically unstable, or even on ECMO support. It is usually successful and helps the patients to survive and to prepare them for other more definitive future procedures.

### 7.8 The Da Silva Cone repair after the Starnes procedure

Although usually successful, the Starnes approach excludes the right ventricle from the pulmonary circulation. So, after the Starnes operation, these patients were traditionally committed to the single ventricle repair pathway [67], which leads to the undesirable long-term complications associated with Fontan palliation [68]. However, we have demonstrated that it is possible to rehabilitate the right ventricle after the Starnes procedure in patients with Ebstein's anomaly and pulmonary atresia, achieving 1.5 or two-ventricle repair [69]. We also have shown that in patients with fetal circular shunt physiology who underwent the Starnes procedure as a newborn, it is possible to rehabilitate the RV and the pulmonary valve, resulting in two-ventricle physiology [70], as demonstrated in **Figure 22**.

Bearing in mind that the cone repair can follow the Starnes procedure, we prefer to use a Gore-Tex patch to exclude the RV in the Starnes procedure, because it causes less adhesions, facilitating its taking down during the cone repair. Furthermore, this patch should be sutured above the TV annulus, and in the Todaro's ligament at the

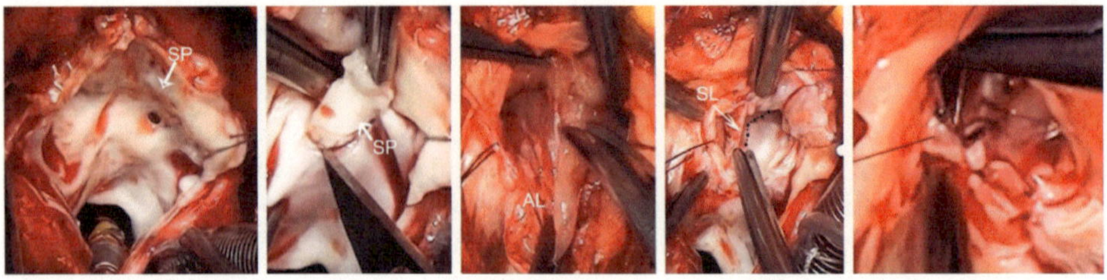


**Figure 22.**
*Intraoperative images of the Da Silva cone repair after the Starnes procedure. (a) Exposure of the tricuspid valve, which is covered with the Starnes patch (SP). (b) Removal of the fenestrated PTFE patch, taking care not to damage the anterior leaflet of the tricuspid valve, which is adjacent to the patch. (c) Extensive tricuspid valve mobilization; this is initiated at the anterior leaflet (AL) hinge line and continues clockwise toward the inferior leaflet; here, the inferior papillary muscle is being cut. (d) A second incision is made near the anteroseptal commissure (arrow); the cut continues counterclockwise to mobilize the medial part of the anterior leaflet and the entire septal leaflet from their proximal attachments. The proximal detachment of the septal leaflet (SL) follows the dotted line. (e) The inferior leaflet is rotated medially, and a vertical interrupted suture unites it with the lateral aspect of the septal leaflet. The resulting cone-shaped structure is sutured to the anatomical tricuspid valve annulus, which completes the cone repair. SP = starnes patch, AL = anterior leaflet, SL = septal leaflet (with permission from reference [58]).*

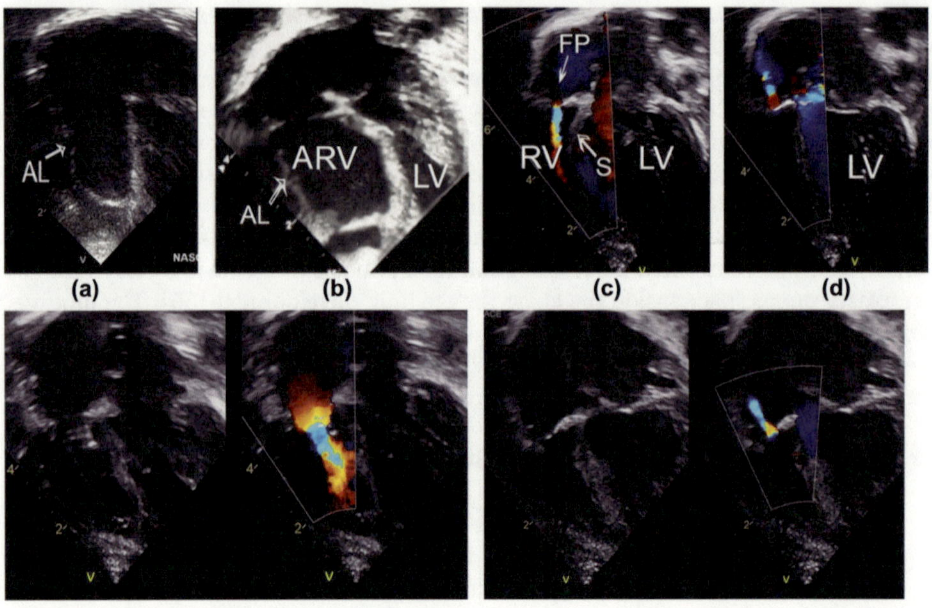


**Figure 23.**
*Serial echocardiograms show cardiac evolution in a four-chamber view. (a, b) Preoperative image shows typical, severe Ebstein's anomaly morphology, with enlarged right heart chambers, and severe downward displacement of septal and inferior leaflets. The ventricular septum is shifted to the left, compressing the left ventricle. (c, d) Postoperative image after the Starnes procedure shows diastolic flow across the fenestration of the right ventricle exclusion patch (FP). Here, the ventricular septum (S) is shifted to the right (arrow); this reduces the area for the right ventricle and provides more space for the left ventricle, which increased in volume and assumed a globular shape. (e, f) Image acquired 3 weeks after biventricular repair shows the results of the Da Silva cone technique; the right ventricle is a good size, and the ventricular septum is in a well-balanced position. (e) The now anatomically positioned tricuspid valve presented good inflow and (f) mild to moderate regurgitation. AL = anterior leaflet of the tricuspid valve, RV = right ventricle, LV = left ventricle, FP = fenestrated polytetrafluoroethylene patch, and S = ventricular septum (**Figure 23c** with permission from reference [70].*

septal area. These technical measures aim to facilitate the patch removal without damaging the TV leaflets or the atrioventricular node at the time of the Da Silva Cone procedure. In **Figure 23**, serial echocardiograms images demonstrate the cardiac evolution of a neonatal Ebstein submitted to the Starnes procedure and later to the Da Silva Cone repair.

## 8. Postoperative care

### 8.1 Hemodynamic management

Neonates may experience low-cardiac-output syndrome after surgical palliation for Ebstein's anomaly. Inotropic support and afterload reduction for support of right ventricular and left ventricular function are necessary. Reduction of right ventricular afterload by decreasing pulmonary vascular resistance protects right ventricular strain and reduces hemodynamically significant tricuspid valve regurgitation. Neonatal patients with Ebstein's anomaly who undergo single ventricular palliation may develop relative pulmonary hypertension or maintain elevated pulmonary vascular resistance and may benefit from inhaled nitric oxide and the use of muscle relaxants, in combination with pain control and sedation. In neonate surgical intervention, leaving an open sternum immediately after cardiopulmonary bypass facilitates ventilation at lower mean airway pressures and decreases right ventricular afterload. The sternum can be closed once improved myocardial function and a decrease in edema have been established.

### 8.2 Left ventricle

Even without associated left ventricular morphological abnormalities, left ventricular function may be compromised due to compression from a dilated atrialized right atrium (**Figure 3b**). Angiographic analysis of 26 patients with Ebstein's anomaly demonstrated seven patients with a decrease in left ventricular diastolic volume (LVEDV <60 ml/m$^2$); 12 patients had increased LVEDV (>80 ml/m$^2$). Eight patients 29 (31%) either with normal or increased LVESV had decreased left ventricular ejection fraction in this study. Patients with a decrease in LVESV had normal left ventricular ejection fraction in this study [71]. Abnormalities of left ventricular morphology involving the myocardium or valves were noted in 39% of Ebstein's anomaly [71], with 18% of patients demonstrating an association with left ventricular non-compaction [72]. Mitral valve prolapse, bicuspid aortic valve, and mitral valve dysplasia, as well as left ventricular systolic dysfunction (7%) and diastolic dysfunction (34%), can be associated with Ebstein's anomaly [72]. A hemodynamically significant left ventricular outflow tract obstruction secondary to the systolic anterior motion of the mitral valve and severe mitral regurgitation was noted in a 52-year-old patient following tricuspid valve replacement and was resolved with esmolol administration [73]. Using three-dimensional models, a global or regional decrease in left ventricular ejection fraction (LVEF) was noted in patients with Ebstein's anomaly (LVEF 41 $\pm$ 7% VS 57 $\pm$ 5%) [74]. In addition, tricuspid regurgitation is negatively correlated with the left ventricular ejection fraction by cardiac magnetic resonance imaging [75]. Rarely, non-apex forming left ventricular anatomy is associated with Ebstein's anomaly, in which, heart transplantation is the only surgical option [76].

### 8.3 Arrhythmia

The downward displacement of the septal leaflet of the tricuspid valve is associated with direct muscular connections in the septal atrioventricular ring resulting in a potential connection for an accessory atrioventricular pathway [77]. Accessory pathways are noted in 10–36% of patients with Ebstein's anomaly [78–80] and most accessory connections are located around the orifice of the malformed tricuspid valve [45, 81]. Delayed ventricular activation with the appearance of a right bundle branch block pattern can be seen in up to 93% of patients with Ebstein's anomaly [80]. In a series of 52 patients with Ebstein's anomaly from Mayo clinic, 34 patients (65%) had arrhythmias preoperatively (supraventricular tachycardia, atrial fibrillation, ventricular arrhythmias, and high-degree atrioventricular block) with perioperative and postoperative arrhythmias noted in 42% of the patients (14 patients had atrial tachyarrhythmia and eight had ventricular arrhythmias) s [82]. Maintenance of sinus rhythm is important to maintaining adequate cardiac output and may necessitate the use of epicardial pacing postoperatively.

### 8.4 Respiratory management

Tanaka et al. reported lung autopsy results from four neonates with Ebstein's anomaly or tricuspid valve dysplasia. Lung hypoplasia or immaturity was not seen in full-term neonates with tricuspid abnormalities unless patients had a concomitant diaphragmatic hernia [83]. Despite an increased cardiothoracic ratio to 92% [83], surgical intervention to relieve tricuspid regurgitation and atrial plication may improve respiratory function by decreasing cardiomegaly and associated lung compression. Strategies to reduce pulmonary vascular resistance and minimize postoperative right ventricular distention and tricuspid regurgitation include the use of supplemental oxygen, inhaled nitric oxide, and ventilation to minimize hypercarbia. Early extubation, if feasible, will reduce intrathoracic pressure and right ventricular afterload.

## 9. Summary

Ebstein's malformation is a condition that results from failure of the septal and inferior leaflets of the tricuspid valve to delaminate from the myocardial wall of the right ventricle which in turn results in the hinge point of the tricuspid valve being located within the right ventricle and not at the annulus. Furthermore, there is variability in the extent to which this failure to delaminate has on the heart. The effects may be limited when this anomaly is mild, but in hearts with more severe Ebstein's anomalies, the rotational appearance of the hinge point of the tricuspid valve is more evident. The clinical presentations vary widely secondary to the abnormal morphology and the tricuspid valve and right ventricle as well as the associated heart defects. Neonatal Ebstein's anomaly is continuous to be challenging. With the improvement in diagnostic methods, surgical treatment, and pre and postoperative care, the patients with a severe form of Ebstein's anomaly still have a chance to undergo two-ventricle repair with good long-term outcomes.

## Acknowledgements

The authors thank Miss Olivia Phillips for her computer assistance in preparing the figures.

## Disclosure

The contributing Authors declare no competing interests in this article.

## Author details

Luciana Da Fonseca Da Silva[1,2], William A. Devine[3], Tarek Alsaied[2,4], Justin Yeh[2,5], Jiuann-Huey Ivy Lin[2,5]* and Jose Da Silva[1,2]

1 Department of Surgery, University of Pittsburgh, Pittsburgh, PA, USA

2 UPMC Children's Hospital of Pittsburgh, Pittsburgh, PA, USA

3 Department of Developmental Biology, University of Pittsburgh, Pittsburgh, PA, USA

4 Division of Pediatric Cardiology, University of Pittsburgh, Pittsburgh, PA, USA

5 Department of Critical Care Medicine and Pediatrics, University of Pittsburgh, PA, USA

*Address all correspondence to: jiuannhuey.lin5@upmc.edu

## References

[1] Attenhofer Jost CH et al. Ebstein's anomaly. Circulation. 2007;**115**(2): 277-285

[2] Ferencz CRJ, Loffredo CA, Magee CA. Epidemiology of congenital heart disease. In: The Baltimore-Washington Infant Study 1981–1989. TX, UK: Futura Publishing Company; 1993. ISBN-10: 0-87993-553-7. ISBN-13: 978-0-87993-553-5

[3] Holst KA et al. Surgical management and outcomes of Ebstein anomaly in neonates and infants: A Society of Thoracic Surgeons congenital heart surgery database analysis. The Annals of Thoracic Surgery. 2018;**106**(3):785-791

[4] Ebstein W. Ueber einen sehr seltenen Fall von Insufficienz der Valvula tricuspidalis, bedingt durch eine angeborene hochgradige Missbildung derselben. Archiv für Anatomie, Physiologie und Wissenschaftliche Medicin. 1866;**33**:238-254

[5] Anderson KR, Lie JT. The right ventricular myocardium in Ebstein's anomaly: A morphometric histopathologic study. Mayo Clinic Proceedings. 1979;**54**(3):181-184

[6] Lamers WH et al. Formation of the tricuspid valve in the human heart. Circulation. 1995;**91**(1):111-121

[7] Sainathan S, da Fonseca da Silva L, da Silva JP. Ebstein's anomaly: Contemporary management strategies. Journal of Thoracic Disease. 2020;**12**(3): 1161-1173

[8] Vettukattil JJ, Bharucha T, Anderson RH. Defining Ebstein's malformation using three-dimensional echocardiography. Interactive Cardiovascular and Thoracic Surgery. 2007;**6**(6):685-690

[9] Saxena A et al. Late noninvasive evaluation of cardiac performance in mildly symptomatic older patients with Ebstein's anomaly of tricuspid valve: Role of radionuclide imaging. Journal of the American College of Cardiology. 1991;**17**(1):182-186

[10] Monibi AA et al. Left ventricular anomalies associated with Ebstein's malformation of the tricuspid valve. Circulation. 1978;**57**(2):303-306

[11] Carpentier A et al. A new reconstructive operation for Ebstein's anomaly of the tricuspid valve. The Journal of Thoracic and Cardiovascular Surgery. 1988;**96**(1):92-101

[12] Anderson KR et al. Morphologic spectrum of Ebstein's anomaly of the heart: A review. Mayo Clinic Proceedings. 1979;**54**(3):174-180

[13] van Engelen K et al. Ebstein's anomaly may be caused by mutations in the sarcomere protein gene MYH7. Netherlands Heart Journal. 2013;**21**(3): 113-117

[14] Hirono K et al. Familial Ebstein's anomaly, left ventricular noncompaction, and ventricular septal defect associated with an MYH7 mutation. The Journal of Thoracic and Cardiovascular Surgery. 2014;**148**(5): e223-e226

[15] Benson DW et al. Mutations in the cardiac transcription factor NKX2.5 affect diverse cardiac developmental pathways. The Journal of Clinical Investigation. 1999;**104**(11):1567-1573

[16] Freud LR et al. Outcomes and predictors of perinatal mortality in fetuses with Ebstein anomaly or

tricuspid valve dysplasia in the current era: A multicenter study. Circulation. 2015;**132**(6):481-489

[17] Patorno E et al. Lithium use in pregnancy and the risk of cardiac malformations. The New England Journal of Medicine. 2017;**376**(23): 2245-2254

[18] Celermajer DS et al. Ebstein's anomaly: Presentation and outcome from fetus to adult. Journal of the American College of Cardiology. 1994; **23**(1):170-176

[19] Freud LR et al. Effect of in utero non-steroidal anti-inflammatory drug therapy for severe Ebstein anomaly or tricuspid valve dysplasia (NSAID therapy for fetal Ebstein anomaly). The American Journal of Cardiology. 2021; **141**:106-112

[20] Booker OJ, Nanda NC. Echocardiographic assessment of Ebstein's anomaly. Echocardiography. 2015;**32**(Suppl. 2):S177-S188

[21] Holst KA, Connolly HM, Dearani JA. Ebstein's anomaly. Methodist DeBakey Cardiovascular Journal. 2019;**15**(2): 138-144

[22] Stephens EH et al. The congenital tricuspid valve spectrum: From Ebstein to dysplasia. World Journal for Pediatric and Congenital Heart Surgery. 2020;**11**(6):783-791

[23] Tsujii N et al. Displacement of the anterior leaflet of the tricuspid valve: Rare variant of Ebstein's anomaly. Pediatrics International. 2016;**58**(8): 775-777

[24] Leung MP et al. Cineangiographic spectrum of Ebstein's malformation: Its relevance to clinical presentation and outcome. Journal of the American College of Cardiology. 1988;**11**(1): 154-161

[25] Eidem BW, O'Leary PW, Cetta F. Echocardiography in Pediatric and Adult Congenital Heart Disease. 3rd edition, PH, USA: LWW; 2014

[26] Celermajer DS et al. Morbid anatomy in neonates with Ebstein's anomaly of the tricuspid valve: Pathophysiologic and clinical implications. Journal of the American College of Cardiology. 1992; **19**(5):1049-1053

[27] Qureshi MY, Sommer RJ, Cabalka AK. Tricuspid valve imaging and intervention in pediatric and adult patients with congenital heart disease. JACC: Cardiovascular Imaging. 2019; **12**(4):637-651

[28] Lianza AC et al. Right ventricular systolic function after the cone procedure for Ebstein's anomaly: Comparison between echocardiography and cardiac magnetic resonance. Pediatric Cardiology. 2020;**41**(5):985-995

[29] Hasan MN et al. Ebstein's anomaly associated with atrial septal defect and Wolff-Parkinson-White (WPW) syndrome. Mymensingh Medical Journal. 2017;**26**(3):676-679

[30] Beroukhim RS et al. Impact of the cone operation on left ventricular size, function, and dyssynchrony in Ebstein anomaly: A cardiovascular magnetic resonance study. Journal of Cardiovascular Magnetic Resonance. 2018;**20**(1):32

[31] Johnson JT et al. Yield of cardiac magnetic resonance imaging as an adjunct to echocardiography in young infants with congenital heart disease. Pediatric Cardiology. 2014;**35**(6): 1067-1071

[32] Arar Y et al. Pre-procedural CT imaging aids neonatal PDA stenting for ductal-dependent pulmonary blood flow with reduction in overall procedural morbidity. Cardiology in the Young. 2021: 1-6. DOI: 10.1017/S1047951121004133

[33] Goodwin JF, Wynn A, Steiner RE. Ebstein's anomaly of the tricuspid valve. American Heart Journal. 1953;**45**(1): 144-158

[34] Gasul BM et al. Angiocardiography in congenital heart disease correlated with clinical and autopsy findings; a five-year clinical and pathological study of thirty-four cases in infants and young children out of a series of eleven hundred patients, and four hundred twenty-five angiocardiograms. A.M.A. American Journal of Diseases of Children. 1953;**85**(4):404-443

[35] Lev M, Gibson S, Miller RA. Ebstein's disease with Wolff-Parkinson-white syndrome; report of a case with a histopathologic study of possible conduction pathways. American Heart Journal. 1955;**49**(5):724-741

[36] Weinberg M Jr et al. Surgical palliation in patients with Ebstein's anomaly and congenital hypoplasia of the right ventricle. The Journal of Thoracic and Cardiovascular Surgery. 1960;**40**:310-320

[37] Barnard CN, Schrire V. Surgical correction of Ebstein's malformation withprosthetic tricuspid valve. Surgery. 1963;**54**:302-308

[38] Hardy KL et al. Ebstein's anomaly: A functional concept and successful definitive repair. The Journal of Thoracic and Cardiovascular Surgery. 1964;**48**: 927-940

[39] Hunter SW, Lillehei CW. Ebstein's malformation of the tricuspid valve; study of a case together with suggestion of a new form of surgical therapy. Diseases of the Chest. 1958;**33**(3): 297-304

[40] Bahnson HT, Bauersfeld SR, Smith JW. Pathological anatomy and surgical correction of Ebstein's anomaly. Circulation. 1965;**31**(Suppl. 1):3-8

[41] Watson H. Natural history of Ebstein's anomaly of tricuspid valve in childhood and adolescence. An international co-operative study of 505 cases. British Heart Journal. 1974;**36**(5): 417-427

[42] Lillehei CW, Kalke BR, Carlson RG. Evolution of corrective surgery for Ebstein's anomaly. Circulation. 1967;**35** (4 Suppl):I111-I118

[43] McFaul RC et al. Ebstein's malformation. Surgical experience at the Mayo Clinic. The Journal of Thoracic and Cardiovascular Surgery. 1976;**72**(6): 910-915

[44] Danielson GK, Maloney JD, Devloo RA. Surgical repair of Ebstein's anomaly. Mayo Clinic Proceedings. 1979; **54**(3):185-192

[45] Danielson GK et al. Operative treatment of Ebstein's anomaly. The Journal of Thoracic and Cardiovascular Surgery. 1992;**104**(5):1195-1202

[46] Kiziltan HT et al. Late results of bioprosthetic tricuspid valve replacement in Ebstein's anomaly. The Annals of Thoracic Surgery. 1998;**66**(5): 1539-1545

[47] Dearani JA, Danielson GK. Surgical management of Ebstein's anomaly in the adult. Seminars in Thoracic and Cardiovascular Surgery. 2005;**17**(2): 148-154

[48] Boston US et al. Tricuspid valve repair for Ebstein's anomaly in young children: A 30-year experience. The Annals of Thoracic Surgery. 2006;**81**(2): 690-695; discussion 695-6

[49] Chauvaud S, Ebstein's malformation. Surgical treatment and results. The Thoracic and Cardiovascular Surgeon. 2000;**48**(4):220-223

[50] Quaegebeur JM et al. Surgery for Ebstein's anomaly: The clinical and echocardiographic evaluation of a new technique. Journal of the American College of Cardiology. 1991;**17**(3): 722-728

[51] Hetzer R et al. A modified repair technique for tricuspid incompetence in Ebstein's anomaly. The Journal of Thoracic and Cardiovascular Surgery. 1998;**115**(4):857-868

[52] Schmidt-Habelmann P et al. Results of valvuloplasty for Ebstein's anomaly. The Thoracic and Cardiovascular Surgeon. 1981;**29**(3):155-157

[53] Sarris GE et al. Results of surgery for Ebstein anomaly: A multicenter study from the European Congenital Heart Surgeons Association. The Journal of Thoracic and Cardiovascular Surgery. 2006;**132**(1):50-57

[54] Silva JP et al. Ebstein's anomaly: Results of the conic reconstruction of the tricuspid valve. Arquivos Brasileiros de Cardiologia. 2004;**82**(3):212-216

[55] Anderson HN et al. Cone reconstruction in children with Ebstein anomaly: The Mayo Clinic experience. Congenital Heart Disease. 2014;**9**(3): 266-271

[56] da Silva JP et al. The cone reconstruction of the tricuspid valve in Ebstein's anomaly. The operation: Early and midterm results. The Journal of Thoracic and Cardiovascular Surgery. 2007;**133**(1):215-223

[57] Silva JP et al. Cone reconstruction in Ebstein's anomaly repair: Early and long-term results. Arquivos Brasileiros de Cardiologia. 2011;**97**(3):199-208

[58] da Silva JP, da Silva Lda F. Ebstein's anomaly of the tricuspid valve: The cone repair. Seminars in Thoracic and Cardiovascular Surgery. Pediatric Cardiac Surgery Annual. 2012;**15**(1):38-45

[59] Chauvaud S et al. Bi-directional cavopulmonary shunt associated with ventriculo and valvuloplasty in Ebstein's anomaly: Benefits in high risk patients. European Journal of Cardio-Thoracic Surgery. 1998;**13**(5):514-519

[60] Malhotra SP et al. Selective right ventricular unloading and novel technical concepts in Ebstein's anomaly. The Annals of Thoracic Surgery. 2009; **88**(6):1975-1981 discussion 1981

[61] Kopf GS et al, Thirty-year follow- up of superior vena cava-pulmonary artery (Glenn) shunts. The Journal of Thoracic and Cardiovascular Surgery, 1990; **100**(5):662-70. discussion 670-1

[62] Quinonez LG et al. Results of the 1.5-ventricle repair for Ebstein anomaly and the failing right ventricle. The Journal of Thoracic and Cardiovascular Surgery. 2007;**133**(5):1303-1310

[63] Liu J et al. Cone reconstruction of the tricuspid valve in Ebstein anomaly with or without one and a half ventricle repair. The Journal of Thoracic and Cardiovascular Surgery. 2011;**141**(5):1178-1183

[64] Pizarro C, Bhat MA, Temple J. Cone reconstruction and ventricular septal defect closure for neonatal Ebstein's anomaly. Multimedia Manual of

Cardio-Thoracic Surgery. 2012;**2012**: mms014

[65] Starnes VA et al. Ebstein's anomaly appearing in the neonate. A new surgical approach. The Journal of Thoracic and Cardiovascular Surgery. 1991;**101**(6): 1082-1087

[66] Reemtsen BL, Starnes VA. Fenestrated right ventricular exclusion (Starnes' procedure) for severe neonatal Ebstein's anomaly. Operative Techniques in Thoracic and Cardiovascular Surgery. 2008;**13**(2):91-100. https://doi.org/10.1053/j.optechstcvs.2008.03.002

[67] Reemtsen BL et al. Current surgical therapy for Ebstein anomaly in neonates. The Journal of Thoracic and Cardiovascular Surgery. 2006;**132**(6): 1285-1290

[68] Kumar SR et al. Single-ventricle outcomes after neonatal palliation of severe Ebstein anomaly with modified Starnes procedure. Circulation. 2016; **134**(17):1257-1264

[69] Da Silva JP et al. The Da Silva cone operation after the Starnes procedure for Ebstein's anomaly: New surgical strategy and initial results. JTCVS Tech. 2020;**3**: 281-283

[70] Lopes LM et al. Critical Ebstein's anomaly with circular shunt: From successful fetal therapy with non-steroidal anti-inflammatory drugs to biventricular repair using Da Silva cone technique. Cardiology in the Young. 2021;**31**(6):1039-1042

[71] Daliento L et al. Angiographic and morphologic features of the left ventricle in Ebstein's malformation. The American Journal of Cardiology. 1997;**80**(8): 1051-1059

[72] Attenhofer Jost CH et al. Left heart lesions in patients with Ebstein anomaly. Mayo Clinic Proceedings. 2005;**80**(3): 361-368

[73] Rafiq I et al. Severe left ventricular outflow tract obstruction immediately after surgical repair of Ebstein's anomaly. JACC: Case Reports. 2020;**2**(5): 725-731

[74] Goleski PJ et al. The shape and function of the left ventricle in Ebstein's anomaly. International Journal of Cardiology. 2014;**171**(3):404-412

[75] Liu X et al. Morphologic and functional abnormalities in patients with Ebstein's anomaly with cardiac magnetic resonance imaging: Correlation with tricuspid regurgitation. European Journal of Radiology. 2016;**85**(9): 1601-1606

[76] Knott-Craig CJ et al. Surgical decision making in neonatal Ebstein's anomaly: An algorithmic approach based on 48 consecutive neonates. World Journal for Pediatric and Congenital Heart Surgery. 2012;**3**(1):16-20

[77] Frescura C et al. Morphological aspects of Ebstein's anomaly in adults. The Thoracic and Cardiovascular Surgeon. 2000;**48**(4):203-208

[78] Hebe J. Ebstein's anomaly in adults. Arrhythmias: Diagnosis and therapeutic approach. The Thoracic and Cardiovascular Surgeon. 2000;**48**(4): 214-219

[79] Brickner ME, Hillis LD, Lange RA. Congenital heart disease in adults. Second of two parts. The New England Journal of Medicine. 2000;**342**(5): 334-342

[80] Iturralde P et al. Electrocardiographic characteristics of patients with Ebstein's anomaly before and after ablation of an accessory atrioventricular pathway.

Journal of Cardiovascular Electrophysiology. 2006;**17**(12):1332-1336

[81] Ho SY et al. The atrioventricular junctions in Ebstein malformation. Heart. 2000;**83**(4):444-449

[82] Oh JK et al. Cardiac arrhythmias in patients with surgical repair of Ebstein's anomaly. Journal of the American College of Cardiology. 1985;**6**(6): 1351-1357

[83] Tanaka T et al. The histology of the lung in neonates with tricuspid valve disease and gross cardiomegaly due to severe regurgitation. Pediatric Cardiology. 1998;**19**(2):133-138

Section 6

# Therapy

Chapter 9

# Pharmacological Treatment of Patent Ductus Arteriosus in Preterm Infants

*Aimann Surak*

## Abstract

The patent ductus arteriosus contribute to many neonatal morbidities. There are different approaches for treatment including conservative, pharmacological and definitive closure. Most commonly, pharmacological therapy is attempted before consideration of surgical intervention.

**Keywords:** preterm infant, PDA, NSAIDs

## 1. Introduction

Patent ductus arteriosus (PDA) was described a long time ago as a pathological entity in preterm babies [1]. From the physiological point of view, and outside the context of ductal-dependent lesions, PDA cannot be physiologically helpful when it comes to neonatal morbidity [2, 3].

In animal studies, there is significant engorgement and increased lymphatic conspicuity, secondary to dilated lymphatic architecture, in lambs with PDAs [4]. In primates, there is data suggesting that closing the PDA early makes a great difference in terms of the ventilation scores [4].

In humans, it takes only 3–7-day exposure to a moderate-large PDA shunt which significantly increases the incidence of bronchopulmonary dysplasia (BPD) [5] and BPD baseline incidence increases in preterm infants exposed to PDA [6].

PDA plays a critical role in the pathophysiology of many neonatal morbidities. This includes pulmonary hemorrhage [7, 8], myocardial changes in shape and size due to volume overload [9, 10], impaired bowel tissue oxygenation and other GI morbidities including necrotizing enterocolitis (NEC) [11–14], increased incidence of renal injury [15], mortality and intraventricular hemorrhage (IVH) [14].

Different approaches exist and vary between centers. In this chapter, we will concentrate on the pharmacological approach.

Role of targeted neonatal echocardiography in detecting hemodynamically significant PDA:

There has not been a standardized consensus to define hemodynamically significant PDA [16, 17].

Clinical assessment on its own was found not sensitive or specific in predicting PDA shunt volume especially in the first few days of life [18]. In addition, ductal size (diameter) only does not define the significance of the ductal shunt. There are large size PDAs that have no hemodynamic significance, and the opposite is true as well.

It appears that a detailed echocardiographic assessment is the key using targeted neonatal echocardiography (TnEcho). This comprehensive assessment includes multiple domains (**Figure 1**). PDA characteristics are crucial to look at, which includes the diameter, PDA flow Doppler pattern as well as PDA shape. It is interesting to think about the morphology of the duct and how is it different in preterm as opposed to less preterm babies. Initially, 5 types of ducts were described from A to E, however, with the increasing number of preterm babies being referred for catheter closure, a 6th type was recognized. The F type (fetal type) ductus is exclusively found in children born prematurely and is long, wide, tortuous and unlikely to close with pharmacological treatments [19].

Assessment of pulmonary circulation is important to establish using multiple parameters (**Figure 1**). Due to poor compliance, assessment of myocardial adaptation to the high shunt load is crucial. In addition, the atrial shunt needs to be assessed and established. Finally, any evidence of systemic compromise should be elaborated as well.

Recently, few biochemical markers were suggested as a part of ductal assessment especially in resource-limited areas. This includes cardiac troponin T (TnT), atrial natriuretic peptide (ANP), brain-type natriuretic peptide (BNP), N-terminal pro-BNP (NTpBNP) and urinary neutrophil gelatinase-associated lipocalin and urinary heart-type fatty acid-binding protein [20–23]. It appears that TnEcho is the proper tool to establish and define hemodynamically significant duct; only then treatment of PDA is shown to have an impact on neonatal outcomes [14, 17, 24, 25].

**PDA characteristics**

1. **PDA diameter**
2. **PDA flow Doppler pattern**
3. **PDA shape**

**Pulmonary over circulation**

1. **Pulmonary vein diastolic velocity**
2. **LA dimensions**
3. **MV E/A ratio**
4. **MV velocity of flow propagation**
5. **LV dimensions**
6. **LV TVI**
7. **LA/AO ratio**
8. **MR peak velocity**
9. **High LVO**
10. **QP:QS**

**Assess atrial shunt**

1. **Diameter trial shunt**
2. **TV E/A ratio**
3. **TV velocity of flow propagation**

**Myocardial adaptation to shunt volume**

1. **MPI (Tei index)**
2. **Systolic function**
3. **Diastolic function**

**Systemic compromise**

1. **SVC flow**
2. **LVO:SVC ratio**
3. **Renal Doppler and RI**
4. **Doppler pattern in celiac artery**
5. **Doppler pattern in SMA**
6. **Doppler pattern in MCA**

**Figure 1.**
*Targeted neonatal parameters needed to establish the hemodynamic significance of PDA.*

## 2. Pharmacological treatment of PDA in preterm infants

Pharmacological treatments induce ductal constriction with good effectiveness overall, whether using non-steroidal anti-inflammatory drugs (NSAIDs) or acetaminophen in different routes of administration [25–29]. However, complete ductal closure or shunt elimination cannot be guaranteed even when combining these agents together; this is in addition to potential adverse side effects [30–32].

## 3. Non-steroidal anti-inflammatory drugs (NSAIDs)

It was known early on that NSAIDs induce ductal constriction and closure [25, 33–35]; this is even in infants who are born prematurely [36, 37]. Early treatment with indomethacin induces ductal closure, however, with concerns about compromising renal function [38]. This is probably due to the vasoconstrictive effects of those agents contributing to the development of renal hypoperfusion, NEC and spontaneous intestinal perforation (SIP), as well as platelet dysfunction and hyperbilirubinemia [39, 40].

A meta-analysis by Ohlsson et al. show that ibuprofen is equal to indomethacin in terms of efficacy in closing PDA with fewer side effects on the kidneys as well as reduced risk for NEC [41]. Rectal ibuprofen has been used as well with similar efficacy to oral ibuprofen [42]. It appears that indomethacin, the most widely used agent, is more prevalent in North America, and ibuprofen is more commonly used in Europe and Asia [43].

Repeated courses of NSAIDs are a common practice when initial treatment wasn't completely successful in closing the PDA, keeping in mind, decreased efficacy with repeated courses [44, 45].

A higher dose of ibuprofen has been attempted as well, and this includes a loading dose of 20 mg/kg, followed by two subsequent doses of 10 mg/kg, 24 hours apart; this is in comparison to the standard dosing regimen which is a loading dose of 10 mg/kg, followed by two subsequent doses of 5 mg/kg, 24 hours apart. It appears that a higher dose of ibuprofen is more effective in closing the PDA, without an obvious increase in the side effects [41, 46].

### 3.1 Acetaminophen

Hammerman et al. reported the first case series of the use of acetaminophen as a therapeutic agent to facilitate ductal closure [27]. Acetaminophen inhibits the POX receptors on the prostaglandin synthesis pathway [29]. In a recent systematic review, Ohlsson et al. included 916 infants in eight studies comparing oral or intravenous acetaminophen to ibuprofen and found similar efficacy for acetaminophen with lower gastrointestinal bleeds, lower serum levels of creatinine, lower serum levels of bilirubin, and higher platelet count but no difference in the neurological outcomes between 18 and 24 months [28].

It is possible that acetaminophen may increase pulmonary vascular resistance [47].

### 3.2 Combination therapy

Another strategy that has been attempted, is combining acetaminophen with NSAIDs specifically ibuprofen which may provide a synergetic effect on the reduction of prostaglandin production, resulting in PDA closure. In a small randomized controlled trial (RCT), Hochwald et al. compared the combination of intravenous ibuprofen and intravenous acetaminophen versus intravenous ibuprofen alone. There was a trend towards increased efficacy with combination therapy but without a statistical difference (83% vs. 42%, $p = 0.08$); also, there was no increase in the side effects [30]. In an observational study by Yurttutan et al., combination therapy with oral ibuprofen and oral acetaminophen was successful in closing the ductus in 9 out of 12 infants who had failed two previous courses with no increase in the side effects [31]. A retrospective cohort by Kimani et al. did not demonstrate any increased adverse effects in the combination group [32].

### 3.3 Other strategies

Diuretics have been used as an adjunct agent to facilitate ductal closure. While diuretics help with symptomatic management of pulmonary over circulation, it appears that it compromises the systemic blood flow and may not provide a significant increase in the closure rates [48]. This is similar to a fluid restriction which may help managing the symptoms of chronic lung disease, but it would worsen the systemic blood flow [49, 50].

## 4. Conclusion

The PDA is common morbidity in preterm infants. There has been a trend towards more conservative management over surgical treatment [51]. The pharmacological treatment causes ductal constriction with good effectiveness overall whether using NSAIDs or acetaminophen in different routes of administration. However, complete ductal closure or shunt elimination cannot be guaranteed even when combining these agents together; this is in addition to potential adverse side effects.

Recently, FDA approved the use of Piccolo device for the purpose of PDA closure in preterm infants which was based of the efficacy and safety of such a device in this fragile population [2]. It appears that this catheter closure approach is becoming more popular as it is feasible, effective, and relatively safe [19, 52]. Whether this approach would result in more favorable neonatal morbidities and outcomes, needs further research.

## Abbreviations

| | |
|---|---|
| BPD | Bronchopulmonary dysplasia |
| NEC | Necrotizing enterocolitis |
| NSAIDs | Non-steroidal anti-inflammatory drugs |
| PDA | Patent ductus arteriosus |
| RCT | Randomized controlled trial |
| SIP | Spontaneous intestinal perforation |
| TnEcho | Targeted neonatal echocardiography |

## Author details

Aimann Surak
Department of Paediatrics, University of Alberta, Edmonton, Alberta, Canada

*Address all correspondence to: aimannsurak@gmail.com

## References

[1] Powell ML. Patent ductus arteriosus in premature infants. The Medical journal of Australia. 1963;**2**:58-60

[2] Vanhaesebrouck S, Zonnenberg I, Vandervoort P, Bruneel E, van Hoestenberghe MR, Theyskens C. Conservative treatment for patent ductus arteriosus in the preterm. Archives of Disease in Childhood: Fetal and Neonatal Edition. 2007;**92**(4):244-247

[3] Semberova J, Sirc J, Miletin J, Kucera J, Berka I, Sebkova S, et al. Spontaneous closure of patent ductus arteriosus in infants ≤1500 g. Pediatrics. 2017;**140**(2)

[4] Alderliesten T, Lemmers PMA, Smarius JJM, van de Vosse RE, Baerts W, van Bel F. Cerebral oxygenation, extraction, and autoregulation in very preterm infants who develop peri-intraventricular hemorrhage. Journal of Pediatrics. 2013;**162**(4):698-704.e2

[5] de Waal K, Kluckow M. Functional echocardiography; from physiology to treatment. Early Human Development. 2010;**86**(3):149-154. DOI: 10.1016/j.earlhumdev.2010.01.030

[6] Datar SA, Johnson EG, Oishi PE, Johengen M, Tang E, Aramburo A, et al. Altered lymphatics in an ovine model of congenital heart disease with increased pulmonary blood flow. American Journal of Physiology - Lung Cellular and Molecular Physiology. 2012;**302**(6):530-540

[7] Chang LY, McCurnin D, Yoder B, Shaul PW, Clyman RI. Ductus arteriosus ligation and alveolar growth in preterm baboons with a patent ductus arteriosus. Pediatric Research. 2008;**63**(3): 299-302

[8] Clyman RI, Liebowitz M, Johng S, Clyman RI, Hills NK. Relationship between duration of infant exposure to a moderate-to-large patent ductus arteriosus shunt and the risk of developing bronchopulmonary dysplasia or death before 36 weeks. American Journal of Perinatology. 2020;**37**(2):216-223

[9] Crump C, Groves A, Sundquist J, Sundquist K. Association of preterm birth with long-term risk of heart failure into adulthood. JAMA Pediatrics. 2021;**175**(7):689-697

[10] Vaisbourd Y, Sharif D, Riskin A, Yaniv L, Dinur G, Amen K, et al. The effect of patent ductus arteriosus on coronary artery blood flow in premature infants: A prospective observational pilot study. Journal of Perinatology. 2020;**40**(9):1366-1374. DOI: 10.1038/s41372-020-0622-4

[11] Lemmers PMA, Toet MC, van Bel F. Impact of patent ductus arteriosus and subsequent therapy with indomethacin on cerebral oxygenation in preterm infants. Pediatrics. 2008;**121**(1):142-147

[12] Palder SB, Schwartz MZ, Tyson KRT, Marr CC. Association of closure of patent ductus arteriosus and development of necrotizing enterocolitis. Journal of Pediatric Surgery. 1988;**23**(5):422-423

[13] McCurnin D, Clyman RI. Effects of a patent ductus arteriosus on postprandial mesenteric perfusion in premature baboons. Pediatrics. 2008;**122**(6):e1262-e1267

[14] Sellmer A, Bjerre JV, Schmidt MR, McNamara PJ, Hjortdal VE, Høst B, et al. Morbidity and mortality in preterm neonates with patent ductus arteriosus

on day 3. Archives of Disease in Childhood: Fetal and Neonatal Edition. 2013;**98**(6):505-510

[15] Chock VY, Rose LA, Mante J, v., Punn R. Near-infrared spectroscopy for detection of a significant patent ductus arteriosus. Pediatric Research. 2016;**80**(5):675-680

[16] El-Khuffash A, James AT, David CJ, Dicker P, Franklin O, Elsayed YN, et al. A patent Ductus arteriosus severity score predicts chronic lung disease or death before discharge. The Journal of pediatrics. 2015;**167**(6):1354-1361.e2. DOI: 10.1016/j.jpeds.2015.09.028

[17] Shepherd JL, Noori S. What is a hemodynamically significant PDA in preterm infants? Congenital Heart Disease. 2019;**14**(1):21-26

[18] Skelton R, Evans N, Smythe J. A blinded comparison of clinical and echocardiographic evaluation of the preterm infant for patent ductus arteriosus. Journal of Paediatrics and Child Health. 1994;**30**(5):406-411

[19] Philip R, Rush Waller B, Agrawal V, Wright D, Arevalo A, Zurakowski D, et al. Morphologic characterization of the patent ductus arteriosus in the premature infant and the choice of transcatheter occlusion device. Catheterization and Cardiovascular Interventions. 2016;**87**(2):310-317

[20] Kluckow M, Evans N. Low superior vena cava flow and intraventricular haemorrhage in preterm infants. Archives of Disease in Childhood: Fetal and Neonatal Edition. 2000;**82**(3):F188-F194

[21] EL-Khuffash A, Molloy E. The Use of N-Terminal-Pro-BNP in Preterm Infants. International Journal of Pediatrics. 2009;**2009**:1-7

[22] Sanjeev S, Pettersen M, Lua J, Thomas R, Shankaran S, L'Ecuyer T. Role of plasma B-type natriuretic peptide in screening for hemodynamically significant patent ductus arteriosus in preterm neonates. Journal of Perinatology. 2005;**25**(11):709-713

[23] Byung MC, Kee HL, Baik LE, Kee HY, Young SH, Chang SS, et al. Utility of rapid B-type natriuretic peptide assay for diagnosis of symptomatic patent ductus arteriosus in preterm infants. Pediatrics. 2005;**115**(3):e255-e261

[24] McNamara PJ, Sehgal A. Towards rational management of the patent ductus arteriosus: The need for disease staging. Archives of Disease in Childhood: Fetal and Neonatal Edition. 2007;**92**:F424-F427

[25] Bussmann N, Smith A, Breatnach CR, McCallion N, Cleary B, Franklin O, et al. Patent ductus arteriosus shunt elimination results in a reduction in adverse outcomes: A post hoc analysis of the PDA RCT cohort. Journal of Perinatology. 2021;**41**(5):1134-1141

[26] Starling MB, Elliott RB. The effects of prostaglandins, prostaglandin inhibitors, and oxygen on the closure of the ductus arteriosus, pulmonary arteries and umbilical vessels in vitro. Prostaglandins. 1974;**8**(3):187-203

[27] Terrin G, Conte F, Oncel MY, Scipione A, McNamara PJ, Simons S, et al. Paracetamol for the treatment of patent ductus arteriosus in preterm neonates: a systematic review and meta-analysis. Archives of Disease in Childhood: Fetal and Neonatal Edition. Mar 2016;**101**(2):F127-F136

[28] Hammerman C, Bin-Nun A, Markovitch E, Schimmel MS, Kaplan M, Fink D. Ductal closure with paracetamol: A surprising new approach to patent

ductus arteriosus treatment. Pediatrics. 2011;**128**(6):e1618-e1621

[29] Ohlsson A, Shah PS. Paracetamol (acetaminophen) for patent ductus arteriosus in preterm or low birth weight infants. Cochrane Database of Systematic Reviews. 2018;**4**(4):CD010061

[30] Jasani B, Weisz DE, McNamara PJ. Evidence-based use of acetaminophen for hemodynamically significant ductus arteriosus in preterm infants. Seminars in Perinatology. 2018;**42**(4):243-252

[31] Hochwald O, Mainzer G, Borenstein-Levin L, Jubran H, Dinur G, Zucker M, et al. Adding paracetamol to ibuprofen for the treatment of patent ductus arteriosus in preterm infants: A double-blind, randomized, placebo-controlled pilot study. American Journal of Perinatology. 2018;**35**(13):1319-1325

[32] Yurttutan S, Bozkaya A, Hüdayioglu F, Oncel MY. The effect of combined therapy for treatment of monotherapy-resistant PDA in preterm infants. Journal of Maternal-Fetal and Neonatal Medicine. 2019;**32**(21):3662-3665

[33] Kimani S, Surak A, Miller M, Bhattacharya S. Use of combination therapy with acetaminophen and ibuprofen for closure of the patent ductus arteriosus in preterm neonates. Paediatrics & Child Health. 2020;**26**(4):e177-e183

[34] Elliott RB, Starling MB, Neutze JM. Medical manipulation of the ductus arteriosus. The Lancet. 1975;**305**(7899):140-142

[35] Sharpe GL, Thalme B, Larsson KS. Studies on closure of the ductus arteriosus. XI. Ductal closure in utero by a prostaglandin synthetase inhibitor. Prostaglandins. 1974;**8**(5):585-596

[36] Coceani F, Olley PM, Bodach E. Lamb ductus arteriosus: Effect of prostaglandin synthesis inhibitors on the muscle tone and the response to prostaglandin E2. Prostaglandins. 1975;**9**(2):299-308

[37] Heymann MA, Rudolph AM, Silverman NH. Closure of the ductus arteriosus in premature infants by inhibition of prostaglandin synthesis. New England Journal of Medicine. 1976;**295**(10):530-533

[38] Friedman WF, Hirschklau MJ, Printz MP, Pitlick PT, Kirkpatrick SE. Pharmacologic closure of patent ductus arteriosus in the premature infant. Obstetrical and Gynecological Survey. 1977;**32**(2):123-138

[39] van Overmeire B, van de Broek H, van Laer P, Weyler J, Vanhaesebrouck P. Early versus late indomethacin treatment for patent ductus arteriosus in premature infants with respiratory distress syndrome. Journal of Pediatrics. 2001;**138**(2):205-211

[40] Betkerur MV, Yeh TF, Miller K, Glasser RJ, Pildes RS. Indomethacin and its effect on renal function and urinary kallikrein excretion in premature infants with patent ductus arteriosus. Pediatrics. 1981;**68**(1):99-102

[41] Kang NS, Yoo KH, Cheon H, Choi BM, Hong YS, Lee JW, et al. Indomethacin treatment decreases renal blood flow velocity in human neonates. Biology of the Neonate. 1999;**76**(5):261-265

[42] Ohlsson A, Walia R, Shah SS. Ibuprofen for the treatment of patent ductus arteriosus in preterm or low birth weight (or both) infants. Cochrane Database of Systematic Reviews. 2020;**2020, 2**(2):CD003481

[43] Demir N, Peker E, Ece İ, Balahoroğlu R, Tuncer O. Efficacy and safety of rectal ibuprofen for patent ductus arteriosus closure in very low birth weight preterm infants. Journal of Maternal-Fetal and Neonatal Medicine. 2017;**30**(17):2119-2125

[44] Irmesi R, Marcialis MA, Anker JVD, Fanos V. Non-steroidal anti-inflammatory drugs (NSAIDs) in the Management of Patent Ductus Arteriosus (PDA) in Preterm Infants and Variations in Attitude in Clinical Practice: A Flight Around the World. Current Medicinal Chemistry. 2014;**21**(27):3132-3152

[45] Olgun H, Ceviz N, Kartal İ, Caner İ, Karacan M, Taştekin A, et al. Repeated courses of oral ibuprofen in premature infants with patent ductus arteriosus: Efficacy and safety. Pediatrics and Neonatology. 2017;**58**(1):29-35

[46] Sangem M, Asthana S, Amin S. Multiple courses of indomethacin and neonatal outcomes in premature infants. Pediatric Cardiology. 2008;**29**(5):878-884

[47] Dani C, Vangi V, Bertini G, Pratesi S, Lori I, Favelli F, et al. High-dose ibuprofen for patent ductus arteriosus in extremely preterm infants: A randomized controlled study. Clinical Pharmacology and Therapeutics. 2012;**91**(4):590-596

[48] Tamir Hostovsky L, Pan J, McNamara PJ, Belik J. Acetaminophen increases pulmonary and systemic vasomotor tone in the newborn rat. Pediatric Research. 2019;**87**:1171-1176. DOI: 10.1038/s41390-019-0725-9

[49] Lee BS, Byun SY, Chung ML, Chang JY, Kim HY, Kim EAR, et al. Effect of furosemide on ductal closure and renal function in indomethacin-treated preterm infants during the early neonatal period. Neonatology. 2010;**98**(2):191-199

[50] de Buyst J, Rakza T, Pennaforte T, Johansson AB, Storme L. Hemodynamic effects of fluid restriction in preterm infants with significant patent ductus arteriosus. Journal of Pediatrics. 2012;**161**(3):404-408

[51] Bell E, Acarregui M. Restricted versus liberal water intake for preventing morbidity and mortality in preterm infants. The Cochrane Database of Systematic Reviews. 2001;**2001**

[52] Sathanandam S, Balduf K, Chilakala S, Washington K, Allen K, Knott-Craig C, et al. Role of Transcatheter patent ductus arteriosus closure in extremely low birth weight infants. Catheterization and Cardiovascular Interventions. 2019;**93**(1):89-96

Chapter 10

# Right Ventricular Outflow Tract Stenting

*Shaad Abqari*

## Abstract

RVOT stenting has gained popularity over the last decade. Conventional treatment of choice in children with cyanotic heart defect with decreased pulmonary blood flow has always been the systemic to pulmonary arterial shunt, but lately, many centres are opting for RVOT stenting as the first choice of palliation. It is associated with fewer post-procedural complications and helps in a more physiological growth of pulmonary arteries, which can significantly impact the definitive repair at later date. Normally, RVOT stenting is performed in the early newborn period but it is not unusual to be done at a later age because of varied reasons. Two-point fixation of the stent ensures its safety against embolization but sparing the valve and covering the infundibular area only protect the child from future trans annular patches, though removing the stent can sometimes be challenging at a later stage. RVOT stenting has now become a safer alternative in centres with early stage of cardiac programmes.

**Keywords:** RVOT stenting, cyanotic heart defect, neonate, aorto-pulmonary shunt, palliation

## 1. Introduction

Cyanotic congenital heart defects continue to be a cause of significant morbidity and mortality among infants and are an important contributor to neonatal mortality. In the new paediatric cardiac programmes, the majority of these defects are being corrected very early in life, but the repair, whether corrective or palliative, sometimes is difficult to achieve, especially in neonates with complex anatomy or those with risk factors. Right ventricular outflow stenting (RVOT) has emerged as the main bridging procedure in infants who require early interventions, such as neonates who are duct dependent or who are severely cyanosed and have poor anatomy of the right ventricular outflow tract and/or pulmonary arterial tree (hypoplastic branch PAs).

## 2. Indications

Neonates with risk factors such as prematurity, low birth weight, infection (sepsis), necrotizing enterocolitis, cerebrovascular event, pulmonary diseases and other conditions requiring noncardiac surgery, which included tracheoesophageal fistula and gastrointestinal anomalies.

Infants and older children with anatomy are not suitable for primary repair or as a bail out procedure in emergent conditions like uncontrolled cyanotic spells.

As reported by various authors, co-morbidities increase the risk of or may delay, primary cardiac repair [1–3]. Blalock–Taussig (BT) shunts performed in infants with these co-morbidities have an increased rate of complications, besides an unpredictable post-op course such as pulmonary over circulation and distortion of pulmonary artery anatomy [4–8].

The unpredictability of pulmonary balloon valvuloplasty combined with the high morbidity/mortality of both modified BT shunt placement and primary repair signalled the need for an alternative palliation option—the RVOT stent. RVOT stenting was initially described by Gibbs et al. [9] but the initial results were not encouraging, and it was re-introduced from 2010 onwards as a mode of palliation.

Sandoval et al., at the Hospital for Sick Children in Toronto [1], performed a detailed retrospective review of their experience managing infants with Tetralogy of Fallot(TOF). Infants were treated in 1 of 4 ways: those with early cyanosis (<3 months of age) were treated with either primary repair (early-PS group in those with pulmonary stenosis, and early-PA group in those with pulmonary atresia) or RVOT stenting (stent group); whereas those without early cyanosis had primary repair electively at an age deemed optimal between 3 and 11 months (surg>3mo group). Risk factors for primary repair were defined as low weight (<2.5 kg), prematurity (<37 weeks' gestational age), pulmonary artery hypoplasia ($Z$ score < −2) and significant noncardiac co-morbidities. The decision to perform early primary repair versus RVOT stenting was based largely on the presence of risk factors. Aortopulmonary shunts and ductal stents were reserved for infants with whom RVOT patency could not be established; that is, RVOT muscular atresia and unsuccessful RVOT intervention, or those with nonconfluent central pulmonary arteries. The early-PS, early-PA, and stent groups all had similar cumulative and postoperative lengths of stay, all significantly longer than that for the surgery >3mo group. Most importantly, the stent group at baseline had significantly smaller pulmonary arteries than the other 3 groups at a median Nakata index of 79 $mm^2/m^2$. After RVOT stenting, there was significant catch-up growth of the pulmonary arteries. Although they remained somewhat smaller at the time of ultimate anatomic repair (median 147 $mm^2/mm^2$ compared with 167 $mm^2/m^2$ in the surg>3mo group), this difference was not statistically significant.

The ideal palliations as described by Glatz in an editorial in 2016 [10] are as follows: 1. Providing a stable and balanced source of pulmonary blood flow; 2. Allowing growth of pulmonary vessels 3. Providing adequate time for subsidence of co-morbidities and to gain weight and 4. Leaving no residue.

Transcatheter techniques in the initial palliation of these patients have previously been attempted [9, 11–13], but did not gain widespread acceptance. Qureshi et al. attempted balloon dilatation as initial palliation in 15 infants with modest results with 10 requiring more than one dilatation [11]. Similarly, Sluysmans T et al. in 1995, published the result of BPV in 19 infants and concluded that it leads to a 30–40% reduction in the need for transannular patches at the time of corrective surgery [12]. Similarly, Gibbs first described RVOT stenting as a palliative procedure in 4 patients with associated co-morbidities [9]. Ballooning of the right ventricular outflow tract has gone out of favour because of dynamic obstruction in patients of TOF.

PDA stenting is gaining popularity in some of the centres but is a technically challenging procedure, besides establishment of pulmonary blood flow is unpredictable and sometimes leads to flooding of pulmonary circulation. Transcatheter RVOT stenting is gaining popularity as this results in a more physiological flow to pulmonary arteries and encourages equal growth of small pulmonary arteries providing a better surgical substrate for subsequent repair.

## 3. Procedure

The procedure as described by Quandt and Stumper et al. [13] include detailed pre-procedure work up and is usually performed under general anaesthesia and mechanical ventilation, since the children are usually hypoxic and sick and can deteriorate fast during the procedure.

Ambient temperature should be maintained by using Bair Hugger to prevent hypothermia.

Prostaglandin infusions are usually continued and all the emergency drugs should be available.

The child is to be positioned on the table with the arms elevated and the area to be painted and draped.

Access is usually via the right femoral vein in a majority of cases but sometimes an internal jugular venous approach is preferred if crossing of RVOT is difficult, especially in smaller children. A right femoral artery cannula is inserted for continuous blood pressure monitoring and for blood gas analysis. Once the right femoral venous sheath (usually 5F) is inserted, 50–100 IU/Kg of Heparin is given. The child also receives a prophylactic antibiotic (Cefazolin) dose.

A right ventricular cineangiogram is performed through an NIH or any other diagnostic catheter placed within the apex of the right ventricle; 30° RAO with 20° cranial tilt and a straight lateral projection are used. Some centres prefer to do angiograms in LAO view instead of lateral view. The intent is to delineate the RVOT, its length and diameter, the diameter of pulmonary valve annulus and the size of branch pulmonary arteries.

Selection of the size and the type of stent to be implanted is guided by the size of the patient, the dimensions of the outflow tract and the anticipated length of palliation.

For smaller children and neonates with short term palliation- coronary stent is preferred.

For older children or those who required medium to longer-term palliation- a bare metal peripheral vascular stent, preferably Cook Formula pre-mounted 414 or 418 stent, may be used.

The advantage of Cooks Formula stent is that it can be re-dilated if required and provided long term palliation. Sometimes, the availability of the specific stent is an issue; in such situations, any peripheral stent may be used. Balloon mounted stents are preferred. However, these stents may require thicker wire (0.035) either Amplatz superstiff or even Teflon wire for the stent delivery. Another disadvantage is that the stiffer wire may precipitate RVOT spasm and the child may have significant desaturation during the procedure.

After the selection of the stent, the appropriate delivery sheath or guide catheter is used. For coronary stents, a 4 French (F) Flexor sheath (Cook Europe, Bjaeverskov, Denmark) or a 60 cm 6 F right Judkins guide catheter (Cordis Corp, Miami Lakes FL) may be used.

A 0.014″ coronary wire is advanced across the RVOT via an end-hole catheter and a stable position is achieved by placing the wire in distal branch pulmonary arteries (PAs). Once the coronary wire is stable in the distal branch pulmonary artery, the selected delivery sheath or guide catheter replaces the diagnostic catheter. In older children where a stiff wire is required, firstly, a softer catheter such as a Glide catheter is passed into the distal branch PAs and then advance a 0.032 Terumo wire and final diagnostic catheter like (Judkins

Right) JR or Multipurpose catheter may be used for replacing the Terumo wire with the stiff wires like Amplatz superstiff. The whole exercise is done due to hypertrophied infundibular area which may not allow the diagnostic catheter to pass over the coronary wire.

Cook Formula stents are implanted through either 5 or 6 F Flexor sheaths or sometimes Mullins sheath may be needed. The disadvantage of using a stiffer sheath is that it normally does not easily crosses the infundibular area, especially in older children who present late and have very hypertrophied RVOT. In these cases, the sheath is placed just below the infundibular area with multiple side arm injections; the stent is negotiated across the RVOT avoiding the annulus. However, if the annulus is small or if there is supravalvular PA narrowing, the stent may be placed across the pulmonary valve achieving a two-point fixation, one at infundibular and another at valve annulus level.

In infants and young children, the pre-mounted stent is placed over the wire but within the delivery sheath and advanced to the intended position within the RVOT and the stent is fully uncovered after checking with test angiograms. When the position of the stent appears satisfactory, (confirming it on echocardiography when necessary), the balloon is inflated. Following placement of the stent, the balloon is slowly deflated whilst the delivery sheath was advanced over the balloon, so as to re-sheath it. The position of the stent is confirmed on the check angiogram (**Figures 1** and 2) via the side arm of the sheath. The position of the stent, opacification of the branch PAs and pulmonary valve movements are recorded on the final angiogram.

Echocardiography is performed for confirmation of the position of the stent, ventricular function, any interference with tricuspid valve function and evidence for effusion. A repeat blood gas analysis is obtained and improvement in PO2 is recorded. When we are confident of the implanted stent, the coronary wire along with the delivery sheath is removed under fluoroscopic monitoring and manual haemostasis is achieved.

The infant/child is transferred to the Neonatal/Paediatric ICU, as appropriate and vital signs are monitored. Patients who experienced an increase of oxygen saturation in excess of 20% are commenced on twice-daily diuretics. Chest X-ray is performed for any evidence of flooding of the lungs. In our experience, a peak gradient in excess of 40 mm Hg across RVOT on Doppler echocardiography post stenting usually does

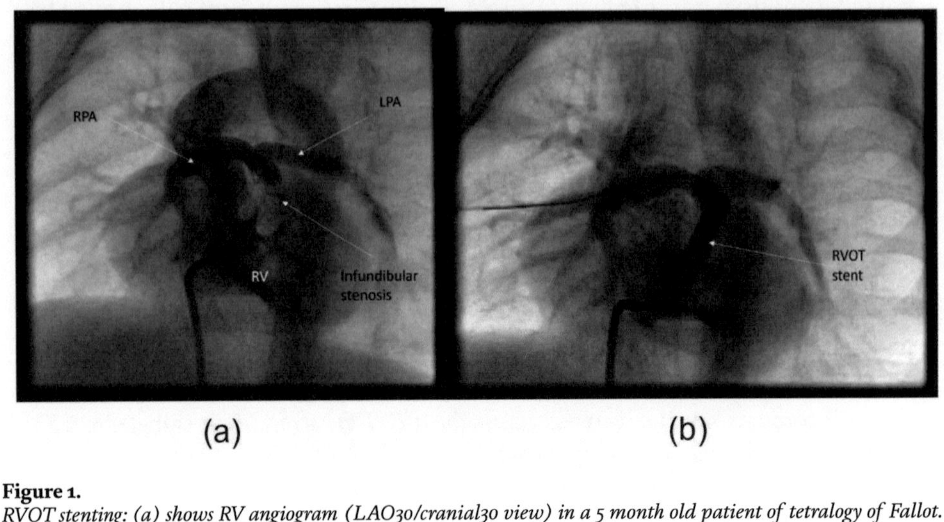


**Figure 1.**
*RVOT stenting: (a) shows RV angiogram (LAO30/cranial30 view) in a 5 month old patient of tetralogy of Fallot. There was severe infundibular and valvular stenosis with diffusely narrow LPA and RPA. RVOT stenting was done using 4 mm × 19 mm bare stent (Evermine) and a RV angiogram was done in a/P view which showed RVOT stent in situ with relief of infundibular stenosis as shown in figure (b).*

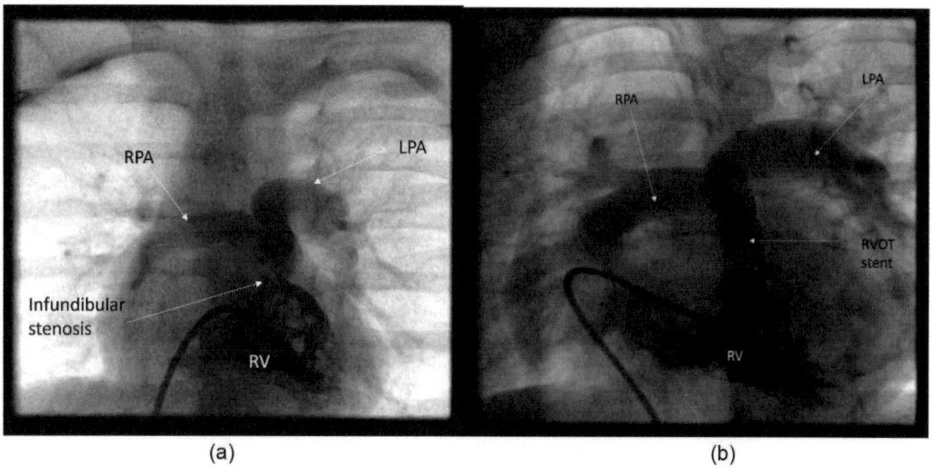


**Figure 2.**
*Successful RVOT stenting: (a) shows RV angiogram done in LAO 30/cranial 30 view in a one year old TOF patient which showed severe infundibular stenosis. RVOT stenting was done in this patient using 8 mm x 37 mm bare stent. (b) shows RV angiogram in the same patient done one year after the RVOT stenting procedure which showed RVOT stent in situ and adequately sized branch PA's.*

not have over circulation. Heparin infusion is continued and replaced with Aspirin (3–5 mg/kg) once the child starts to take it orally and the aspirin is continued till the child undergoes complete repair. RVOT stenting usually leads to a uniform growth of branch pulmonary arteries as shown in **Figure 2** where a repeat angiogram one year post procedure showed adequate sized pulmonary arteries amiable for complete repair.

## 4. Modifications

The use of a long sheath as described by Quandt et al. [13] is mainly performed to minimise the tricuspid valve apparatus injury and to achieve a stable stent position by repeated test angiograms. However, the use of a long delivery sheath may be associated with haemodynamic instability, particularly in smaller and sicker patients due to tricuspid valve splinting open leading to compromised cardiac output and extreme cyanosis.

Linnane et al. have used periventricular approach in 4 patients weighing ≤2 kg through a small subxiphoid incision [14]. This approach provided a more direct route to the RVOT and the stent was deployed under Trans Thoracic Echocardiography (TTE) guidance.

Linnane et al. [15] also described a method for avoiding long delivery sheath during the stent deployment by crossing the tricuspid valve and RVOT with an angled glide catheter to facilitate placement of the guidewire in the branch pulmonary arteries and doing 3–4 clockwise rotations to create some backwards tension on the wire during stent advancement. The authors utilised TTE to guide the stent placement rather than angiography.

## 5. Complications

Malposition or migration- of the stent may occur due to more proximal deployment of the stent. If the stent does not achieve 2 point fixation, it remains unstable. The commonest site of embolization is descending aorta (**Figure 3**). The use of a long delivery sheath for confirming the position and preventing the slippage of the stent

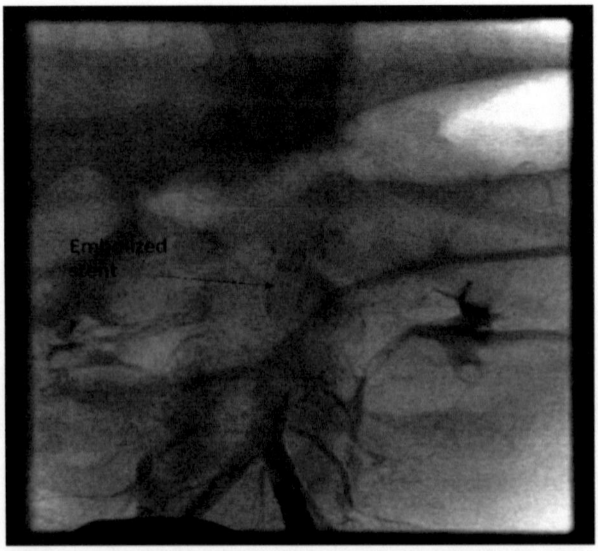

**Figure 3.**
*Stent embolization: Figure shows stent (4 mm × 20 mm, Encurse) had embolized into the abdominal aorta at the level of left renal artery.*

minimises the risk. Sometimes, distal deployment of the stent can lead to migration of stent into branch pulmonary arteries.

Other Complications include balloon rupture, dissection, stent induced pulmonary oedema, arrhythmias, injury to adjoining structures and injury to tricuspid valve leading to tricuspid regurgitation, hypotension and hemodynamic instability during the procedure.

## 6. Challenges

The procedure is a technically difficult procedure with a significant learning curve and is difficult to execute in a new program.

Requirement of re-interventions, especially if performed in early neonatal period with very hypoplastic pulmonary arteries.

Difficult corrective surgery post stenting- Removal of stent can be challenging with increased cardiopulmonary bypass time, sometimes the posterior aspect of stent is left in situ, and concerns of injury to adjoining structures like aortic and tricuspid valve can complicate the post-op recovery.

Long term data on RVOT stenting is lacking, especially RV dilatation, growth of pulmonary vessels and need for re-interventions.

## 7. Outcomes

The immediate outcome in children undergoing RVOT stenting is quite favourable with saturations improving immediately after the procedure. In a yet unpublished data from the authors more than 30 children had undergone RVOT stenting majority of which were more than one year of age, there was significant improvement in the saturations and children were shifted out of PICU within 24 hrs. There were two instances of stent embolization which happened in the initial phase of the learning curve with no in-hospital mortality. The children were discharged on antiplatelets and no episode of stent thrombosis or fracture was noted on follow up.

In a retrospective study by Sandoval et al. at the Hospital for Sick Children in Toronto [1] which divided the children undergoing treatment for TOF into four categories as described earlier, it was found that the RVOT stent group had significantly smaller pulmonary arteries as compared to other 3 groups (median Nakata index of 79 $mm^2/m^2$) with a comparable post-operative stay, thereby implying that the procedure can be done in children with very unfavourable anatomy.

## 8. Summary

Transcatheter RVOT stenting is increasingly preferred over other palliative procedures as aorto-pulmonary shunts have a very unpredictable course post-operatively, especially neonatal BT shunts. The risks of shunt thrombosis or pulmonary over circulation can influence the post-operative recovery, shunt leads to disruption and distortion of the pulmonary arteries which can significantly impact the definitive repair at a later date. RVOT stenting establishes a more physiological flow to pulmonary arteries and encourages equal growth of small pulmonary arteries providing a better surgical substrate for subsequent repair.

## 9. Conclusion

With increasing expertise and modifications like avoidance of long sheath and reducing procedure time, RVOT stenting is emerging as a safer alternative to other palliative procedures. However, many centres are opting for early primary repair. The RVOT stenting procedure is likely to gain more and more acceptance among other palliative options as the institutes increase their experience.

## Author details

Shaad Abqari
Division of Paediatric Cardiology, Department of Paediatrics, Jawaharlal Nehru Medical College, Aligarh Muslim University, Aligarh, India

*Address all correspondence to: drshaadabqari@gmail.com

## References


[1] Sandoval JP, Chaturvedi RR, Benson L, Morgan G, Van Arsdell G, Honjo O, et al. Right ventricular outflow tract stenting in tetralogy of Fallot infants with risk factors for early primary repair. Circulation: Cardiovascular Interventions. 2016;**9**:e003979

[2] Dohlen G, Chaturvedi RR, Benson LN, Ozawa A, Van Arsdell GS, Fruitman DS, et al. Stenting of the right ventricular outflow tract in the symptomatic infant with tetralogy of Fallot. Heart. 2009;**95**:142-147. DOI: 10.1136/hrt.2007.135723

[3] Barron DJ, Ramchandani B, Murala J, Stumper O, De Giovanni JV, Jones TJ, et al. Surgery following primary right ventricular outflow tract stenting for Fallot's tetralogy and variants: Rehabilitation of small pulmonary arteries. European Journal of Cardio-Thoracic Surgery. 2013;**44**:656-662. DOI: 10.1093/ejcts/ezt188

[4] Kirsch RE, Glatz AC, Gaynor JW, Nicolson SC, Spray TL, Wernovsky G, et al. Results of elective repair at 6 months or younger in 277 patients with tetralogy of Fallot: a 14-year experience at a single center. The Journal of Thoracic and Cardiovascular Surgery. 2014;**147**:713-717

[5] Gladman G, McCrindle BW, Williams WG, Freedom RM, Benson LN. The modified Blalock-Taussig shunt: Clinical impact and morbidity in Fallot's tetralogy in the current era. The Journal of Thoracic and Cardiovascular Surgery. 1997;**114**:25-30

[6] Kanter KR, Kogon BE, Kirshbom PM, Carlock PR. Symptomatic neonatal tetralogy of Fallot: Repair or shunt? The Annals of Thoracic Surgery. 2010;**89**:858-863. DOI: 10.1016/j.athoracsur.2009.12.060

[7] Nakashima K, Itatani K, Oka N, Kitamura T, Horai T, Hari Y, et al. Pulmonary annulus growth after the modified Blalock-Taussig shunt in tetralogy of Fallot. The Annals of Thoracic Surgery. 2014;**98**:934-940

[8] Petrucci O, O'Brien SM, Jacobs ML, Jacobs JP, Manning PB, Eghtesady P. Risk factors for mortality and morbidity after the neonatal Blalock-Taussig shunt procedure. The Annals of Thoracic Surgery. 2011;**92**:642-651

[9] Gibbs JL, Uzun O, Blackburn ME, et al. Right ventricular outflow stent implantation: An alternative to palliative surgical relief of infundibular pulmonary stenosis. Heart. 1997;**77**:176-179

[10] Glatz CA. Right ventricular outflow tract stenting. The ideal palliative option in the management of high-risk cyanotic infants with tetralogy of fallot? Circulation: Cardiovascular Interventions. 2016;**9**(12):1-3. DOI: 10.1161/CIRCINTERVENTIONS.116.004721

[11] Qureshi SA, Kirk CR, Lamb RK, Arnold R, Wilkinson JL. Balloon dilatation of the pulmonary valve in the first year of life in patients with tetralogy of Fallot: A preliminary study. British Heart Journal. 1988;**60**(3):232-235

[12] Sluysmans T, Neven B, Rubay J, et al. Early balloon dilation in infants with tetralogy of Fallot: Risks and benefits. Circulation. 1995;**91**:1506-1511

[13] Quandt D, Penford G, Ramchandani B, Bhole V, Mehta C, Stumper O. Stenting of the right ventricular outflow tract as primary palliation for Fallot-type lesions. Journal of Congenitive Cardiology. 2017;**1**(1):3

[14] Linnane N, Walsh KP, McGuinness J, Kenny D. Evolution of approach to right venticular outflow tract stenting in infants ≤2 Kgs. Structural Heart Disease. 2018;**4**(2):50-55

[15] Linnane N, Nasef MA, McMahon CJ, et al. Right ventricular outflow tract stenting in symptomatic infants without the use of a long delivery sheath. Catheterization and Cardiovascular Interventions. 2021;**98**:E275-E281

Chapter 11

# Advances in the Management of Congenital Malformations of the Aortic Valve

*Si Hui Wong, Daniel Nento, Harinder Singh and Arpit Agarwal*


## Abstract

Congenital aortic valve disease is a life-long condition that can require multiple interventions. It is one of the most common causes of congenital heart defect, with bicuspid aortic valve present in at least 1–2% of the general population. Surgical management of congenital aortic valve disease consists of either valve repair or replacement. While aortic valve replacement using the Ross procedure can be considered the gold standard management in the pediatric population, advancements in aortic valve repair techniques have proved its usefulness as an initial management approach as it prevents prosthesis-related complications and patient-prostheses mismatch while the patient grows. Overall, all techniques have their benefits and limitations in terms of growth potential, durability of repair, freedom from reoperation and anticoagulation, infection risk, and mortality. Each patient will require an individualized judiciously selected management plan to minimize the number of interventions over their lifetime. The aim of this review is to discuss the merits and drawbacks of the major techniques currently used in both aortic valve repair and replacement.


**Keywords:** aortic valve, congenital, Ozaki procedure, balloon valvuloplasty, surgical valvulotomy

## 1. Introduction

The appropriate management of patients with aortic valve disease is perhaps one of the most debated topics. Unlike the mitral valve, management of aortic valve disease is a more delicate process as poor decisions can lead to chronic strain on the left ventricle, development of aortic insufficiency, high re-intervention rates, morbidity, and mortality. For many patients, the first arguable decision is between balloon valvuloplasty and surgical repair. Balloon valvuloplasty has evolved over many decades and is a reliable and straightforward procedure for any patient who needs immediate relief of a stenosed aortic valve. On the other hand, emerging aortic valve repair techniques have also shown satisfactory results for the management of aortic valve disease. However, repairs in severely dysplastic unicuspid and bicuspid valves are still evolving, and though promising results are seen in some studies, its utility long-term, especially in the pediatric population, is still unknown. Aortic valve replacement techniques have also improved throughout the years and have been the method of choice for some irreparable dysplastic valves. As more technically challenging repair and reconstruction techniques are developed throughout the years, it is imperative to understand if repair or replacement is a better option for certain patient populations.

This chapter will review current literature and attempt to address the following gaps: 1) Is balloon valvuloplasty or surgical valvulotomy more superior? 2) What repair techniques are available for management of aortic valve disease? 3) What are the available options for aortic valve replacement? 4) Is aortic valve repair superior to replacement, or is it just another way to delay aortic valve replacement?

## 2. Balloon valvuloplasty vs. surgical valvulotomy

The debate of whether balloon valvuloplasty or surgical valvulotomy is the superior initial management for aortic stenosis remains controversial. In balloon valvuloplasty, it is imperative to balance reducing the aortic valve gradient while limiting the amount of aortic regurgitation produced [1]. The challenge interventionalists face is having to make the decision of leaving a patient with residual aortic stenosis (AS) or acute aortic regurgitation (AR) when an ideal outcome is not possible. Both outcomes can pose as risk factors for poor long-term results and further reinterventions [2]. On the other hand, surgical valvulotomy for aortic stenosis is an emerging approach with continuous technique improvements to decrease mortality. However, it is not offered at many institutions as it can be technically challenging, especially for neonates. Hence, it is important to analyze the outcomes for both techniques in terms of the age of presentation – critical neonatal aortic stenosis vs. noncritical aortic stenosis.

### 2.1 Critical aortic stenosis of neonates

Patients under one month of age with aortic stenosis are classified as having critical neonatal aortic valve stenosis [1]. These patients are usually symptomatic, ductal dependent for survival, and have other associated cardiac congenital anomalies [3]. Most patients will have a smaller valve annulus with either a bicuspid or unicuspid aortic valve, although many are too dysplastic to differentiate [1, 3].

Balloon valvuloplasty has been the preferred method for the management of critical neonatal aortic valve stenosis for many decades. When balloon valvuloplasty is performed on patients with bicuspid or unicuspid valves, the tendency to cause a tear in the fused leaflet is high, causing prolapse of the leaflet, regurgitation, and a need for further intervention [4]. Hence, improvements in surgical valvulotomy techniques have raised the question of which is the superior management option for this patient population.

Donald et al. reviewed literature comparing the outcomes of both approaches in neonates and concluded that mortality is higher for balloon valvuloplasty (56%) compared to surgical valvulotomy (19%). They also concluded that undergoing either procedure during the neonatal period is a risk factor itself for poor outcomes [5]. A similar conclusion was reached by Siddiqui and colleagues who reported that for the group who underwent surgical valvulotomy, freedom from reintervention at 10 years for neonates and infants was 53.9% and 75%, respectively. Freedom from reintervention at 10 years for neonates who underwent balloon valvuloplasty was 17% compared to 50% in infants. They further reported that besides balloon valvuloplasty and age < 1 month, other factors associated with reintervention include unicuspid valve morphology, presence of endocardial fibroelastosis and presence of an atrial septal defect [6]. Zain et al. compared both approaches by performing a retrospective analysis on 25 neonates who underwent both balloon valvuloplasty and surgical valvulotomy. The majority of patients had a bicuspid aortic valve morphology, and one patient had unicuspid aortic valve morphology. Like the previous studies, they also concluded that patients who underwent balloon valvuloplasty had a higher reintervention rate. When comparing other long-term results like development of moderate to severe aortic regurgitation, balloon dilation was still the inferior option [7].

There are other studies that focused on the outcomes of balloon valvuloplasty mentioning neonatal intervention as a risk factor for mortality and high reintervention rates [1, 8–11]. However, many of these studies included patients before the year 1998, when the Norwood procedure was introduced. When excluding patients after the year 1998, mortality from balloon valvuloplasty decreased significantly. Another limitation that is not always mentioned in these studies, especially in retrospective studies, is that neonates who underwent balloon valvuloplasty tend to be more complex or ill at the time of intervention, hence resulting in a biased comparison [12].

Surgical repair techniques for aortic stenosis can range from a simple blade commissurotomy, to leaflet reconstruction with pericardial patches [13]. Although techniques for the repair of critical neonatal aortic stenosis are evolving, this approach is not adopted at many centers and most still prefer balloon valvuloplasty as the initial palliative method of choice [14]. In patients with tricuspid aortic valve morphology, most repairs consist of a simple blade commissurotomy where the extent of repair is largely within the surgeons' control [7, 15], unlike balloon valvuloplasty which is a blind technique, and the degree of damage is unknown at the time of intervention [7]. Some have argued that leaflet debridement should also be done for better long-term results during the surgical procedure [6, 14, 16]. For bicuspid and unicuspid aortic valves, surgical repair techniques are more complex as they can range from simple repairs or complete reconstruction of the aortic valve. Repair techniques will be discussed in a later section.

Alexiou et al. analyzed 18 neonates who underwent open valvulotomy for critical isolated aortic stenosis and concluded that operative mortality for surgical repair in this patient population has been decreasing over time as repair techniques improve. They performed simple commissurotomy to the aortic annulus and also excised obstructive nodules on the aortic valvular surfaces if present. Patients with bicuspid aortic valve morphology were not converted to tricuspid morphology. This study yielded excellent results where there was no early mortality and freedom from aortic reintervention was 85% at 5 years. However, the sample size was small and the study excluded patients with complex repairs [15]. Hraska and colleagues agreed with the previous study and stated that surgical valvulotomy in neonates can produce predictable and reliable long-term results for any valve morphology. They analyzed 34 neonates with various valve morphology and achieved a 100% freedom from aortic valve replacement at 20 years for patients with tricuspid valve morphology. They concluded that the underlying morphology and function of the LV are more important compared to the method of repair for determining outcomes. However, the long-term preservation of an acceptable function of the native aortic valve seems to depend on the method and the cusp anatomy. They believe that it is important to achieve tricuspid morphology in a dysplastic trileaflet valve during the repair for a better outcome, but valve reconstruction into a tricuspid morphology from a bicuspid or unicuspid morphology will not yield the same result [16]. Vergnat and colleagues adopted a 2-step approach for 103 neonates with critical neonatal aortic stenosis. It consists of leaflet remodeling and apparatus rehabilitation, and an attempt to achieve a tricuspid arrangement without leaflet reconstruction. They also highlighted the importance of leaflet debridement, which is only possible with surgical repair, to preserve the native valve as balloon dilation resulted in early stenosis [14].

In summary, although preliminary results seem to favor surgical repair of critical neonatal aortic stenosis, there are many other factors to consider. Patients in this population are often very ill and require immediate intervention for survival. This would have contributed to the high mortality rate for balloon valvuloplasty. Additionally, in most studies where the surgical repair was possible, they usually consist of simple surgical techniques like commissurotomy and debridement. Complex repairs are technically demanding and rarely performed in neonates and infants. Therefore, a non-bias method is needed to accurately compare the two approaches. This will be difficult as every patient presents differently and will have specific needs [16]. In terms of replacement options in this population, the Ross–Konno procedure may be the only option because of the small aortic annulus [17]. The Ross procedure will be discussed in a later section.

### 2.2 Noncritical aortic stenosis

Patients who present after the neonatal period generally have fewer dysplastic valves and adequate aortic annulus size, making surgical repair more feasible [3, 18]. Similar to critical aortic stenosis, surgical repair seems to be preferred in this patient population.

Hill and colleagues performed a meta-analysis to compare both techniques and reported that most literature either determined surgical valvulotomy as the more superior method or found no difference between the two. The meta-analysis consisted of 2368 patients with mean age of 2.9 months. Overall, at 10 years, the survival rate was 87% for balloon valvuloplasty and 90% for surgical valvulotomy. There was a significant difference for freedom from reintervention at 10 years, with balloon valvuloplasty at 46% and surgical valvulotomy at 73%; however, no significant difference for freedom from replacement was found. In a subgroup analysis for infants <1 year of age, the results were similar and only differences for freedom of reintervention were found with balloon valvuloplasty at 40% and surgical valvulotomy at 60% [19].

Brown et al. also concluded that surgical repair is the superior option after performing analysis on 158 patients older than 2 months of age. They reported that the surgical method resulted in greater gradient reduction and significantly less regurgitation. There was also a longer interval for reintervention for the surgical approach [18]. Brown et al. performed a retrospective analysis on 509 patients who underwent balloon valvuloplasty and concluded that patients older than 11 years of age have an increased risk of developing moderate to severe aortic regurgitation after balloon valvuloplasty [20]. Hence, it appears there may be certain age groups where balloon valvuloplasty should be avoided to minimize the possibility of reintervention.

Overall, it appears that surgical repair is superior to balloon valvuloplasty for patients with noncritical aortic stenosis by comparing freedom from reintervention rates. However, without standardization for the definition of successful management, thresholds for reintervention and replacement, or ballooning and repair techniques, it is difficult to compare the two modalities accurately without biases in both critical and noncritical aortic stenosis patients. Furthermore, most studies cover a diverse age group, span over different amounts of follow-up time, or cover different time periods, making the comparison even harder [5, 11, 12]. Since each patient's anatomy, physiology, and age of presentation are different, the management plan should be tailored for each individual to minimize complications [7, 9]. A successful outcome also depends on the options available and skills of the surgeons and interventionalists [9].

Balloon valvuloplasty has improved and become safer over the past decade [9]. Having a standardized progression may be helpful for this blind technique in minimizing complications. Porras et al. performed a study to investigate the utility of a Standardized Clinical Assessment and Management Plan (SCAMP) algorithm for the management of congenital aortic stenosis. They used the cut-off of ≤35 mmHg residual aortic stenosis and the degree of aortic regurgitation present after each ballooning to determine the option for further intervention. Following the algorithm, they managed to ensure that all patients achieve a final gradient of ≤35 mmHg without causing greater aortic regurgitation after the ballooning procedure [21]. However, it is worth noting that the study sample size only consisted of 23 patients and 92 controls, and follow-up duration was only 10 years.

There are other studies that agree with Porras et al. that acute residual aortic stenosis gradient and post-dilation aortic regurgitation were factors most strongly related to the decision for long-term aortic valve replacement [2, 10, 12, 20]. Rao and colleagues concluded that the most important factors leading to restenosis are immediate post-valvuloplasty aortic valve stenosis and patients ≤3 years of age at the time of procedure. They also commented that many studies found a linear relationship between follow-up time duration and post-procedural aortic insufficiency, however, no definite causative factors were found [12]. Brown et al. also concluded that a residual aortic stenosis gradient of ≤35 mmHg was associated with greater freedom from aortic valve replacement and stated that having a lower aortic stenosis gradient might be more important than ensuring minimal aortic regurgitation [20]. However, Sullivan et al. disagreed and reported that acute post-procedural aortic regurgitation is associated with a greater risk instead. They discovered that patients with moderate or severe acute aortic regurgitation post-procedure with residual aortic stenosis gradients <30 mmHg had three times greater long-term risk for aortic valve replacement compared to those with mild or less aortic regurgitation and > 30 mmHg residual gradient. However, they did note that the study population consisted of more neonates, and age could be a modifier [2].

Since reinterventions and replacement might be inevitable due to recurrent stenosis or progressive aortic regurgitation [11, 22], balloon valvuloplasty can be considered as an initial palliative option for ill patients [7, 11]. Zain et al. proposed that balloon valvuloplasty should be done for bicuspid valves with equal size leaflets, while surgery should be reserved for thick, nodular dysplastic valves or unicuspid valves with small aortic annulus to prevent the need for multiple interventions [7, 11]. Ballooning in highly dysplastic valves distributes circumferential force unevenly, causing tears in the weakest part of the aortic valve and may therefore disrupt the cusps unevenly leading to poorer outcomes [11, 18]. On the other hand, surgical repair allows for direct inspection of the valve where surgeons can have better control of the extent of commissurotomy and more precise repair [7, 15]. Nonetheless, repeat balloon valvuloplasty should still be considered as the first option in most patients after restenosis as it can still yield excellent results [12].

## 3. Aortic repair

Many aortic repair techniques have evolved since their first introduction resulting in improved mortality and reintervention rates. However, its place in the management of patients with aortic valve disease is still controversial. Another big debate is whether aortic repair or replacement is superior, despite most agreeing that aortic valve replacement is inevitable in patients with congenital aortic valve disease.

The aortic repair can range from simple techniques such as commissurotomy to complex ones such as aortic valve neocuspidization. To perform a precise aortic valve repair, it is imperative to understand that the aortic valve operates as a unit consisting of the ventriculo-aortic (VAJ) and sino-tubular junction (STJ). These provide a framework for a functional annulus and cusps (**Figure 1**). Hence, both the annulus and cusps need to be considered at the time of surgery to ensure a proper repair [4, 23–26]. The ideal goal of any aortic valve repair is to restore the leaflets and functional aortic annulus to their normal geometry while ensuring normal mobility of the valve cusps [24].

A repair-oriented functional classification was developed to improve understanding of the pathophysiology and communication between physicians [27, 28]. With this classification, an algorithm can be established to guide physicians to the correct procedure. Type 1 refers to defects in the functional annulus, and it is divided into several subtypes. Type 1a refers to dilation in the STJ and ascending aorta, type 1b indicates dilation is in the STJ, sinuses of Valsalva, and the VAJ, and lastly type 1c refers to pure dilation of the VAJ. Depending on the subgroup, the regurgitant jet differs and physicians will be able to determine the type of annuloplasty that is appropriate [24, 26–30]. Type 2 refers to aortic insufficiency caused by cusp prolapse due to excessive motion of the aortic cusps [24, 26–28]. These are generally managed by resuspension, free margin plication, or triangular resection techniques [27–29]. Lastly, there is type 3 aortic insufficiency where cusp motion is restricted, possibly due to thickening and fibrosis. This is potentially the most challenging pathology for repair procedures as an additional patch augmentation is frequently needed which can result in structural degradation [24, 26–28, 31]. Other aortic valve pathologies that are not classified are cusp perforation and aortic stenosis. Cusp perforations are generally repaired directly with a patch [28]. Materials for leaflet

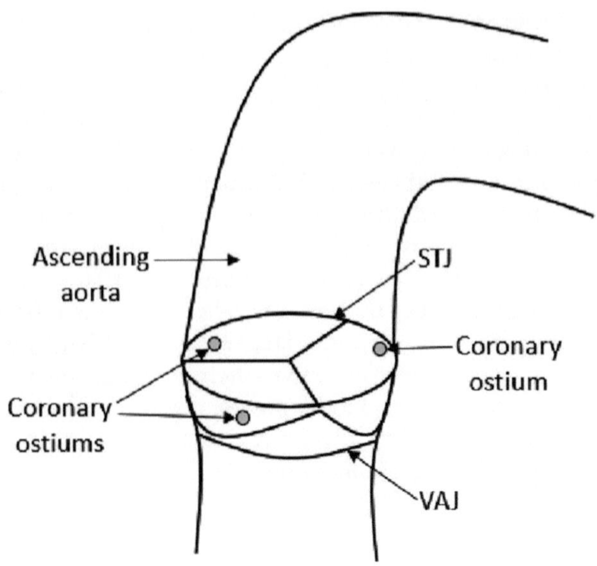


**Figure 1.**
*Anatomy of the aortic valve.*

and patch repair will be discussed in a later section. Aortic stenosis is commonly managed with commissurotomy [29] or reconstruction, depending on the complexity, if the repair route is chosen.

Since bicuspid aortic valves are the most prevalent aortic valve disease, these are also the most commonly repaired morphology [29]. They often present with defects that are combined from the subgroups listed above, with the most common being prolapse of the fused cusp with dilation in the annulus [24, 28, 32]. Cusp configuration of bicuspid aortic valves uses a different classification first proposed by Sievers and Schmidtkes (**Table 1**). The most common, type 1, refers to a bicuspid valve with a median raphe and asymmetrical aortic sinuses, and type 0 refers to a symmetrical bicuspid valve with no raphe present [24, 27]. Repairs for type 0 valves are usually straightforward and performed in a similar fashion to tricuspid valves, where the nonprolapsed cusp is used as the reference height for plication or resuspension. In type 1 repairs, patch augmentation may be required depending on the amount of native cusp tissue left after shaving or debridement [24]. For patients where annulus dilation is present, a valve-sparing reimplantation technique for annuloplasty might be preferred as it carries less risk for recurrent dilation. Although reimplantation is a more technically challenging procedure, compared to a subcommisural annuloplasty, both techniques are similar in terms of morbidity [24, 33]. Hence, surgeons who have the expertise should consider performing valve-sparing implantation for better long-term outcomes. The overall goal in the repair of bicuspid valves should meet the following two criteria to ensure an optimal aortic root geometry: 1) the basal ring diameter should be reduced to less than 25 mm, 2) effective cusp height should be restored to above 8 mm. This will lead to better long-term valve stability and minimize degradation rate of the tissues [28].

Unicuspid aortic valves were previously classified under the Sievers classification for BAV as Type 2 due to the presence of two raphes; however many now consider it as a separate entity due to its unique anatomy [32, 34]. There are two main types of unicuspid aortic valves – either unicommissural (most common) where an eccentric slit-like orifice is present with one commissural attachment, or a commissural where there is a pinhole orifice with no commissural attachment [34–37]. Management of unicuspid aortic valve remains a challenge since patients often have dysplastic and severely calcified cusps with no functional native tissue [28]. Therefore, the aortic replacement has been the main method of management for a unicuspid aortic valve for many decades; however, more are turning to repair first and delaying replacement to prevent complications from valve replacement [38].

| **Sievers and Schmidtkes classification** | | | |
|---|---|---|---|
| **Types** | **Type 0** | **Type 1** | **Type 2 (unicuspid)** |
| Number of raphes (shown as dotted lines) | 0 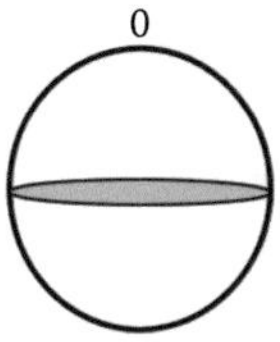 | 1 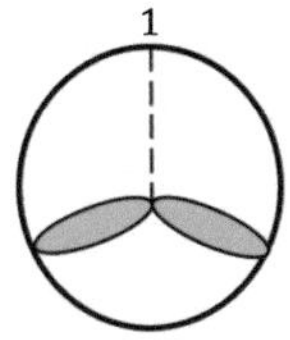 | 2 or more 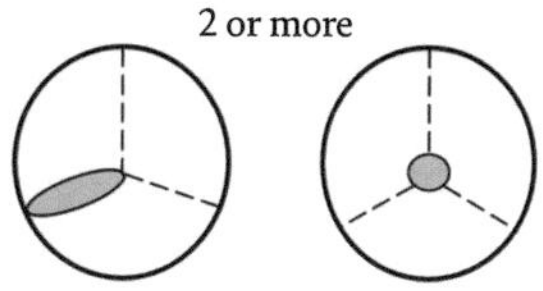 |

**Table 1.**
*Sievers and Schmidtkes classification for bicuspid aortic valve.*

### 3.1 Bicuspidization

Schäfers et al. proposed the first unicuspid aortic valve bicuspidization repair technique which consisted of a reconstructive approach for unicommissural unicuspid aortic valve with aortic regurgitation or dilatation [34, 36]. The technique utilized stay sutures on the commissure with normal height, as well as one placed at the same height above the rudimentary anterior commissure to indicate the location of the new commissure. The fused cusp tissue was then incised anteriorly. Glutaraldehyde-treated autologous pericardium was then used to fill the gap between the rudimentary cusp and new commissure, and also for the defect of the fused cusp so that it is in the position of the rudimentary cusp [36]. This ultimately leads to a standard asymmetric BAV configuration with 2 normal commissures [34]. The key parameter in this repair was an effective cusp height of 8 mm in pediatric and 10 mm in adult repairs to ensure a near-normal geometry to guarantee consistency and reliable results. The technique was performed on 20 patients with a mean age of 26. Schafers et al. reported good initial functional results with satisfactory hemodynamics post repair. At 4 years following repair, freedom from moderate or more aortic regurgitation was 77%, freedom from reoperation was 67%, and freedom from aortic valve replacement was 100%. However, the durability of autologous pericardium for cusp extension was not explored in this study. Furthermore, due to the short follow-up period, cusp configuration as a patient grows is also unknown [36].

Aicher et al. investigated hemodynamic effects and overall stability differences between the asymmetric reconstruction technique proposed by Schafers et al. previously, and a similar symmetric bicuspidization cusp reconstruction. The study consisted of 118 patients at a mean age of 27 years with either aortic stenosis, aortic regurgitation, or both. Glutaraldehyde-treated autologous pericardium was used for both groups, and both the effective and geometric heights were kept consistent at 10 mm and > 20 mm, respectively. Overall, there was no significant difference in reoperation rates between the configurations; however, the symmetric configuration yielded better hemodynamics with lower mean and peak gradients, especially during exercise [39]. Furthermore, Aicher et al. and Franciulli et al. combined the repair technique to include root remodeling to address aneurysm of ascending aorta and aortic roots which occur commonly in the unicuspid aortic valve. Dilation of the VAJ had previously been identified as a risk factor for repair failure [40]. Both studies reported improvement in the durability comparted to isolated aortic valve repair. Additionally, Franciulli et al. reported postoperative hemodynamics similar to age-matched patient population with tricuspid aortic valve.

Kolesar et al. extended the symmetrical cusp repair technique to 17 patients with stenotic unicuspid aortic valve and a mean age of 23 years. They also agreed on the importance of ensuring a standardized cusp effective height to minimize the risk of reoperation. Kolesar and colleagues also performed open extra-aortic ring implantation using a Dacron tubular graft in patients with annulus ≥25 mm, given the high risk of aortic annulus dilatation in unicuspid aortic valve. They reported that performing a ring annuloplasty in valve-sparing aortic valve repair significantly increases freedom from valve-related reoperation and freedom from moderate or worse aortic regurgitation. Freedom from valve-related reoperation was 100%, although the follow-up period was too short (about 2 years). Similar to the previous studies, they also highlighted the importance of creating a symmetrical orientation with the new commissure. One difference between the repair techniques proposed by Kolesar and Schafer is that Kolesar used equine pericardium instead of autologous pericardium.

Despite this, Kolesar reported no statistically significant difference in freedom of reoperation between the two patch materials [37].

Matsushima et al. [41] proposed that management of unicuspid aortic valve, whether aortic stenosis or regurgitation, should be a three-stage approach - firstly, balloon aortic valvulotomy during infancy or neonatal period, then bicuspidization with cusp augmentation, and lastly aortic valve replacement mainly with a pulmonary autograft later in life if needed. They also used a symmetrical bicuspidization technique and involved 60 patients who are 18 years old or younger in the study. These authors reported an overall survival of 96% at 5 and 10 years. However, 33% of patients required aortic valve reoperation, mainly due to patch degeneration. The authors also agreed with Kolesar et al. that an external suture annuloplasty is necessary during the repair to improve cusp coaptation, reduce cusp stress and prevent suture dehiscence especially if the aortic root is dilated.

The authors also noted that bicuspidization using their technique can be done even after a balloon aortic valvuloplasty is performed during neonatal period. Their repair technique can tolerate cusp tear which occurs commonly during balloon valvuloplasty. Therefore, initial balloon valvulotomies are not a contraindication for their bicuspidization cusp repair technique. In balloon dilation for unicuspid aortic valve, tears commonly occur opposite to the normal commissure, which in this case is removed for this bicuspidization technique, hence avoiding the controversial debate on initial management plan [41]. They utilized three different patch materials for cusp augmentation – glutaraldehyde-treated autologous pericardium, decellularized xenogenic tissue, and expanded polytetrafluoroethylene (ePTFE) membrane. For each material, freedom from aortic valve reoperation using autologous pericardium was 72% and 52% at 5 and 10 years respectively. 50% of patients with ePTFE membrane required aortic valve reoperation later in life; however, this sample size was small (2 out of 4 patients). None of the patients with decellularized xenogeneic tissue required aortic valve reoperation. They concluded that each patch material had its own limitations. For example, patch augmentation with glutaraldehyde-fixed autologous pericardium was more prone to patch degeneration, and suture dehiscence was more commonly seen when using the ePTFE membrane. Overall, decellularized xenopericardial patch yielded the best durability, however, a longer follow-up period is required to compare appropriately with autologous pericardium [41].

Other studies have also investigated the utility of different materials in aortic valve repair of various valve morphology. Nezhard et al. compared the repair of various aortic valve malformations with either bovine or non-treated autologous pericardium. They concluded that non-treated autologous pericardium was preferred in easy and less technical repairs, such as perforation patching, and the bovine pericardium was preferred in complex repairs or when autologous pericardium was not available. Overall, the bovine pericardium is comparable with autologous pericardium, however, it still does not compare with native valve tissue and should be avoided if possible [42]. Nordmeyer et al. investigated the durability of decellularized bovine pericardial patch material for aortic valve reconstruction. Despite the reported advantages of the material and excellent short-term results, the authors disagreed with Matsushima and reported concerns regarding long-term durability of the material. Patients with decellularized bovine pericardial patches had thickened leaflets with reduced mobility at 3 years and required further reintervention. Therefore, the search for an optimal patch material is still ongoing [43].

Si et al. addressed the issue of patch degeneration by proposing a bicuspidization unicuspid aortic valve repair with primary leaflet reconstruction and geometric annuloplasty ring repair. They studied patients with aortic regurgitation and attempted to create cusps using primarily the patient's native leaflet tissue. Using this technique supported with an appropriately sized annuloplasty ring, they created cusps with equal free-edge length, geometric, and effective heights. The authors reported excellent results and concluded that most unicuspid aortic valve variations can be repaired using this standard technique. However, the study was limited due to its small sample size and short follow-up durations. More importantly, the repair technique was limited by the smallest available ring size, which is currently around 19 mm, making the technique inappropriate for repair in infants or children [44].

### 3.2 Tricuspidization/reconstruction

A recently emerging repair technique for unicuspid, as well as bicuspid aortic valves, is tricuspidization by reconstructing all three leaflets [45]. Reconstruction of aortic valves was first proposed by Duran et al.; these authors reported 51 patients with a mean age of 31.2 years who underwent reconstruction of all three leaflets using a single strip of rectangular glutaraldehyde-treated autologous pericardium [46]. Despite some success, the authors concluded that a standardized procedure is needed to ensure technique reproducibility and that further research is needed to determine the best material for reconstruction [46]. Most recent literature includes various valve morphologies in their studies, with the majority being bicuspid aortic valves.

Ozaki et al. proposed another technique that consisted of the reconstruction of each leaflet independently using glutaraldehyde-treated autologous pericardium [47]. This technique is also known as aortic neocuspidization (AVNeo). Since the technique involves complete resection of all three dysplastic leaflets, it can be applied to any congenital aortic valve malformation, even when root reimplantation is required in patients with annulo-aortic ectasia [47]. The authors performed this technique in over 404 patients with unicuspid, bicuspid, tricuspid, and quadricuspid aortic valves. They believe that an aortic valve should be considered as a collection of different-size cusps, and by measuring the distance between the commissure, one should be able to determine the area of each cusp and perform individual cusp reconstruction. With this technique, reconstruction can more effectively preserve the natural motion of the annulus and the coordination between the structures surrounding the aortic valve. At 4 years of follow-up, the survival rate was 87.7% and freedom from reoperation was 96.2% [48]. In another study, Ozaki and associates focused the technique on bicuspid and unicuspid valve morphology in patients under 60 years and noted commendable hemodynamics in all patients, especially those under 40 years. There were also no signs of calcification, as well as natural motion of all three cusps [49]. Ozaki and colleagues later updated their procedure, and the biggest change was seen in the repair of patients without trileaflet aortic valves. They decided that tricuspidization with three equal-size cusps was preferred for an even movement of the cusps [50].

Previously, AVNeo was performed largely in the adult population, where the predominant pathology was acquired calcific aortic stenosis associated with bicuspid valves. In the pediatric population, patients who require further intervention usually are diagnosed with congenital aortic valve stenosis and have previously undergone balloon aortic valvuloplasty resulting in regurgitation. Therefore, since AVNeo requires excision of all leaflets, it is applicable in most pediatric patients as well [45]. The AVNeo procedure was reproduced by Baird and colleagues on the pediatric population with a variety of congenital aortic valve morphologies. Due to the prevalence of bicuspid and unicuspid valve morphology in the pediatric population that required intervention, the authors noted technical differences in the pediatric population when creating the 3 equal leaflets. They also highlighted a need to augment the noncoronary sinus leaflet to accommodate 3 equal leaflets creating similar annular and STJ, given the small aortic valve dimensions [51]. Overall, they found satisfactory post-reconstruction hemodynamics and the possibility for annular growth. They also concluded that the Ozaki procedure is promising for pediatric patients, however, it can be technically challenging in patients with smaller aortic annuli and roots and should only be performed by experienced surgeons [45]. Wiggins and associates also utilized AVNeo, as well as a single leaflet reconstruction technique for tricuspidization in pediatric patients who were unable to undergo either a mechanical replacement or the Ross procedure. They were able to successfully perform the procedure in patients with annular sizes as small as 6.7 mm with resultant favorable post-surgical hemodynamics. The authors also commented on the benefit of increased free margin length in AVNeo, and the advantages of preserving annular hemodynamics to allow growth and further reconstruction surgeries if required [22].

### *3.2.1 Reconstruction materials*

Another controversial topic in the reconstruction of aortic valves is the preferred material for the AVNeo procedure [45]. While autologous pericardium is the most widely used for the procedure due to its availability, convenience, and low cost [4, 52]. Recent studies have shown it to be less favorable due to its poor biomechanical properties, high rates of calcification, and lack of growth potential [4, 45, 51].

The autologous pericardium has been considered the "gold standard" material for aortic valve repair and reconstruction for many decades. Treatment with glutaraldehyde produces autologous pericardium that is more resistant to retraction and degeneration [52]. It can also increase the tensile strength to four times greater than noncalcified native aortic leaflets [50]. However, varying reoperation rates ranging from 15 to 33% have been reported in different studies. Many previous studies focused on the durability of glutaraldehydetreated autologous pericardium in AVNeo performed in the adult population, but its durability in younger patients has not been studied and needs to be further investigated since there is an increased risk of degeneration [22].

The first studies investigating materials for aortic valve reconstruction were by Duran et al., where they compared bovine and autologous pericardium. They determined that autologous pericardium was more favorable as it did not show fibrocalcific deterioration, unlike bovine pericardium. They also concluded that the durability of pericardium will depend on its implanted position and the pretreatment process [53].

Several types of treated bovine pericardium have since been introduced for valve leaflet reconstruction. An example is CardioCel®, where bovine pericardium is treated with glutaraldehyde, as well as by further anti calcification tissue-engineering techniques, prior to reconstruction [45, 51]. Mazzitelli and colleagues utilized CardioCel® for three pediatric AVNeo procedures and reported that there were no reoperations at early follow-up [54]. Despite promising results, long-term follow-up is not available and is needed due to concerns about developing calcification [22, 45, 51]. Another example is the Photofix®, a bovine pericardium that undergoes photo-oxidation fixation. Compared to the glutaraldehyde-treated bovine pericardium, it is more resistant to calcification and inflammation, making it a more durable option. However, Photofix® showed signs of annular separation that are of concern [45, 51]. Lastly, there is also the Matrix®, an untreated equine pericardium, which has shown satisfactory preliminary results. Furthermore, its thin thickness may be advantageous for smaller pediatric patients [45]. Another interesting theory that is yet to be explored is the remodeling characteristics of extracellular matrix scaffolds. It has been proven in some tissues that degradation occurs due to host remodeling responses to naturally occurring biologic extracellular matrix scaffolds. Hence, durable valve leaflets can potentially be produced if extracellular matrix scaffolds are seeded with mesenchymal stem cells to be differentiated into valve leaflets. However, this theory has yet to be proven [4].

### 3.3 Unicuspid aortic valve: bicuspidization or tricuspidization?

In unicuspid aortic valves, it is debatable whether a symmetrical bicuspidization technique is superior to a tricuspidization method. This may have been related to the variability in commissural height and interrelation of three coaptation lines in tricuspid aortic valves [39].

Kawase et al. performed trileaflet reconstruction on 9 unicommissural unicuspid aortic valve patients. They utilized glutaraldehyde-treated autologous pericardium to independently construct each leaflet so that coordination of the valve leaflets is maximized. These authors reported that tricuspidization is superior to bicuspidization as it produces a longer total length of the free margin of the aortic valve leaflets, resulting in a better full opening of the aortic valve. However, the study was only performed on adults with a mean age of 48.9, and the average follow-up time was 18 months. Hence, a larger and wider study population, and long-term results are needed [38]. Kohei and associates discussed tricuspidization of 2 patients with unicuspid aortic valves and performed aortic valvuloplasty and root construction using autologous pericardium and a prosthetic graft. They agree that bicuspidization is hemodynamically inferior to tricuspidization as it adds stress to the leaflets and restricts opening. However, long-term results are also unavailable to determine the durability of this approach [55]. Therefore, it appears that tricuspidization is an area of repair that yet to be explored for unicuspid aortic valve repair. Both studies discussing tricuspidization techniques were performed on adults with a small sample size, hence durability results in pediatric population and long-term results are lacking.

## 4. Aortic valve replacement

Before the emergence of surgical repair as an option to delay aortic valve replacement, the common management plan for most patients with isolated aortic stenosis was to perform balloon valvuloplasty until a replacement is needed. Isolated aortic valve replacement is generally associated with low mortality and morbidity especially if performed worsening the myocardial function [56]. However, the decision of which type of aortic valve replacement to choose is complex as it depends on many factors such as patient characteristics, medication compliance, access to care, etc. [57]. In younger patients, it is important to choose a valve replacement that is resistant to degeneration, infection, and has growth potential [56]. Whereas, in the older population, the priority lies in minimizing the need for anticoagulation due to potential thromboembolism complications [57, 58].

Tissue aortic valves can be either bioprosthetic with bovine or porcine valves, homografts, or allografts. They are generally preferred in older patients due to their low thromboembolism risk [57–59]. However, tissue valves are prone to a high risk of degeneration and structural failure which translates to high reoperation rates [56, 59–62], hence their use needs to be carefully evaluated [58]. Additionally, they often come in sizes larger than 19 mm, lack growth potential, and are prone to patient-prosthesis mismatch (PPM) as the recipient grows. One of the few pediatric populations, where tissue replacement can be considered is teenage females who wish to be pregnant in the future due to lack of anticoagulation. However, if accompanying conditions such as atrial fibrillation, previous emboli, or an enlarged left atrium are present, the need for anticoagulation may still be warranted [56, 58, 62, 63]. Homografts may sometimes be available in smaller sizes suitable for younger children, and they are associated with excellent hemodynamics. They are also resistant to infection, which makes them preferred for patients with invasive endocarditis. However, the limitation of rapid valve deterioration leading to recurrent stenosis and regurgitation outweighs these benefits, hence its use is often discouraged [61].

The most attractive aspect of mechanical aortic valves is its superb durability. However, its biggest drawbacks are the need for anticoagulation which can significantly impact quality of life, and the lack of growth potential [58, 64, 65]. In older patients, this can lead to drug interactions and increased thromboembolic risks. In children, there can be possible compliance issues and difficulty with activity restraints, though children seem to have an overall lower risk of bleeding and thromboembolism [58]. Newer generation mechanical valves have been explored to prevent the need for warfarin and an INR goal >2.5, however, eliminating anticoagulation completely is still unattainable in mechanical valves [57]. In children with mechanical valves, the use of antiplatelet drugs instead of warfarin for anticoagulation can be considered [63]. Reoperations are uncommon in patients who have received mechanical valve replacements, and they are mainly due to PPM or subvalvular obstruction, both more prevalent in the younger recipients [58, 61, 64]. Overall, the freedom from reoperation for this subgroup is over 92% at 20 years in both adults and children [64].

The Ross procedure utilizes the patient's own pulmonary valve to replace the diseased aortic valve and a tissue valve for the pulmonary valve [59]. Though this procedure is more technically demanding than the other replacement methods, it produces better hemodynamics, fewer complications, and allows growth potential in the aortic valve [58, 59, 66]. Since the pulmonary autograft is relatively resistant to calcification or degeneration, trans-valvular gradients mostly remain unchanged from the immediate post-operative period. Additionally, having better post-replacement hemodynamics places less strain on the left ventricle, overall resulting in improved mortality [59].

The biggest disadvantage to this approach is that it results in a double valve disease where both valves will be at risk for reoperation and degeneration [60]. Some argue that most reoperations after a Ross procedure occur on the pulmonary conduit [60, 67], and this results in a higher total reoperation rate if both valves are considered, compared to mechanical replacement [60, 66, 68]. Many alternatives for the pulmonary valve have been investigated but none were superior to a homograft. The only exception was in young infants since homografts have poor durability [66].

The preferred age groups for the Ross procedure are older children and young adults, especially those with normal-sized aortic annulus due to procedure complexity [65, 66]. Infants less than age 1 generally have a high mortality rate of up to 20%, but this decreases as patient age increases and falls to almost 1% for children above 1 year old [58, 60, 69]. It is also important to note that patients who require the Ross procedure as an infant generally have critical stenosis with failed previous repair or balloon valvuloplasty which may have contributed to the high mortality [69]. Besides mortality, pulmonary valve reoperations were also reported to be higher in neonates and infants compared to older children [60, 69].

The most common complication of the Ross procedure is aortic root dilation causing regurgitation [58, 70]. Reoperation rates due to dilation can range from 8 to 30% within 10 years after surgery [66, 70]. Several methods to prevent dilation and improve durability have been explored. The most common strategy is to place external support, using either a Dacron (DuPont, Wilmington, DE) graft or a Gelweave (Vascutek Ltd., Renfrewshire, United Kingdom) sinus of Valsalva graft around the aortic root. Excellent results have been reported for this technique – freedom from dilatation for standard Ross at 3 years was 52%, and is 90% for supported Ross [58, 66, 68, 71, 72]. External stabilization using a strip of Daron at the STJ has also been explored and is considered a standard Ross procedure in some institutions for older children [66, 73]. Another common approach is to wrap the native aortic root around the pulmonary autograft for extra stabilization [70, 71]. However, this approach is limited by the size of the aortic root. In patients with bicuspid aortic valve and aortic insufficiency, their aortic roots are usually already dilated and hence will be unable to provide adequate support. On the other hand, patients with bicuspid aortic valves with aortic stenosis tend to have small aortic roots which are not feasible for this method of stabilization [73].

Despite promising results with different supported Ross procedures, these stabilization techniques should only be used for older children or young adults because it eliminates the growth potential which is a crucial benefit of the Ross procedure as a replacement option [14, 68, 71–73]. A new supported Ross technique with Konno annular enlargement using a subcoronary technique has been explored to extend the procedure to younger children. However, this procedure becomes extremely complicated, and long-term results are needed to prove its durability [72].

Between tissue and mechanical aortic valve replacements, mechanical replacements seem superior overall. Tissue valves do not require anticoagulation and can be available in smaller sizes; however, their high rate of valve degeneration and reintervention makes it a poor valve replacement option for young patients. On the other hand, mechanical valves have better durability and higher freedom from reoperation rates [64, 69]. Despite better long-term benefits, its impact on quality of life due to anticoagulation needs to be evaluated when considering this replacement option.

Both tissue replacement and the Ross procedure share similar immediate post-operative hemodynamic and are both resistant to infections. Furthermore, they are both available in small sizes and do not require anticoagulation. In terms of surgical technicality, tissue replacements are generally easier since it does not involve the pulmonary valve. However, tissue valves are associated with rapid valve deterioration, resulting in higher mortality and reoperation rates. Therefore, though it can be an option if resources are available, it is less preferred in the younger patients [59, 60, 69, 74].

Overall, there is no statistically significant difference in reoperation rates between mechanical replacement and the Ross procedure [65, 69]. However, surgeries involving the mechanical valve are less complicated since it does not involve the pulmonary valve or the aortic root procedures [64]. The Ross procedure may have superiority since it allows for growth potential and does not involve anticoagulation, resulting in more favorable cardiac and valve-related mortality [59, 60, 65, 69]. Nonetheless, it is difficult to compare these two approaches since the Ross procedure is usually performed on younger patients for congenital causes, whereas the mechanical replacement is favored in older patients with connective or rheumatic tissue pathologies, or preoperative aortic regurgitation [75].

Ultimately, all approaches to replacement have their own risk and benefits. To properly evaluate the best option, it is important to first consider the age of the patient, the need for growth potential, and the possible need for reoperations in the future. The second important point is then to assess for possible complications and comorbidities.

### 4.1 Repair vs. replacement

The topic of whether aortic valve repair or replacement is the preferred approach to the management of aortic valve pathology is again controversial. Both aortic valve repair and replacement have produced similar results and shown their respective benefits and limitations [76]. Many institutions have started to express their preference to repair valves and delay replacement for as long as possible. Burrato and associates noted an increase in durability when the Ross procedure is done as a reoperation after valve repair and attributed this to the presence of postoperative scarring aiding in natural stabilization [77]. Similarly, favorable results were also reported by Popov et al. regarding mechanical valve replacement after previous repair [61].

There are subgroups of patients in whom repair has been shown to be a superior approach to replacement. Etnel et al. performed a meta-analysis and concluded that replacement is a suboptimal option in the pediatric population [60]. Generally, the repair is preferred in younger patients as it allows for growth potential, where most replacement options are unable to accommodate growth and will require multiple reoperations. Repair also avoids anticoagulation complications and activity restrictions [23, 78]. Danial et al. compared repair and the Ross procedure and concluded that both options were similar in terms of mortality and freedom from reintervention. However, aortic valve repair pulled ahead in terms of surgical morbidity and complications. They also noted that in patients who require immediate intervention, repair with a patch is the preferred option since it yields better short-term outcomes [64]. It is important to note that both young age and unicuspid valve morphology were identified as the greatest risk factors for poor outcomes in repairs [31]. Additionally, pediatric patients who present with an aortic valve deformity usually have complex pathology that requires multiple interventions. Hence, these risks and repair complexity should be weighed against the limitations of having a replacement [79]. It is possible that aortic valve repair should be considered for neonates and infants, whereas both aortic valve repair and the Ross procedure can be options for older children [78]. Ultimately, replacement may be unavoidable for patients who present with aortic valve disease at a young age.

Another population where a repair can be more favorable is in adults where replacement is contraindicated or those who are already undergoing other cardiac procedures at the same time [23, 27]. Regardless of the patient population, the surgeon's comfort level and experience in performing the aortic valve repair can also deter the decision as well [23, 80]. Another thought is to choose the management approach depending on whether the pathology is aortic stenosis, insufficiency, or mixed disease. Valve repair has shown satisfactory low reintervention rates for patients with aortic stenosis. However, the repair had a higher reintervention rate for patients with mixed disease or aortic insufficiency. This could however be institution dependent as repair outcomes depend largely on the surgeon's experience and expertise [81].

In conclusion, it is difficult to compare both modalities without bias as repair techniques are still evolving and there is still a lack of long-term data available.

Additionally, many complex repair techniques, especially for children, are only available at several specialized institution whereas aortic valve replacement techniques have been around for many decades and are known to be safe and successful among most surgeons [23]. Studies that focused solely on either repair or replacement usually consist of different patient populations with varying aortic valve pathology [29].

To increase the widespread practice of aortic valve repair techniques, there needs to be a standardized range of techniques to help guide surgeons through variations in valve deformities. More surgeons will need to be trained and familiarized with these techniques so that they will have the expertise to explore repair instead of relying on the reliable replacement option [23, 81]. An example algorithm was proposed by Danial and colleagues, where repair should be preferred if native cusps with good mobility can be achieved after shaving and/or debridement, there is at least one functional commissure, and a cusp-free margin that is composed of half native tissue. However, if the aortic annulus is less than two standard deviations, both repair and replacement can be done together with the Konno procedure [67, 81]. Another management pathway that was suggested for the pediatric population depended on peak systolic gradient or Doppler mean gradient [82].

## 5. Conclusion

There are many decisions to make when managing a patient with aortic valve disease, and it is crucial to conscientiously evaluate each decision as they can all have a huge impact on the patient's life. Regardless of the management approach, it is certain that young age of intervention, especially for neonates and babies under the age of 1, is the main risk factor for poor outcomes. For the pediatric population, an attempt to preserve the native valves for as long as possible is important to minimize reintervention rates. A possible basic algorithm for patients with aortic stenosis could be to either perform balloon valvuloplasty or simple surgical valvulotomy as an initial step and to delay replacement for as long as possible. The choice between balloon or surgery will be dependent on the age, condition severity, and symptoms at presentation. If replacement is then needed at a later age, a supported or non-supported Ross procedure may be the most appropriate. Unfortunately, the management of patients with aortic regurgitation or mixed disease is a lot more complex. Many promising repair techniques have been developed for highly dysplastic bicuspid or unicuspid valves, however, long-term and age-matched results for durability and morbidity are still lacking.

## Conflict of interest

The authors declare no conflict of interest.

**Author details**

Si Hui Wong[1], Daniel Nento[2], Harinder Singh[2] and Arpit Agarwal[2*]

1 The Children's Hospital of San Antonio, San Antonio, USA

2 Baylor College of Medicine, The Children's Hospital of San Antonio, San Antonio, USA

*Address all correspondence to: arpit.agarwal@bcm.edu

## References

[1] Boe BA, Zampi JD, Kennedy KF, Jayaram N, Porras D, Foerster SR, et al. Acute success of balloon aortic valvuloplasty in the current era: A National Cardiovascular Data Registry study. JACC: Cardiovascular Interventions. 2017;**10**(17):1717-1726. DOI: 10.1016/j.jcin.2017.08.001

[2] Sullivan PM, Rubio AE, Johnston TA, Jones TK. Long-term outcomes and re-interventions following balloon aortic valvuloplasty in pediatric patients with congenital aortic stenosis: A single-center study. Catheterization and Cardiovascular Interventions. 2017;**89**(2):288-296. DOI: 10.1002/ccd.26722

[3] Jonas R. Comprehensive Surgical Management of Congenital Heart Disease. CRC press; 2002. ISBN-13: 978-1444112153. ISBN-10: 1444112155

[4] Baird CW, Myers PO, Pedro J. Aortic valve reconstruction in the young infants and children. In: Seminars in Thoracic and Cardiovascular Surgery: Pediatric Cardiac Surgery Annual. Elsevier. 2012;**15**(1):9-19. DOI: 10.1053/j.pcsu.2012.01.004

[5] Donald JS, Konstantinov IE. Surgical aortic valvuloplasty versus balloon aortic valve dilatation in children. World Journal for Pediatric and Congenital Heart Surgery. 2016;7(5):583-591. DOI: 10.1177/2150135116651091

[6] Siddiqui J, Brizard CP, Galati JC, Iyengar AJ, Hutchinson D, Konstantinov IE, et al. Surgical valvotomy and repair for neonatal and infant congenital aortic stenosis achieves better results than interventional catheterization. Journal of the American College of Cardiology. 2013;**62**(22):2134-2140. DOI: 10.1016/j.jacc.2013.07.052

[7] Zain Z, Zadinello M, Menahem S, Brizard C. Neonatal isolated critical aortic valve stenosis: Balloon valvuloplasty or surgical valvotomy. Heart, Lung and Circulation. 2006;**15**(1):18-23. DOI: 10.1016/j.hlc.2005.02.003

[8] Crespo D, Miró J, Vobecky SJ, Poirier N, Lapierre C, Zhao NN, et al. Experience in a single Centre with percutaneous aortic valvoplasty in children, including those with associated cardiovascular lesions. Cardiology in the Young. 2009;**19**(4):372-382. DOI: 10.1017/S1047951109990308

[9] Torres A, Vincent JA, Everett A, Lim S, Foerster SR, Marshall AC, et al. Balloon valvuloplasty for congenital aortic stenosis: Multi-center safety and efficacy outcome assessment. Catheterization and Cardiovascular Interventions. 2015;**86**(5):808-820. DOI: 10.1002/ccd.25969

[10] Maskatia SA, Ing FF, Justino H, Crystal MA, Mullins CE, Mattamal RJ, et al. Twenty-five year experience with balloon aortic valvuloplasty for congenital aortic stenosis. The American Journal of Cardiology. 2011;**108**(7):1024-1028. DOI: 10.1016/j.amjcard.2011.05.040

[11] Fratz S, Gildein HP, Balling G, Sebening W, Genz T, Eicken A, et al. Aortic valvuloplasty in pediatric patients substantially postpones the need for aortic valve surgery: A single-center experience of 188 patients after up to 17.5 years of follow-up. Circulation. 2008;**117**(9):1201-1206. DOI: 10.1161/CIRCULATIONAHA.107.687764

[12] Rao PS. Role of balloon aortic valvuloplasty in the management of aortic stenosis. Journal of Clinical Cardiology and Cardiovascular Interventions. 2021;**4**(12). DOI: 10.31579/2641-0419/171

[13] Donald JS, Wallace FR, d'Udekem Y, Konstantinov IE. Congenital aortic valve stenosis: To dilate or operate? Heart, Lung & Circulation. 2019;**28**(4):519-520. DOI: 10.1016/j.hlc.2019.02.001

[14] Vergnat M, Asfour B, Arenz C, Suchowerskyj P, Bierbach B, Schindler E, et al. Aortic stenosis of the neonate: A single-center experience. The Journal of Thoracic and Cardiovascular Surgery. 2019;**157**(1):318-326. e1. DOI: 10.1016/j.jtcvs.2018.08.089

[15] Alexiou C, Langley SM, Dalrymple-Hay MJ, Salmon AP, Keeton BR, Haw MP, et al. Open commissurotomy for critical isolated aortic stenosis in neonates. The Annals of Thoracic Surgery. 2001;**71**(2):489-493. DOI: 10.1016/S0003-4975(00)02232-3

[16] Hraška V, Sinzobahamvya N, Haun C, Photiadis J, Arenz C, Schneider M, et al. The long-term outcome of open valvotomy for critical aortic stenosis in neonates. The Annals of Thoracic Surgery. 2012;**94**(5):1519-1526. DOI: 10.1016/j.athoracsur.2012.03.056

[17] McLean KM, Lorts A, Pearl JM. Current treatments for congenital aortic stenosis. Current Opinion in Cardiology. 2006;**21**(3):200-204. DOI: 10.1097/01.hco.0000221581.63996.da

[18] Brown JW, Rodefeld MD, Ruzmetov M, Eltayeb O, Yurdakok O, Turrentine MW. Surgical valvuloplasty versus balloon aortic dilation for congenital aortic stenosis: Are evidence-based outcomes relevant? The Annals of Thoracic Surgery. 2012;**94**(1):146-155. DOI: 10.1016/j.athoracsur.2012.02.054

[19] Hill GD, Ginde S, Rios R, Frommelt PC, Hill KD. Surgical valvotomy versus balloon valvuloplasty for congenital aortic valve stenosis: A systematic review and meta-analysis. Journal of the American Heart Association. 2016;**5**(8):e003931. DOI: 10.1161/JAHA.116.003931), 10.1161/JAHA.116.003931)

[20] Brown DW, Dipilato AE, Chong EC, Lock JE, McElhinney DB. Aortic valve reinterventions after balloon aortic valvuloplasty for congenital aortic stenosis: Intermediate and late follow-up. Journal of the American College of Cardiology. 2010;**56**(21):1740-1749. DOI: 10.1016/j.jacc.2010.06.040

[21] Porras D, Brown DW, Rathod R, Friedman K, Gauvreau K, Lock JE, et al. Acute outcomes after introduction of a standardized clinical assessment and management plan (SCAMP) for balloon aortic valvuloplasty in congenital aortic stenosis. Congenital Heart Disease. 2014;**9**(4):316-325. DOI: 10.1111/chd.12142

[22] Wiggins LM, Mimic B, Issitt R, Ilic S, Bonello B, Marek J, et al. The utility of aortic valve leaflet reconstruction techniques in children and young adults. The Journal of Thoracic and Cardiovascular Surgery. 2020;**159**(6):2369-2378. DOI: 10.1016/j.jtcvs.2019.09.176

[23] Rimmer L, Ahmad MU, Chaplin G, Joshi M, Harky A. Aortic valve repair: Where are we now? Heart, Lung and Circulation. 2019;**28**(7):988-999. DOI: 10.1016/j.hlc.2019.02.007

[24] El Khoury G, de Kerchove L. Principles of Aortic Valve Repair. Elsevier. 2013;**145**(3):S26-S29. DOI: 10.1016/j.jtcvs.2012.11.071

[25] Boodhwani M, El Khoury G. Aortic valve repair. Operative Techniques in Thoracic and Cardiovascular Surgery.

2009;**14**(4):266-280. DOI: 10.1053/j.optechstcvs.2009.11.002

[26] Bisleri G. Aortic valve repair. Current Opinion in Cardiology. 2016;**31**(6):581-584. DOI: 10.1097/HCO.0000000000000334

[27] Ribeiro IB, Boodhwani M. Aortic valve repair. In: Cardiac Surgery. Berlin, Heidelberg: Springer; 2020. pp. 325-343. ISBN: 978-3-642-12206-4. DOI: 10.1007/978-3-030-24174-2_36

[28] Girdauskas E, Petersen J, Sachweh J, Kozlik-Feldmann R, Sinning C, Rickers C, et al. Aortic valve repair in adult congenital heart disease. Cardiovascular Diagnosis and Therapy. 2018;**8**(6):789. DOI: 10.21037/cdt.2018.11.01

[29] Fok M, Shaw M, Sancho E, Abello D, Bashir M. Aortic valve repair: A systematic review and meta-analysis of published literature. Aorta. 2014;**2**(01):10-21. DOI: 10.12945/j.aorta.2014.14-003

[30] Boodhwani M, de Kerchove L, Glineur D, Poncelet A, Rubay J, Astarci P, et al. Repair-oriented classification of aortic insufficiency: Impact on surgical techniques and clinical outcomes. The Journal of Thoracic and Cardiovascular Surgery. 2009;**137**(2):286-294. DOI: 10.1016/j.jtcvs.2008.08.054

[31] Poncelet AJ, El Khoury G, De Kerchove L, Sluysmans T, Moniotte S, Momeni M, et al. Aortic valve repair in the paediatric population: Insights from a 38-year single-Centre experience. European Journal of Cardio-Thoracic Surgery. 2017;**51**(1):43-49. DOI: 10.1093/ejcts/ezw259

[32] Ehrlich T, de Kerchove L, Vojacek J, Boodhwani M, El-Hamamsy I, De Paulis R, et al. State-of-the art bicuspid aortic valve repair in 2020. Progress in Cardiovascular Diseases. 2020;**63**(4):457-464. DOI: 10.1016/j.pcad.2020.04.010

[33] Boodhwani M, de Kerchove L, Glineur D, Rubay J, Vanoverschelde J-L, Noirhomme P, et al. Repair of regurgitant bicuspid aortic valves: A systematic approach. The Journal of Thoracic and Cardiovascular Surgery. 2010;**140**(2):276-284. e1. DOI: 10.1016/j.jtcvs.2009.11.058

[34] Gorton AJ, Anderson EP, Reimer JA, Abdelhady K, Sawaqed R, Massad MG. Considerations in the surgical Management of Unicuspid Aortic Stenosis. Pediatric Cardiology. 2021;**42**(5):993-1001. DOI: 10.1007/s00246-021-02541-0

[35] Pan J. Unicuspid aortic valve: A rare congenital anomaly. Cardiology. 2022;**147**:207-215. DOI: 10.1159/000521623

[36] Schäfers H-J, Aicher D, Riodionycheva S, Lindinger A, Rädle-Hurst T, Langer F, et al. Bicuspidization of the unicuspid aortic valve: A new reconstructive approach. The Annals of Thoracic Surgery. 2008;**85**(6):2012-2018. DOI: 10.1016/j.athoracsur.2008.02.081

[37] Kolesar A, Toporcer T, Bajmoczi M, Luczy J, Candik P, Sabol F. Aortic valve repair of a stenotic unicuspid aortic valve in young patients. The Annals of Thoracic Surgery. 2018;**105**(5):1351-1356. DOI: 10.1016/j.athoracsur.2017.12.031

[38] Kawase I, Ozaki S, Yamashita H, Uchida S, Nozawa Y, Matsuyama T, et al. Aortic valve reconstruction of unicuspid aortic valve by tricuspidization using autologous pericardium. The Annals of Thoracic Surgery. 2012;**94**(4):1180-1184. DOI: 10.1016/j.athoracsur.2012.05.016

[39] Aicher D, Bewarder M, Kindermann M, Abdul-Khalique H, Schäfers H-J. Aortic valve function after bicuspidization of the unicuspid aortic valve. The Annals of Thoracic Surgery. 2013;**95**(5):1545-1550. DOI: 10.1016/j.athoracsur.2013.02.030

[40] Aicher D, Schneider U, Schmied W, Kunihara T, Tochii M, Schäfers H-J. Early results with annular support in reconstruction of the bicuspid aortic valve. Elsevier. 2013;**145**:S30-S34. DOI: 10.1016/j.jtcvs.2012.11.059

[41] Matsushima S, Heß A, Lämmerzahl JR, Karliova I, Abdul-Khaliq H, Schäfers H-J. Unicuspid aortic valve repair with bicuspidization in the paediatric population. European Journal of Cardio-Thoracic Surgery. 2021;**59**(1):253-261. DOI: 10.1093/ejcts/ezaa285

[42] Mosala Nezhad Z, de Kerchove L, Hechadi J, Tamer S, Boodhwani M, Poncelet A, et al. Aortic valve repair with patch in non-rheumatic disease: Indication, techniques and durability. European Journal of Cardio-Thoracic Surgery. 2014;**46**(6):997-1005. DOI: 10.1093/ejcts/ezu058

[43] Nordmeyer S, Murin P, Schulz A, Danne F, Nordmeyer J, Kretzschmar J, et al. Results of aortic valve repair using decellularized bovine pericardium in congenital surgery. European Journal of Cardio-Thoracic Surgery. 2018;**54**(6):986-992. DOI: 10.1093/ejcts/ezy181

[44] Si M-S, Conte JV, Romano JC, Romano MA, Andersen ND, Gerdisch MW, et al. Unicuspid aortic valve repair using geometric ring annuloplasty. The Annals of Thoracic Surgery. 2021;**111**(4):1359-1366. DOI: 10.1016/j.athoracsur.2020.04.147

[45] Baird CW, Marathe SP, Del Nido PJ. Aortic valve neo-cuspidation using the Ozaki technique for acquired and congenital disease: Where does this procedure currently stand? Indian Journal of Thoracic and Cardiovascular Surgery. 2020;**36**(1):113-122. DOI: 10.1007/s12055-019-00917-9

[46] Duran CM, Gometza B, Kumar N, Gallo R, Martin-Duran R. Aortic valve replacement with freehand autologous pericardium. The Journal of Thoracic and Cardiovascular Surgery. 1995;**110**(2):511-516. DOI: 10.1016/S0022-5223(95)70248-2

[47] Ozaki S, Kawase I, Yamashita H, Uchida S, Nozawa Y, Matsuyama T, et al. Aortic valve reconstruction using self-developed aortic valve plasty system in aortic valve disease. Interactive Cardiovascular and Thoracic Surgery. 2011;**12**(4):550-553. DOI: 10.1510/icvts.2010.253682

[48] Ozaki S, Kawase I, Yamashita H, Uchida S, Nozawa Y, Takatoh M, et al. A total of 404 cases of aortic valve reconstruction with glutaraldehyde-treated autologous pericardium. The Journal of Thoracic and Cardiovascular Surgery. 2014;**147**(1):301-306. DOI: 10.1016/j.jtcvs.2012.11.012

[49] Ozaki S, Kawase I, Yamashita H, Nozawa Y, Takatoh M, Hagiwara S, et al. Aortic valve reconstruction using autologous pericardium for patients aged less than 60 years. The Journal of Thoracic and Cardiovascular Surgery. 2014;**148**(3):934-938. DOI: 10.1016/j.jtcvs.2014.05.041

[50] Ozaki S, Kawase I, Yamashita H, Uchida S, Takatoh M, Kiyohara N. Midterm outcomes after aortic valve neocuspidization with glutaraldehyde-treated autologous pericardium. The Journal of Thoracic and Cardiovascular Surgery. 2018;**155**(6):2379-2387. DOI: 10.1016/j.jtcvs.2018.01.087

[51] Baird CW, Cooney B, Chávez M, Sleeper LA, Marx GR, Pedro J. Congenital aortic and truncal valve reconstruction using the Ozaki technique: Short-term clinical results. The Journal of Thoracic and Cardiovascular Surgery. 2021;**161**(5):1567-1577. DOI: 10.1016/j.jtcvs.2020.01.087

[52] Halees ZA, Shahid MA, Sanei AA, Sallehuddin A, Duran C. Up to 16 years follow-up of aortic valve reconstruction with pericardium: A stentless readily available cheap valve? European Journal of Cardio-Thoracic Surgery. 2005;**28**(2):200-205. DOI: 10.1016/j.ejcts.2005.04.041

[53] Duran CM, Gometza B, Shahid M, Al-Halees Z. Treated bovine and autologous pericardium for aortic valve reconstruction. The Annals of Thoracic Surgery. 1998;**66**(6):S166-S169. DOI: 10.1016/S0003-4975(98)01030-3

[54] Mazzitelli D, Nöbauer C, Rankin JS, Vogt M, Lange R, Schreiber C. Complete aortic valve cusp replacement in the pediatric population using tissue-engineered bovine pericardium. The Annals of Thoracic Surgery. 2015;**100**(5):1923-1925. DOI: 10.1016/j.athoracsur.2014.06.052

[55] Abe K, Kawazoe K, Ito J, Yamasaki M, Kuwauchi S, Misumi H. Tricuspidization and reimplantation procedure for unicuspid aortic valve with annuloaortic ectasia. The Annals of Thoracic Surgery. 2015;**99**(3):1095-1096. DOI: 10.1016/j.athoracsur.2014.10.071

[56] Solymar L, Rao PS, Mardini MK, Fawzy ME, Guinn G. Prosthetic valves in children and adolescents. American Heart Journal. 1991;**121**(2):557-568. DOI: 10.1016/0002-8703(91)90726-X

[57] Henn MC, Moon MR. Mechanical prosthetic valves. In: Cardiac Surgery. Cham: Springer; 2020. pp. 291-298. ISBN: 978-3-030-24174-2. DOI: 10.1007/978-3-030-24174-2_32

[58] Alsoufi B. Aortic valve replacement in children: Options and outcomes. Journal of the Saudi Heart Association. 2014;**26**(1):33-41. DOI: 10.1016/j.jsha.2013.11.003

[59] Bouhout I, El-Hamamsy I. The Ross procedure. In: Cardiac Surgery. Cham: Springer; 2020. pp. 351-357. DOI: 10.1007/978-3-030-24174-2_38

[60] Etnel JR, Elmont LC, Ertekin E, Mokhles MM, Heuvelman HJ, Roos-Hesselink JW, et al. Outcome after aortic valve replacement in children: A systematic review and meta-analysis. The Journal of Thoracic and Cardiovascular Surgery. 2016;**151**(1):143-152. e3. DOI: 10.1016/j.jtcvs.2015.09.083

[61] Popov AF, Coskun KO, Tirilomis T, Schmitto JD, Hinz J, Kriebel T, et al. Mechanical aortic valve replacement in children and adolescents after previous repair of congenital heart disease. Artificial Organs. 2009;**33**(11):915-921. DOI: 10.1111/j.1525-1594.2009.00886.x

[62] Rao PS, Solymar L, Fawzy ME, Guinn G. Reassessment of usefulness of porcine Heterografts in mitral position in children. Pediatric Cardiology. 1991;**12**:164-169. DOI: 10.1007/BF02238524

[63] Rao PS, Solymar L, Mardini MK, Fawzy ME, Guinn G. Anticoagulant therapy in children with prosthetic valves. The Annals of Thoracic Surgery. 1989;**47**:589-592. DOI: 10.1016/0003-4975(89)90440-2

[64] Karamlou T, Jang K, Williams WG, Caldarone CA, Van Arsdell G, Coles JG, et al. Outcomes and associated risk factors for aortic valve replacement in 160

children: A competing-risks analysis. Circulation. 2005;**112**(22):3462-3469. DOI: 10.1161/CIRCULATIONAHA.105.541649

[65] Mazine A, David TE, Rao V, Hickey EJ, Christie S, Manlhiot C, et al. Long-term outcomes of the Ross procedure versus mechanical aortic valve replacement: Propensity-matched cohort study. Circulation. 2016;**134**(8):576-585. DOI: 10.1161/CIRCULATIONAHA.116.022800

[66] Ruzmetov M, Vijay P, Rodefeld MD, Turrentine MW, Brown JW. Evolution of aortic valve replacement in children: A single center experience. International Journal of Cardiology. 2006;**113**(2):194-200. DOI: 10.1016/j.ijcard.2005.11.011

[67] Danial P, Neily A, Pontailler M, Gaudin R, Khraiche D, Osborne-Pellegrin M, et al. Ross procedure or complex aortic valve repair using pericardium in children: A real dilemma. The Journal of Thoracic and Cardiovascular Surgery. 2022;**163**(3):1180-1191. e6. DOI: 10.1016/j.jtcvs.2021.02.093

[68] Jacobsen RM, Earing MG, Hill GD, Barnes M, Mitchell ME, Woods RK, et al. The externally supported Ross operation: Early outcomes and intermediate follow-up. The Annals of Thoracic Surgery. 2015;**100**(2):631-638. DOI: 10.1016/j.athoracsur.2015.04.123

[69] Sharabiani MT, Dorobantu DM, Mahani AS, Turner M, Peter Tometzki AJ, Angelini GD, et al. Aortic valve replacement and the Ross operation in children and young adults. Journal of the American College of Cardiology. 2016;**67**(24):2858-2870. DOI: 10.1016/j.jacc.2016.04.021

[70] Bradley SM. Aortic valve insufficiency in the teenager and young adult: The role of prosthetic valve replacement. World Journal for Pediatric and Congenital Heart Surgery. 2013;**4**(4):397-402. DOI: 10.1177/2150135113488781

[71] Al Rashidi F, Bhat M, Höglund P, Meurling C, Roijer A, Koul B. The modified Ross operation using a Dacron prosthetic vascular jacket does prevent pulmonary autograft dilatation at 4.5-year follow-up. European Journal of Cardio-Thoracic Surgery. 2010;**37**(4):928-933. DOI: 10.1016/j.ejcts.2009.11.008

[72] Tweddell JS. The root replacement remains the gold standard for the Ross procedure. European Journal of Cardio-Thoracic Surgery. 2021;**59**(1):234-235. DOI: 10.1093/ejcts/ezaa366

[73] Riggs KW, Colohan DB, Beacher DR, Alsaied T, Powell S, Moore RA, et al. Mid-term outcomes of the supported Ross procedure in children, teenagers, and young adults. In: Seminars in Thoracic and Cardiovascular Surgery. Elsevier; 2020. pp. 498-504. DOI: 10.1053/j.semtcvs.2019.10.020

[74] Lupinetti FM, Duncan BW, Lewin M, Dyamenahalli U, Rosenthal GL. Comparison of autograft and allograft aortic valve replacement in children. The Journal of Thoracic and Cardiovascular Surgery. 2003;**126**(1):240-245. DOI: 10.1016/S0022-5223(03)00041-2

[75] Alsoufi B, Al-Halees Z, Manlhiot C, McCrindle BW, Al-Ahmadi M, Sallehuddin A, et al. Mechanical valves versus the Ross procedure for aortic valve replacement in children: Propensity-adjusted comparison of long-term outcomes. The Journal of Thoracic and Cardiovascular Surgery. 2009;**137**(2):362-370. e9. DOI: 10.1016/j.jtcvs.2008.10.010

[76] Quader MA, Rosenthal GL, Qureshi AM, Mee RB, Mumtaz MA,

Joshi R, et al. Aortic valve repair for congenital abnormalities of the aortic valve. Heart, Lung and Circulation. 2006;**15**(4):248-255. DOI: 10.1016/j.hlc.2006.05.005

[77] Buratto E, Konstantinov IE. Aortic valve surgery in children. The Journal of Thoracic and Cardiovascular Surgery. 2021;**161**(1):244-250. DOI: 10.1016/j.jtcvs.2020.06.145

[78] Buratto E, Konstantinov IE. Commentary: Aortic valve surgery in children: Repair now, Ross procedure later. The Journal of Thoracic and Cardiovascular Surgery. 2022;**163**(3):1193-1194. DOI: 10.1016/j.jtcvs.2021.03.064

[79] Bouhout I, Ba PS, El-Hamamsy I, Poirier N. Aortic valve interventions in pediatric patients. In: Seminars in Thoracic and Cardiovascular Surgery. Elsevier; 2019. pp. 277-287. DOI: 10.1053/j.semtcvs.2018.10.009

[80] Hawkins JA, Minich LL, Shaddy RE, Tani LY, Orsmund GS, Sturtevant JE, et al. Aortic valve repair and replacement after balloon aortic valvuloplasty in children. The Annals of Thoracic Surgery. 1996;**61**(5):1355-1358. DOI: 10.1016/0003-4975(96)00018-5

[81] Pozzi M, Quarti A, Colaneri M, Oggianu A, Baldinelli A, Colonna PL. Valve repair in congenital aortic valve abnormalities. Interactive Cardio Vascular and Thoracic Surgery. 2010;**10**(4):587-591. DOI: 10.1510/icvts.2009.224097

[82] Coskun KO, Popov AF, Tirilomis T, Schmitto JD, Coskun ST, Hinz J, et al. Aortic valve surgery in congenital heart disease: A single-center experience. Artificial Organs. 2010;**34**(3):E85-E90. DOI: 10.1111/j.1525-1594.2009.00958.x

Section 7

# International Issues

Chapter 12

# Management of Congenital Heart Disease in Low-Income Countries: The Challenges and the Way Forward

*Osama Elshazali, Murtada Ibrahim and Abdelmoniem Elseed*


## Abstract

In this article, we will discuss the management of congenital heart disease in low-income and low-middle income countries. First, we will review the epidemiology of congenital heart disease in the low-income and low-middle income countries and compare it to that in the high-income countries; cardiac disease is the commonest cause of death globally. The challenges that are facing the delivery of pediatric cardiac services will be discussed and some solutions will be suggested to improve these services. Pediatric cardiac services face huge economic, financial, social, and health care system delivery challenges. Collaboration between countries and non-governmental and philanthropy organizations is strongly needed to improve delivery of pediatric cardiac services in low-income and low-middle income countries. Planning of pediatric cardiac services in these countries should consider the context of each country or region; some countries managed to transform their pediatric cardiac services to be better.


**Keywords:** congenital heart disease, pediatric, low-income countries, low-middle income countries, management, children

## 1. Introduction

Congenital heart disease (CHD) is the most common among all birth defects, occurring in about nine per 1000 live births globally. Fortunately, most of the CHD lesion are simple lesions, but 25% are critical lesions [1], which need urgent intervention within the first six months of age.

Each year about 1.35 million children are born with CHD; the majority of them are born in low-income countries (LICs). LICs have a higher fertility rate of 4.6 per woman compared to 1.6 per woman in high-income countries (HICs). The birth rate in LICs is 22 per 1000 population compared to 10 per 1000 population in HICs [2]. Each year around 140 million babies are born globally [3]; of these 1.4 million are born with CHD. Ninety percent of those born with CHD are born in a place with inadequate resources for pediatric cardiac care [4].

CHD is one of the main seven causes of death globally and has a significant socio-economic impact on the community [5].

The past 50 years have witnessed massive breakthrough advances in cardiovascular care such as improvements in diagnosis, surgical treatment, catheter interventions, and Intensive care management. Survival of newborns with CHD has improved dramatically in HICs. Unfortunately, however, this is not the case in many low and low –middle-income countries where the burden is the heaviest and rates of death and disability continue to increase [6, 7].

Management of CHD requires significant resources, namely, highly developed infrastructure, equipment and highly skilled professionals who need years of training. This makes cardiovascular care in children very costly, and it needs a long time to be established. HICs have perfected the treatment of CHD over the past 50 years and are now able to provide adequate treatment to their population. LICs are only starting to build a structure to deliver such care. Even in HICs, the management of some complex CHD lesions is challenging, but in LICs the management of even simple lesions can be a challenge [8].

In LICs, 90% of children with CHD do not have access to pediatric cardiac services, even in the same country, there is a disparity in the access to the services between rural and urban, rich and poor. The challenges include poor financial and human resources and lack of infrastructure [9].

There is a huge disparity in pediatric cardiac resources between HICs and LICs, to put this difference into prospective we can compare the number of pediatric cardiac surgeons between HICs and LICs; in HICs, there are 1.67 pediatric cardiac surgeons per million population compared to 0.03 in LICs [10].

Pediatric cardiac services are expensive and need resources and large investments in the infrastructure. There is a positive correlation between the economic status of the country and the access to pediatric cardiac services [10].

The challenges and obstacles leading to suboptimal delivery of cardiac care for children with CHD in LICs, and potential solutions to improve access to cardiac care in LICs must be considered within the context of each country or region and social, economic, political and health care systems [11].

Need for greater awareness of CHD, increased education and training for in-country program clinicians, strategic health care planning at governmental and policy levels, and innovative solution for financing cardiac services in LICs are needed to help improve pediatric cardiac services [12].

As mentioned earlier, CHD is the commonest congenital anomaly, representing 28% of all congenital anomalies [13]. Studies from different parts of the world showed variation in the reported prevalence of CHD, some of the differences are due to the study methodology and setting i.e., hospital-based studies show higher prevalence compared to population studies. The prevalence figure of 8–10 per 1000 which came from HICs is generally taken as the approximate prevalence worldwide [8].

Significant geographical differences in the prevalence of CHD were reported. The lowest reported prevalence was in Africa (1.9 per 1000 live birth), the highest was in Asia (9.3 per 1000 live birth), while the prevalence in Europe was 8.2 per 1000 live birth [7].

The reported prevalence figures of CHD in Africa, especially in low-income countries, is not usually accurate and thought to be an underestimate owing to a paucity of data, poor health care system, difficulty in accessing health care system, poor health infrastructure, limited resources and early mortality [6]. CHD occur worldwide and although the incidence and prevalence may vary according to genetic and environmental factors there is no reason to think that they are lower in LICs compared to HICs [6].

In Africa, CHD is starting to become a major public health concern as the pediatric population represents 50% of the total population [14, 15] and due to the scarce availability of pediatric cardiac services, the affected population is starting to accumulate. CHD has now surpassed rheumatic heart disease (RHD) as the commonest cause of pediatric heart disease in some parts of Africa; presumably, this is related to increased awareness and better diagnostic facilities [16].

Delayed diagnosis is a major problem in LICS; this is due to low awareness of the families and medical professionals about CHD. In HICs, the diagnosis of CHD is established by 1 week of age in 40–50% of patients and by 1 month in up to 60% [7]. In addition, the fetal diagnosis is not well developed in LICs, with only 1% of cases detected antenatally [17], while in HICs prenatal diagnosis is routinely used to detect most of CHD cases before birth. Screening for CHD is not routinely practiced in LICs [1], this combined with low awareness contributes to late diagnosis. Often, late-stage presentation with complications such as pulmonary hypertension and myocardial dysfunction, few benefits from surgical treatment. Because of delayed diagnosis, lack of skilled personnel and non-availability of treatment facilities, the problem is further exacerbated [11].

## 2. Challenges

### 2.1 Economic and financial resources

The world bank classifies countries according to their incomes into four groups; in 2022 there are 27 countries in low-income economy (LICs) with Gross National Income (GNI) per capita of $1045 or less, 55 countries with Lower Middle-income economy (LMICs) with GNI per capita range of $1046–$4095, 55 countries in Upper Middle-income economy (UMICs) with GNI per capita range of $4096–$12,695, and 80 countries in high-income economy (HICs) with GNI per capita of $12,696 or more [18].

The majority of LICs are struggling to meet the basic primary health problems such as vaccination, malnutrition, and infectious diseases, making it very hard to provide tertiary pediatric cardiovascular services [6]. Due to lack of awareness, some policymakers and even medical professionals in LICs consider pediatric cardiac services as a luxury and not an essential service [19].

LICs are struggling to provide the health services investment required for life-saving CHD interventions. A study exploring associations between risk-adjusted CHD surgical mortality from 17 LMICs and global development indices [20] found a statistically significant positive correlation between under-five mortality and surgical mortality rate, and a negative correlation between specialist surgical workforce and CHD mortality: as specialist surgical workforce increases, congenital heart surgery mortality decreases, suggesting that adequate workforce is vital to quality congenital heart surgical capacity [20].

The association between outcome of CHD surgery and GNI per capita is well established; in LMICs, surgical mortality for CHD was found to be higher in countries with lower GNI per capita [21]. In addition, low health care expenditure per capita, poverty, malnutrition, and high under-five mortalities also play a significant role [20].

CHD is the second cause of mortality under 1 year of age, the first being infections [22].

There is a huge difference in mortality of CHD between HICs and LICs; in HICs, the mortality is 3–7% compared to 20% in LICs. Mortality figures from CHD in LICs are likely to be underestimated since access to the health services is difficult and the available data is not reliable most of the time. Most of the available data is from patients in tertiary centres rather than community-based studies [8].

#### *2.1.1 Solutions and moving forward*

We recommend that LICs governments should look for innovative ways to finance pediatric cardiac services, using partnership models. Targeting potential partners such as private sector, insurance companies, nonprofit organizations and international organizations [11]. The system should be flexible to finance mainly the needed sectors in the community; this will ensure the funds will go a long way in helping many children.

Economic efficiency could be improved by the following measures:

Comprehensive care through dedicated cardiovascular programs and centres, these centres will have important roles including improving awareness, prevention, treatment, staff training and research. These centres will have a high-volume workload and this is likely to lead to more efficient manpower management and cheaper consumables.

The cost of consumables and drugs may also be reduced by tax breaks and by encouraging the production of some of these items locally [11] or purchasing the items in bulk.

At the cardiac centre level, prioritization of intervention types is crucial in the context of severe resource limitations; palliative, staged and off-pump operations may be more suitable and safer than complex interventions [11]; of course, this will raise an ethical and philosophical dilemma when a decision is reached not to intervene in patients with complex congenital defects such as single ventricle palliation [23].

Many studies from LMICs demonstrated that it is more cost-effective to adopt early screening programs [1, 24], streamlining of referral pathways, maintaining a balanced case mix with focus on correctable lesions and provide cost-effective intensive care management through the implementation of clinical protocols and best practices as well as to minimize the use of expensive drugs or treatment modalities [25, 26].

### 2.2 Health care system challenges

For a health system to be effective, it has to be staffed by well trained and efficient medical, nursing, allied, and administrative staff. To be sustainable, it requires a robust infrastructure, real leadership, good governance, and continuing education program. In LICs the health system is usually not well planned due to a lack of information and unawareness of the local health needs and priorities. The health care system support usually comes from the government with some input from academic institutions and NGOs [21].

Poorly supported health care delivery systems remain a major problem in LICs, which can lead to poor management of CHDs in LICs. There is a clear disparity between the poor and affluent as well as urban and rural settings. In LICs more than 60% of the population reside in rural setting. In LICs the health services are struggling to provide support for other services and some of these deficiencies could have an adverse effect on the pediatric cardiac services such as poor antenatal care, poorly controlled diabetes in pregnancy, and congenital rubella syndrome. Since the vaccination program is not well-established congenital rubella is still seen in LICs [8].

For a health care system to be functioning well and delivering good service, it has to be affordable, accessible and the population has to be aware of the services [27]. Unfortunately, the health care delivery system in LICS is struggling with all of these three factors.

The costs are excessive for most families [21]. Affordability is one of the main reasons for delayed interventions and the associated high morbidity and mortality [21]. Most of the LICs are trying to provide pediatric cardiac services in public hospitals either free or for a reduced cost but such hospitals lack funding and resources and are extremely busy and overwhelmed [19, 21].

LICs have very few pediatric cardiac centres [26], and they are always located in the main cities. Patients who live in non-urban setting sometimes have to travel long journeys to access such services. Inaccessible services will lead to late presentation and delayed diagnosis, and both are associated with high morbidity and mortality [21, 27].

Awareness of the parents, allied health workers and the health care professionals in LICs is not adequate about pediatric cardiac disease. Parents in HICs are aware and well informed about pediatric cardiac disease. The robust health system in HICs also has several safety mechanisms in the system to detect and diagnose pediatric cardiac disease early such as fetal diagnosis [24], routine neonatal check post-delivery, oxygen saturation screening [1], routine primary health check, and routine school health screening. Lack of awareness in LICs is one of the most important factors contributing to late presentation, missed and delayed diagnosis [6, 27].

In the poorest parts of Africa and Asia, the pediatric cardiovascular services are limited. Some of the larger cities have facilities for diagnosis and intervention of selected and straightforward conditions in older children but infant and newborn services are limited.

The preoperative phase requires earlier detection. Fetal echocardiography and screening programs are not readily available in LICs which leads to delay diagnosis. One study from Sudan showed the antenatal diagnosis was 1% compared to the figures of 10–15% in the HICs [17].

There are many barriers to accessibility and affordability in the process from diagnosis to management [5]. The waiting list in the cardiac centres in LICs is getting longer because of the increase workload and the inability of the existing centres to cope. The waiting list is especially long for stable patients who tend to be pushed down in the list because of the urgent and sick cases.

Postoperative critical care has witnessed slow but steady progress in the developing programs. Cardiac intensive care remains a bottleneck for the waiting list in LICs due to increased length of stay for patients secondary to increased morbidity. In developing programs, the cardiac intensive care unit (CICU) is usually integrated with the general pediatric ICU [5]. While this is useful in terms of reducing the cost and sharing of financial and human resources, this could create a problem for bed availability as pediatric ICU patients may occupy the cardiac ICU beds affecting the waiting list adversely. The teamwork philosophy approach has had a major positive effect on the outcome of cases [25].

The poor economic and financial situation will have a detrimental effect on attracting and retaining trained cardiac physicians and nursing staff [5]. The team that looks after pediatric cardiac disease consists of surgeons, physicians, nurses and technicians, all are highly trained and receive specialized training that is lengthy and expensive. The LICs must invest in them so the respective countries can develop and maintain pediatric cardiac services. This staff will require continuing job training and reasonable pay and benefits. Unfortunately, most of the time this does not happen and the staff either start working in the private sector, usually in adult centres or migrate abroad to richer countries leading to a brain drain which is a major problem in the LICs [6, 28].

*2.2.1 Solutions*

The health care systems in LICs need to be reformed to improve the delivery of primary and secondary health care. Pediatric cardiac services are very specialized that need a health system with robust infrastructure [11].

Antenatal care services providers, pediatricians and primary care providers should have increased awareness of aforementioned health care issues. Programs targeting CHD include, screening programs such as fetal echocardiography, oxygen saturations in the newborn prior to discharge, and neonatal examinations should be established.

Creative solutions to tackle access and geographic barriers to care have been used in countries such as India, Brazil, Vietnam, and Morocco. These in-country programs operate mobile health care units that are staffed with trained cardiac clinicians and equipped with portable electrocardiogram and echocardiogram equipment. These units provide outreach services to non-urban communities increasing accessibility to the services, raise awareness of CHD, provide education to local clinicians, and screen children for structural heart disease [8].

Pediatricians with an interest in cardiology, especially in non-urban areas should be provided with support from pediatric cardiologists such as telemedicine facilities and satellite clinics. These services should be easily accessible to the residents of non-urban areas and could improve the care of the children by providing early diagnosis and referral to specialized centres. The above approach is cost-effective since the training is shorter compared to the pediatric cardiology training.

Human resources are the most valuable asset; there is a great need for healthcare workers to be trained, sustained, and retained in LICs [6, 28].

## 3. Centers of excellence

Every country should strive to establish their own cardiac centres. These dedicated Centers of Excellence (COE) would provide clinical, educational, training, research, and administrative support to the services and the programs within the country in addition to their role in providing patient care [5].

These COEs would lead the service development and be a centre for data gathering, research and development and may serve as a hub for medical missions [11]. The COEs can also lead and coordinate the partnership with global cardiovascular organizations and forums; such partnership can help enormously in establishing cardiac services for children in LICs [9].

If appropriately organized, COEs are economically and financially efficient and can save resources especially if their patient volume is large [5].

The cost of these centres may be shared with the adult cardiology programs to save the resources. The COEs would provide the greatly needed training. They also provide a hub for visiting humanitarian missions [29] which may promote high standards of practice and training.

COEs may have a major role in education and training of the local teams while visiting teams will train the pediatric cardiac personnel including surgeons, physicians, anesthetists, Intensivists, perfusionists, and nurses. For sustaining the skills, the local team's training may have to be augmented by training abroad. However, training abroad is expensive, and the trainee may not get good hands-on training. Recently, there is a move toward long-term embedding projects, where experienced cardiologists and/or surgeons spend one to 12 months in host programs. This has great value both medically and financially [30, 31].

## 4. Voluntary and humanitarian initiatives

Voluntary organizations' partnerships with the local governments can help bridge the gap in pediatric cardiac services [29, 31]. The long-term strategy should be a building of capacity and empowerment of the local team [6]. The twinning program model between local centres and visiting centres is a successful one to follow [26, 31].

## 5. Research and Development

There is currently no reliable data on epidemiology and pattern of pediatric cardiac disease in LICs; such information would improve the awareness and help in planning and prioritizing the pediatric cardiac services [8, 32].

## 6. Conclusion

Pediatric cardiac services are a burden and a challenge to LICs. Currently, the services available in most LICs are not accessible, not affordable and there is still a lack of awareness about the need for quality pediatric cardiac services. Health planners should be aware that pediatric cardiac services are essential services and not a luxury.

Collaboration and partnerships between international organizations, national and local governments, non-governmental organizations, and patient and family advocates are needed to ensure that children around the world have access to quality and sustainable pediatric cardiac care.

There are some shining examples of countries that managed to transform pediatric cardiac services with strategic planning and leadership, for example, Cuba, India and China.

Capacity building toward the ultimate goal of self-sufficient LIC and LMIC programs will require a paradigm shift in the recognition by the leadership, greater collaboration among stakeholders, encouragement of data sharing, and research development.

## Conflict of interest

The authors declare no conflict of interest.

## Author details

Osama Elshazali[1*], Murtada Ibrahim[2] and Abdelmoniem Elseed[1]

1 Department of Paediatrics and Child Health, University of Khartoum, Sudan

2 Department of Paediatric Cardiac Surgery, Ahmed Gasim Cardiac Centre, Khartoum, Sudan

*Address all correspondence to: o.elshazali@uofk.edu

## References

[1] Mahle WT, Newburger JW, Paul Matherne G, Smith FC, Hoke TR, Koppel R, et al. Role of Pulse Oximetry in Examining Newborns for Congenital Heart Disease the Council on Cardiovascular Disease in the Young, Council on Cardiovascular Nursing, and Interdisciplinary Council on Quality of Care and Outcomes Research; and the American Academy of Pediatrics Section on Cardiology and Cardiac Surgery, and Committee on Fetus and Newborn. 2009 Available from: http://www.americanheart.org/presenter.jhtml? [cited 2019 Sep 4]

[2] World Bank. Fertility Rate, Total (Births per Woman). 2021. Available from: https://data.worldbank.org/indicator/SP.DYN.TFRT.IN

[3] World-Death-and-Birth-Rate. Available from: https://statisticstimes.com/demographics/world-death-and-birth-rate.php

[4] Zheleva B, Atwood JB. The invisible child: childhood heart disease in global health. The Lancet. Jan 2017;**389**(10064):16-18

[5] Nguyen N, Pezzella A. Pediatric cardiac surgery in low-and middle-income countries or emerging economies: A continuing challenge. World Journal for Pediatric and Congenital Heart Surgery. 2015;**6**(2):274-283

[6] Musa NL, Hjortdal V, Zheleva B, Murni IK, Sano S, Schwartz S, et al. The global burden of paediatric heart disease. Cardiology in the Young. 2017;**27**:S3-S8

[7] van der Linde D, Konings EEM, Slager MA, Witsenburg M, Helbing WA, Takkenberg JJM, et al. Birth prevalence of congenital heart disease worldwide. Journal of the American College of Cardiology. 2011;**58**(21):2241 LP-2242247 Available from: http://www.onlinejacc.org/content/58/21/2241.abstract

[8] Bernier P, Stefanescu A, Samoukovic G, Tchervenkov C. The challenge of congenital heart disease worldwide: Epidemiologic and demographic facts. Seminars in Thoracic and Cardiovascular Surgery. Pediatric Cardiac Surgery Annual. 2010;**13**:26-34

[9] Nguyen N, Jacobs J, Dearani J, Weinstein S, Novick W, Jacobs M, et al. Survey of nongovernmental organizations providing pediatric cardiovascular care in low-and middle-income countries. World Journal for Pediatric and Congenital Heart Surgery. 2014;**5**(2):248-255

[10] Vervoort D, Meuris B, Meyns B, Verbrugghe P. Global cardiac surgery: Access to cardiac surgical care around the worlde. The Journal of Thoracic and Cardiovascular Surgery. 2020;**159**(3):987-996

[11] Murala J, Karl T, Pezzella A. Pediatric cardiac surgery in low-and middle-income countries: Present status and need for a paradigm shift. Frontiers in Pediatrics. 2019;**7**:214

[12] Saxena A. How to deliver the best: A call for action for congenital heart disease treatments in India. Future Cardiology. 2014;**10**(3):359-366

[13] Dolk H, Loane M, Garne E. Congenital heart defects in Europe: Prevalence and perinatal mortality, 2000 to 2005. Circulation. 2011;**123**(8):841-849

[14] Mocumbi AO, Lameira E, Yaksh A, Paul L, Ferreira MB, Sidi D. Challenges on the management of congenital

heart disease in developing countries. International Journal of Cardiology. 2011;**148**(3):285-288

[15] Ellis J, Martin R, Wilde P, Tometzki A, Senkungu J, Nansera D. Echocardiographic, chest X-ray and electrocardiogram findings in children presenting with heart failure to a Ugandan paediatric ward. Trop Doctor. 2007;**37**:149-150

[16] Okoromah CA, Ekure E, Ojo O, Animasahun B, Bastos M. Structural heart disease in children in Lagos: Profile, problems and prospects. The Nigerian Postgraduate Medical Journal. 2008;**15**(2):82-88

[17] Elshazali Osama H, Abdullahi H, HES O. Assessment of quality of counselling for down syndrome in Sudan. Journal of Pediatrics and Neonatal Care. 2018;**8**(5):232-234 Available from: http://medcraveonline.com

[18] World Bank Country and Lending Groups. World Bank Data Help Desk. 2022. Available from: https://datahelpdesk.worldbank.org/knowledgebase

[19] Jivanji S, Lubega S, Reel B, Qureshi S. Congenital heart disease in East Africa. Frontiers in Pediatrics. 2019;7:250

[20] Rahman S, Zheleva B, Cherian K, Christenson J, Doherty K, de Ferranti D, et al. Linking world bank development indicators and outcomes of congenital heart surgery in low-income and middle-income countries: Retrospective analysis of quality improvement data. BMJ Open. 2019;**9**(6):e028307

[21] Rahman S, Cherian KM, Christensen J, Doherty K, De Ferranti D, Gauvreau K, et al. Congenital heart disease congenital heart disease survival in low and middle income countries: Linking investment and outcomes presentation number: 1208-370. Journal of the American College of Cardiology. 2018;**71**(11S):A607-A607

[22] WHO. The Top 10 Causes of Death-Fact Sheet. Geneva: WHO; 2020 Available from: https://www.who.int/news-room/fact-sheets/detail/the-top-10-causes-of-death

[23] Iyer K. Treating hypoplastic left heart syndrome in emerging economies: Heading the wrong way? Annals of Pediatric Cardiology. 2013;**6**(1): 12-14

[24] Sharland G. Fetal cardiac screening and variation in prenatal detection rates of congenital heart disease: Why bother with screening at all? Future Cardiology. 2012;**8**(2):189-202

[25] Kumar R. Teamwork in pediatric heart care. Annals of Pediatric Cardiology. 2009;**2**(2):140-145

[26] Dearani J, Neirotti R, Kohnke E, Sinha K, Cabalka A, Barnes R, et al. Improving pediatric cardiac surgical care in developing countries: Matching resources to needs. Seminars in Thoracic and Cardiovascular Surgery. Pediatric Cardiac Surgery Annual. 2010;**13**(1):35-43

[27] Bode-Thomas F. Challenges in the Management of Congenital Heart Disease in developing countries. In: Rao PPS, editor. Congenital Heart Disease - Selected Aspects. London, UK: InTech; 2012. pp. 472-476

[28] Peñaloza B, Pantoja T, Bastías G, Herrera C, Rada G. Interventions to reduce emigration of health care professionals from lowand middle-income countries. Cochrane Database of Systematic Reviews. 2011;**9**:CD007673

[29] Cardarelli M, Vaikunth S, Mills K, DiSessa T, Molloy F, Sauter E, et al. Cost-effectiveness of humanitarian Pediatric cardiac surgery programs in low- and middle-income countries. JAMA Network Open. 2018;**1**(7):e184707

[30] Vervoort D, Swain JBD, Pezzella AT, Kpodonu J. Cardiac surgery in low- and middle-income countries: A state-of-the-art review. The Annals of Thoracic Surgery. 2021;**111**(4):1394-1400

[31] Dearani J, Jacobs J, Bolman IR, Swain J, Vricella L, Weinstein S, et al. Humanitarian outreach in cardiothoracic surgery: From setup to sustainability. The Annals of thoracic surgery. 2016;**102**(3):1004-1011

[32] Jacobs J, Maruszewski B, Kurosawa H, Jacobs M, Mavroudis C, Lacour-Gayet FG, et al. Congenital heart surgery databases around the world: Do we need a global database? Seminars in Thoracic and Cardiovascular Surgery: Pediatric Cardiac Surgery Annual. 2010;**13**(1):3-19

Chapter 13

# Establishing Sustainable Pediatric Cardiac Surgery Program in Nigeria: Challenges and Prospects

*Ikechukwu Andrew Nwafor, Josephat Maduabuchi Chinawa, John Chukwuemeka Eze and Fidelis Anayo Onyekwulu*


## Abstract

Unlike in the Western world, the delivery of cardiovascular services to children and adults born with congenital heart defects (CHDs) in Nigeria is grossly inadequate. There are problems all through the ages of these unfortunate patients. Accurate statistical data of CHD in Nigeria is lacking, but it is comparable to 8 per 1000 live births as seen in other countries. The burden is presently being ameliorated by medical tourisms and foreign cardiac surgery missions, but such services are still inadequate. There is a need for the government to share resources between this noncommunicable (CHD) and communicable diseases. When this is done with assistance of international partners and humanitarian organizations, a sustainable pediatric cardiac surgery program will be established that will definitely enhance the care of these patients at childhood, adolescent, and adult stages of their lives.


**Keywords:** pediatric, surgery, program, congenital, sustainable, medical tourism

## 1. Introduction

Unlike in developed countries, the delivery of cardiovascular services to children born with congenital heart defects in Nigeria is inadequate. There are problems at both pediatric and adult ages with high morbidity and mortality on account of inadequate surgical care. The country initially lacked both manpower and infrastructure so that many souls of congenital pediatric patients departed their bodies with their pathologies undiagnosed and untreated. Pioneers of cardiac surgery in Nigeria were not decisive of separate pediatric cardiac program while they engaged the government. Presently, with many trained personnel, there is a need for structured pediatric cardiac team with requisite infrastructure to work. This will bring the desired success.

## 2. Historical aspects

In Nigeria, a foreign cardiac team with a local team performed the first open heart surgery in our institution, University of Nigeria Teaching Hospital (UNTH),

Enugu, in 1974. UNTH is the teaching hospital for the Federal Government of Nigeria and is affiliated to University of Nigeria, Nsukka. Foreign cardiac team was led by a British-Egyptian Surgeon, Sir (Dr) Magdi Yacoub, and indigenous team was led by late Professor Fabian Udekwu. This singular act added to many others attracted the attention of the Federal Military Government of Nigeria, which designated it the National Cardiothoracic Center of Excellence (NCTCE) in 1984.

Adult cardiac surgery was the main focus of the program. The hospital stood by her deeds and was able to establish itself, as the leader in open heart surgery not only in Nigeria but also in West African subregion [1]. Afterward, the center's activities decreased due to poor military governance and corruption. The near total neglect of healthcare system (HCS) in the country led to the collapse of the center due to brain drain and inadequate facilities such that between 1974 and 2000, only a total of 102 open heart operations were carried out, mainly by local team [1].

With return to civilian rule in Nigeria in 1999, efforts were made to improve the center through Foreign Cardiac Mission Model. The first mission was by International Children Heart Foundation (ICHF) in 2003 under the sponsorship of Kanu Heart Foundation. Incidentally, that mission was the first pediatric mission, and William Novick (International Cardiac Foundation) was the lead surgeon. The team visited once and performed mainly pediatric cases for the first time at the center. Other international cardiac missions started visiting 10 years later and became regular with more frequent visits every year [2]. Options considered toward sustenance of pediatric cardiac surgery were staff training and equipment procurement. One way to achieve the desired training in emerging country like ours is by regular and frequent visits to centers such as NCTCE by foreign cardiac teams and performing the surgery alongside the local team (cardiac mission model) [3–5]. Other options include sending the local team to established centers, for example, India for hands-on training for a period not less than 2 years. Furthermore, members of the local team individually went for training abroad on their personal arrangement at different times and in different established centers.

The cardiac mission model would not even have been possible without the aids from some agencies of the Federal Government of Nigeria, Nigerians in Diaspora, public spirited individuals, and foreign organizations as shown in **Table 1**. Most of the countries in West African subregion are very poor, and a study by Edwin F et al. showed that no existing cardiac center in the subregion came into being without huge governmental support [6].

Good things that go for foreign mission team include high technical skill and team work in contrast to what is obtainable on the ground. Treating patients locally in this method is cheaper and serves as workshop and training session for different categories of workers at minimal cost to the institution. However, model of cardiac missions is not a sustainable one because a lot of effort and expenditure are allocated toward surgery on a few patients [7].

The adoption of cardiac mission model by developing countries such as Nigeria as a way of helping indigent patients with both congenital and acquired heart diseases is good. However, that method is like giving someone a fish anytime he demands it. The best way is to incorporate teaching the person how to fish, that is, developing and equipping local team. It is only in this way will establishing pediatric cardiac center across the low- and middle-income countries become sustainable.

Pediatric cardiology and pediatric cardiac surgery practices in Nigeria are taxing [8, 9]. Getting all the requirements to cater for the surgical needs of a very

| S/N | Name of organization | Local or foreign | Aid provided |
|---|---|---|---|
| 1 | Federal Ministry of Health (FMOH) | Local | Payment of salaries and allowances of local team members. Provided infrastructure |
| 2 | UNTH | Local | When UNTH moved to new site, a ward was restructured for cardiac surgery and ICU. Sponsorship for both foreign and local training of local team. Also, provided air tickets, local transportation, feeding and security for foreign cardiac teams as well as sourcing for disposables. |
| 3 | TET fund (University of Nigeria) | Local | Equipment (Cath Lab, six ventilators, two theater tables, two theater lights, eight ICU beds, six monitors, etc.) |
| 4 | Kanu Heart foundation (KHF) | Local | Sponsorship of International Children Heart Foundation (ICHF) visit in 2003. Brought equipment and disposables |
| 5 | Enugu State Government | Local | Logistics for foreign team and fees for some patients |
| 6 | Innova Hospital, Hyderabad, India in 2009 | Foreign | UNTH sent two cardiac anesthetists, two cardiothoracic surgeons, two medical laboratory scientists for perfusion, two pediatric cardiologists, three nurses, two physiotherapists, and a technician for training as staff build up to her restart of open-heart surgery in 2013. It was tuition-free |
| 7 | VOOM Foundation from 2013 | Diaspora (USA) | Foreign team, equipment, and disposables severally |
| 8 | Save-a-Heart Nigeria started with VOOM but separated later. | Diaspora (UK) | Foreign team, equipment, and disposables severally |
| 9 | Rotary Club of Nigeria | Local | Payment of surgical fees for some patients |
| 10 | Opubic of Italy | Foreign | Free pediatric cardiac surgery with disposables severally |
| 11 | Novic Cardiac Alliance of USA with VOOM Foundation | Foreign | Foreign team, equipment, and disposables |
| 12 | Cardiostat of USA with VOOM Foundation | Foreign | Foreign team, equipment, and disposables |
| 13 | Public spirited individuals, businesses | Local | Payment of surgical fees and blood donation |
| 14 | Bigard Seminary, Enugu (Seminarians were donors) | Local | Free blood donation severally |
| 15 | Santarina of India | Foreign | |
| 16 | UNEC medical students | | Free blood donations |

**Table 1.**
*Some collaborations took place both locally or outside your country in helping capacity building but help will also be needed in some aspect.*

large number of children with congenital heart defects with its attendant financial constraints, poor funding from the government is really a huge task.

Pediatric cardiology and pediatric cardiac surgery training in Nigeria involve the management of different cardiac diseases in children. This covers children with both congenital and acquired heart disease [10]. This also includes arrhythmias and coronary heart diseases. Besides, interventional cardiology practice is really at the primordial phase with less than three teaching hospitals providing the skills and competences all over the country [10].

Even the foreign missions that come occasionally could not provide the necessary skills of all the surgical intervention as they spend few days and may not inculcate such skills to the local surgeons within few days of stay.

**Infrastructure problems, non-availability of high technology**: The equipment used for heart surgery in Nigeria is imported from other countries. Virtually all the drugs are also imported. Prostheses and other consumables are imported, and their cost is quoted in US Dollars or Naira equivalent. With the heavy devaluation of Nigerian currency, many of these items are lacking or beyond reach. Therefore, the team has to improvise, but this state of affairs leads to poor outcome.

**Human resources, team members**: The practice is a team work, and the team members include pediatric cardiac surgeons, pediatric cardiologists, pediatric cardiac anesthetists, cardiac interventional radiologists, clinical perfusionists, medical laboratory scientists, and pharmacists. Other members are physiotherapists, perioperative nurses, cardiothoracic nurses, intensive care unit nurses, and equipment technicians. Human resources are not adequate locally trained and pediatric cardiac surgeons are not sufficiently skilled to handle complex congenital cardiac defects.

**Training/skill acquisition**: Every member in this team requires some skill to fit into the team, but our local training program leaves room for vital overseas exposure. Currently, there is neither perfusion school nor equipment training center in Nigeria that will produce manpower that will operate high-tech equipment or trouble shoot malfunction, respectively. Surgical management of heart disease is not a trial-and-error program. Every member of the team is expected to be proficient in his/her area. If mistake is made, the patient suffers. Only correct actions at every stage of the management will produce good outcome. There is need for further training or continuing education, research, workshop, seminar, and recertification. In the absence of these, the workers will become outdated. No member of the team should grow weary of this exercise, and this is where a leader with vision is needed.

Pediatric cardiac surgery program requires enormous resources and commitment to establish. Training of cardiac anesthetist like every other personnel in the team requires enormous funds. This is because the training is done abroad [11].

Training and retraining are also necessary in order to prevent attrition. Attrition therefore constitutes a big problem as the volume of cardiac surgery carried out in Nigeria is very small compared with the burden of pediatric cardiac disease in the country. Training or upgrading the education of the pediatric cardiac team, massive training of core personnel for pediatric cardiac surgery and pediatric cardiologist will enable the work to be self-sustaining as their services will be patronized by both locals and foreigners. Funds will be generated as is done in other heart centers in India, America, etc.

There are three main methods of acquiring training. It could be by an institution sending a team to undergo training in another institution. The second option involves inviting experts to come and train the local personnel on the job while the third option is for individuals to scout for training positions anywhere by themselves.

Another good alternative is to engage a cardiac team from a good cardiac center to work with the locals on continuous basis until skill transfer is achieved. This will be cost-effective, and more patients will receive care while skill acquisition will take place smoothly [11].

**Financing of equipment/supply of equipment**. Equipment is usually procured through tenders by government, but one noticeable problem is the dumping of unserviceable and outdated equipment at the hospital, by fraudulent contractors and their collaborators. The end user more often than not is not in the picture although the pediatric cardiac surgery is equipment-driven. Many of the equipment in use now are computer-based, but computer illiteracy is pervasive, resulting in poor handling and subsequent breakdown of these sophisticated and expensive machines.

Monitoring in cardiac anesthesia is pivotal to the success of cardiac surgery [12]. Monitoring equipment is expensive, and for a country such as Nigeria, acquisition of these equipment is difficult to come by. This equipment ranges from anesthesia work station, ultrasound, transesophageal echocardiography, multiparameter monitor, cardiac output monitor, I-Stat machine for point of care test in the operation theater, and intensive care unit. Other equipment include syringe pump, infusion pumps, blood warmer, etc.

**Disposables/consumables** are equally as important as non-availability of central venous catheters, arterial cannula, transducers; pressure tubing, etc., can prevent successful surgery. These consumables can be secured by the hospital management if she is committed to the sustainability of the program. Non-availability of drugs is also an impediment to cardiac surgery in Nigeria as some of the required drugs are not approved by the National Food and Drug Administration agency (NAFDAC). Some opioids and inotropes are not readily available, and this makes patient management difficult.

Procurements through competitive bidding: The prices are usually overinflated owing to the fact that contractors are owed for a period between 1 and 2 years. This adds to the high cost of pediatric cardiac surgery in Nigeria. Some cardiac missions such as Cardiostart International, William Novick cardiac Alliance, VOOMF, Save-a-heart Nigeria, ICHF/Kanu Heart foundation brought consumables during visits. These are, however, not usually enough.

## 3. Challenges accruing from establishing pediatric cardiac surgery

NCTCE has some challenges emanating from poor funding, incomplete treatment of patients, and late presentation by patients as well as poor equipment maintenance. It is thought that successful creation of Nigeria Cardiac Foundation where every Nigerian contributes 0.20–0.25% monthly salary will impact significantly in funding cardiac surgery. Another alternative is to incorporate pediatric cardiac surgery into National Health Insurance (NHIS). This will also address the challenges of late presentation. As can be seen, the Cardiac Surgery Intersociety Alliance (CSIA) or any other body can assist our center in providing appropriate training for pediatric cardiac surgeons, anesthetists, perfusionists, nurses, etc., among other helps that are needed. Donation of consumables and equipment will be of immense benefit to the program. CSIA model is what NCTCE needs at this time in addition to what others may offer.

## 4. Why the initial efforts were unsustainable?

These initial efforts were not sustained owing to the following factors: poor funding and total neglect of health sector, brain drain syndrome, reliance on medical tourism, and competing double burden of diseases as well as corruption, nepotism. Other issues were poor social infrastructures such as public power and water supply, poor remuneration of health workers with incessant strike actions, and insecurity in the land and inter-professional conflicts [1].

### 4.1 Poor funding and neglect of health sector

Low government health spending over the last two decades has limited the expansion of highly cost-effective interventions, stunted health outcomes and exposing large shares of the population to catastrophic health expenditures. Nigeria spends less on health than nearly every country in the world. In 2016, government health spending was 0.6% as a share of GDP or just $US11 per capita. As a result, Nigeria significantly underperforms on key health outcomes. Maternal mortality at 576 deaths per 100,000 live births is one of the highest in the world (2.6 times the global average); one in eight children dies before reaching their fifth birthday; and 25% of households spend more than 10% of their household consumption on health [13].

### 4.2 Brain drain syndrome

The migration of health professionals from Nigeria to high-income countries—medical brain drain, deserves critical attention due to its adverse effects on the healthcare system (HCS) for developing nations, which indirectly impacts population health outcomes and creates greater inequity among vulnerable populations. This international migration of medical doctors (MDs) has created a great challenge for public health systems; it worsens already weak healthcare systems, which widens the health inequalities gap worldwide. Globally, Nigeria ranks among the worst countries in regard to maternal health outcomes. Although it represents 2% of the global population, it disproportionately contributes to nearly 10% of global maternal deaths [14]. With the current new world order, where the world is a global village, it is very easy and fashionable for members of the team to migrate and work in other parts of the world. With the skill, training, exposure, vigor, endurance, and other qualities, the tested professional can easily leave the service and country and comfortably settle and earn hard currency. The attraction to brain drain is always there for members of this team, and this has adversely affected the growth of pediatric cardiac surgery and other programs in UNTH, in particular, and Nigeria in general. Unless something urgent is done, this trend will continue, and Nigeria will be the loser.

## 5. Political issues with changing governments

Political instability in the country and frequent widespread violence combine to limit the number of foreign agencies that participate in the surgical management of heart disease in Nigeria. Some of these charities have personnel and equipment. Some foreign physicians want experience in treating types of heart disease that are no longer common in their countries. However, even charitable organizations cannot take their safety for granted. Furthermore, political decisions that affect the treatment of heart disease vary with each political leader, and these leaders change very often. Their successors do not maintain continuity. Some emphasize primary health care to the detriment of the treatment of heart disease.

*Intensive labor*: The practice is labor-intensive at no incentive. Safety of patients guides the staff activity rather than welfare of the worker. More often than not, the treatment of patient usually exceeds expected period of time. This can easily lead to frustration if the involved personnel have not prepared for any extra time on duty post. Majority of the staff are based in the intensive care unit with the attendant stress.

**High cost of treatment/low sponsorship**: As a result of heavy outlay in the provision of surgical treatment, patients are made to pay higher than an average patient in the hospital. Many of these patients are indigent and therefore cannot afford the bill. Moreover, there is no universal health insurance coverage for the citizens, which would have sponsored patients for this kind of treatment. We have a situation where the government has succeeded in providing infrastructure, but the patient cannot benefit from the available services. When compared with the cost of treatment abroad, it is still far cheaper to provide this locally.

**Inter-professional conflict**: It is an established fact that our healthcare field has been experiencing inter-professional conflicts. The surgical team managing the heart disease is inclusive. These conflicts rob the patients the united attention that would have helped in overcoming their predicament. Some members of the team keep to the legality of the duty but are morally bankrupt, and this causes problem. Other causes of problem are pride, envy, jealousy, inferiority/superiority complex, and cheating.

**Others**: Public utilities such as water and electric power are not readily available, and they are very essential in this business. Hospital resorts to alternative source of power outside the national grid, and this is more expensive, thereby increasing the cost of treatment. Non-payment of salary as and when due and stagnation in service add to the challenges in the management of their patients.

## 6. Burden

It is important to note that lack of facilities for sustainable pediatric cardiac services and pediatric cardiology practice in Nigeria results in preventable deaths and suffering. Regrettably, about 15 million children are noted to have died and had some morbidities from potentially treatable cardiac diseases [15].

The practice of pediatric cardiac surgery had been ignored for long, as this has now evoked major concern to governmental and nongovernmental organizations and cardiovascular specialists [1]. In some areas in West African province, it is noted that only 20% of the parents of children who are less than 15 years and who needed pediatric surgical intervention are able to finance the operation within 12 months of diagnosis [1, 16].

Early diagnosis and treatment are very necessary to enhance the survival of children with cardiac disease [1]. This can be achieved by the provision of affordable human resources, diagnostic and surgical as well as other interventional facilities at each level of care in the country.

## 7. Challenges incurred in establishing pediatric cardiology practice

The practice of pediatric cardiology and pediatric cardiac services in Nigeria is faced with several challenges. The cost of pediatric cardiac services is very exorbitant and unaffordable for most developing nations. Nigeria gives priority to other disease burdens other than cardiac disease during budget allocations. The current COVID-19 pandemic, HIV/AIDS pandemic, poor health infrastructure and referral systems, malaria, pneumonias, and malnutrition have made the situation worse and dampen the importance of pediatric cardiac service.

The population of children with uncorrected congenital heart disease in Nigeria in particular and Africa in general is considerable. This is due to the fact that most pediatric services are centered on diagnosis and management of infectious diseases, shortage of trained personnel who diagnose congenital heart defects, resulting in late diagnosis and referral. Besides, the number of facilities for pediatric cardiac surgery is meager with attendant paucity of pediatric cardiac surgeons [16].

In Africa, pediatric cardiac surgery is usually performed in adults than in younger children, due to lack of manpower [17, 18]. The country no longer completely lacks facility and skills in carrying out stage procedures for cyanotic congenital cardiac disease or palliative surgery such as pulmonary artery banding or systemic-pulmonary shunt as earlier reported [19].

The challenges encountered in the establishment of pediatric surgery for cardiovascular diseases in African could be resolved through capacity building and inculcating expertise in the diagnosis and management of congenital heart diseases; training and retraining of local pediatric cardiologist and pediatric cardiac surgeon in the management of cardiac disease tailored to our sociocultural background; getting state-of-the-art equipment and facilities that will enhance the management of cardiovascular diseases in children; public enlightenment and campaign on preventive measures on emerging and reemerging cardiac disease, creating endowment funds and financial support where there will be community participation; making policies that establish pediatric cardiac training in Nigeria that will be sustainable and achievable; reinforcement of skills in terms of professional competences, exchange program, knowledge, innovative surgical techniques, new technologies, equipment, and human resources; granting financial aid to take care of the poorest of the poor by public, governmental, or private initiatives; establishment of number of centers of excellence dedicated to training, retraining, research, and clinical care in pediatric heart surgery in sub-Saharan Africa; developing international cooperation through foundations and nongovernmental organizations, and through banking firms and grants; and seeking the support of pharmaceutical industries and medical equipment [20–22].

## 8. Prospects

In short, we want to outline and describe what it took to overcome some of the obstacles we faced in developing or expanding pediatric cardiac care.

### 8.1 Successes achieved

After the ICHF/KHF mission in our center in 2003, pediatric cardiology and surgery activities in our center dwindled owing to dilapidated equipment, poor workers' remuneration, and brain drain as well as poor leadership, coupled with government directive to move UNTH to the permanent site without any building for pediatric cardiac surgery activities. In 2007, UNTH moved to the permanent site and then came a change in the leadership of NCTCE. Through continuous appropriate dialog and advocacy, NCTCE benefitted from TETFUND program. With advice from Prof. Tom Pezzella of ICHF, USA, a training center was found in India (ICHH, Hyderabad India), with institutional collaboration. With this development, pediatric cardiac anesthetists and intensivists, technicians, ICU and perioperative nurses including pediatric cardiologists got training within periods ranging from 6 months to 2 years.

There was the arrangement for pediatric cardiac surgeons to do 1 year training at the Indian center with the Indian team coming to our center to see a smooth takeoff of sustainable pediatric cardiac surgery program. However, that arrangement did not materialize because cardiac mission model was adopted. This cardiac mission model started in February 2013 and ended in October 2019. During the period, William Global Cardiac Alliance, Vincent Ohaju Memorial Foundation, Save-A-Heart-Nigeria, Cardiostart International, O'Pobic, Santarina all visited our center and performed operations in 113 in pediatric patients over 7 year period [23, 24].

Currently, our cardiologists can adequately handle all echocardiographic investigations. In addition, our adult cardiologists are able to handle all forms of cardiac pacemaker insertions, coronary angiography, and some coronary artery stenting and angioplasties. Our cardiothoracic surgeons with anesthesiologists and other theater staff can handle all non-open heart surgical procedures and some open-heart surgical procedures such as repair of atrial septal defects (ASD), repair of some ventricular septal defects (VSD), excision of some types of intracardiac tumors, and replacement of the mitral valve. We are still not able to do intracardiac repair for the blue babies in addition to some other types of congenital cardiac anomalies as well as some types of valve repair/replacement and coronary artery bypass procedures.

The COVID-19 pandemic has slowed the engagement of a resident foreign pediatric cardiac surgeon (GhanianModerl–ref) at NCTCE by the present UNTH/NCTCE management to equip the local surgeon with adequate skills that will make the program very sustainable.

## Author details

Ikechukwu Andrew Nwafor[1]*, Josephat Maduabuchi Chinawa[2], John Chukwuemeka Eze[1] and Fidelis Anayo Onyekwulu[3]

1 Faculty of Medical Sciences, Department of Surgery, University of Nigeria, Enugu, Nigeria

2 Faculty of Medical Sciences, Department of Pediatrics, University of Nigeria, Enugu, Nigeria

3 Faculty of Medical Sciences, Department of Anaesthesia, University of Nigeria, Enugu, Nigeria

*Address all correspondence to: igbochinanya2@yahoo.com; ikechukwu.nwafor@unn.edu.ng

## References

[1] Eze JC, Ezemba N. Open heart surgery in Nigeria; indications and challenges. Texas Heart Institute Journal. 2007;**34**(1):8-10

[2] Nwafor I, Eze JC. Status of congenital heart defects in Nigeria: The role of cardiac surgery. World Journal of Cardiovascular Surgery. 2013;**09**(07):63-72

[3] Cox JL. Presidential address: Changing boundaries. The Journal of Thoracic and Cardiovascular Surgery. 2001;**122**(30):413-418

[4] Pezzalla AT. Progress in international cardiac surgery: Emerging strategies. The Annals of Thoracic Surgery. 2001;**71**(2):407-408

[5] Ghosh P. Setting up an open surgical program in a developing country. Asian Cardiovascular & Thoracic Annals. 2005;**13**(4):299-301

[6] Edwin F, Tettey M, Aniteye E, Tematey M, Serebroe L, et al. Development of cardiac surgery in West Africa. The Pan African Medical Journal. 2011;**9**:15

[7] Falase B, Sanusi M, Majekodunmi A, Animasahun B, Ajose I, Idowu A, et al. Open heart surgery in Nigeria; a work in progress. Journal of Cardiothoracic Surgery. 2013;**8**:6. DOI: 10.1186/1749-8090-8-6

[8] Chinawa JM, Chinawa AT, Obu HA, Chukwu BF, Eke CB. Performance of medical students in pediatric examinations and associated factors. Current Pediatric Research. 2013;**17**:101-105

[9] Rao SG. Pediatric cardiac surgery in developing countries. Pediatric Cardiology. 2007;**28**:144-148

[10] Budzee A, Tantchou Tchoumi JC, Ambassa JC, Gimberti A, Cirri S, Frigiola A, et al. The Cardiac Center of Shisong Hospital, the first cardio-surgical center in West and Central Africa is inaugurated in Cameroon. The Pan African Medical Journal. 2010;**4**:4

[11] Eze JC, Nwafor IA, Onyekwulu FA, Arodiwe I, Etukokwu K, Ezemba N, et al. Pattern and outcome of congenital heart defects managed at Innova Children Heart Hospital, Hyderabad, India as a skill acquisition center. Chirurgia, Italy. 2017;**30**(1):1-5

[12] Eze JC, Ikechukw AN, Fidelis AO, Kenneth CE, Ndubueze E, Ijeoma A, et al. The pattern and Outcome of congenital heart defects managed over a year period at Innova Children Heart hospital, Hyderabad India, as a skill acquisition center. Journal of Chirurgia. 2017;**30**(1):1-5

[13] Onyekwulu FA, Nwafor IA, Ezemba N, Ogudua F. Establishing an indigenous cardiac Anaesthesia Service in Enugu: Report of two cases of atrial septal defect (ASD) closure. Ibom Medical Journal. 2020;**13**(3):214-217

[14] Reem H. Nigeria Health Financing System Assessment. World Banks Group (Health, Nutrition and population). April 2018

[15] Imafidon J. One Way Traffic: Nigeria Medical Brain Drain, a Challenge for Maternal Health & Public Health System in Nigeria. Los Angeles: University of Carlifornia; 2018

[16] Frimpong-Boateng K. The Beginnings of Cardiothoracic Surgery in Ghana. In Deep Down My Heart. 1st ed. Accra: Woeli Publishing Services; 2000

[17] Edwin F, Tettey M, Aniteye E, Tamatey M, Sereboe L, et al. The development of cardiac surgery in West Africa-the case of Ghana. Pan African Medical Journal. 2011;**9**(1):1-15

[18] Roheena ZP, Awais A, Muhammad MA. Earlier surgical intervention in congenital heart disease results in better outcome and resource utilization. BMC Health Services Research. 2011;**11**:353. Available from: https://www.ncbi.nlm.nih.gov/pmc/articles/PMC3277492/

[19] Okoromah CA, Ekure EN, Ojo OO, Animasahun BA, Bastos MI. Structural heart disease in children in Lagos: Profile, problems and prospects. The Nigerian Postgraduate Medical Journal. 2008;**15**(2):82-88

[20] Antunes MJ. Current status of surgery for congenital heart disease in infancy. South African Medical Journal. 1985;**67**(10):359-362

[21] Pinho P, von Oppell UO, Brink J, Hewitson J. Pulmonary artery banding: Adequacy and long-term outcome. European Journal of Cardio-Thoracic Surgery. 1997;**11**(1):105-111

[22] Yacoub MH. Establishing pediatric cardiovascular services in the developing world: A wake-up call. Circulation. 2007;**116**:1876-1878

[23] Pediatric Cardiothoracic Program-Cedars-Sinai. Available from: http://www.cedars-sinai.edu/Patients/Programs-and-Services/Heart-Institute/Centers-and-Prog [Assessed: August 12, 2013]

[24] Ikechukwu N, Eze JC, Osemobor K. The status of congenital heart defects in Nigeria and challenges of surgical treatment: 6 year review. Journal of Vascular Medicine and Surgery. 2021;**S4**:002